BRONCHITIS

Edited by **Ignacio Martín-Loeches**

Bronchitis
Edited by Ignacio Martín-Loeches

Published by InTech
Janeza Trdine 9, 51000 Rijeka, Croatia

Publishing Process Manager Petra Zobic

Technical Editor Teodora Smiljanic

Cover Designer InTech Design Team

Additional hard copies can be obtained from orders@intechopen.com

Bronchitis, Edited by Ignacio Martín-Loeches
p. cm.
ISBN 978-953-307-889-2

For EU product safety concerns:
IN TECH d.o.o., Prolaz Marije Krucifikse Kozulić 3, 51000 Rijeka, Croatia,
info@intechopen.com or visit our website at intechopen.com.

Meet the editor

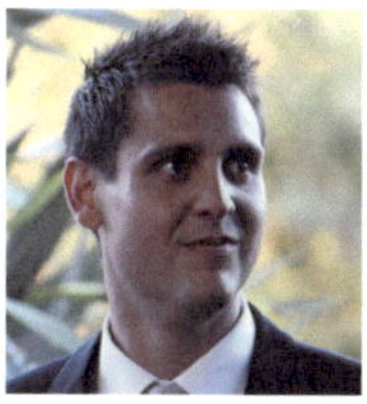

Dr. Ignacio Martin-Loeches received his medical degree from the Autonomous University of Madrid, Spain and trained in Intensive Care Medicine from Doctor Negrín University Hospital, Las Palmas de Gran Canaria, Spain. Dr Martin-Loeches completed an additional year of fellowship training in Critical Care Medicine at Mater Misericordiae University Hospital, Dublin. He was appointed Consultant Intensivist in St James University Hospital, Dublin after he return to Spain. He completed a PhD through the University of Las Palmas de Gran Canaria, Spain on genetics and severe Community Acquired pneumonia in 2008. He is currently working as a Consultant Intensivist at Parc Taulí Hospital-Sabadell, Barcelona, Spain. He has published several articles in international journals and chapters in scientific books, and serves as a reviewer for peer–reviewed journals of intensive care medicine, amongst others. His interests are critically ill infection, sepsis and translational medicine.

Contents

Preface

Lung parenchyma has been extensively investigated. Nevertheless, the study of bronchial small airways is much less common. In addition, bronchitis represents, in some occasions, an intermediate process that easily explains the damage in the lung parenchyma. The main target of this book is to provide a bronchial small airways original research from different experts in the field. Different points of views have been included searching the most interesting and state-of-the art topics. COPD, impact of obesity, critical care and toxicity among others have been extensively reported. Other vanguard topics, such as traditional medicine or the impact of environment have been included in the present preface. The editors would like to thank the authors for their contribution and we hope this book might increase the interest in the field.

Ignacio Martin-Loeches
Critical Care Center,
Parc Taulí Hospital-Sabadell,
Spain

Part 1

Comorbid States and Enviroment

1

The Impact of Obesity and Metabolic Syndrome in COPD

Francesco Sava, Francois Maltais and Paul Poirier
Centre de recherche de l'Institut de cardiologie et de pneumologie de Québec, Université Laval, Québec, Canada

1. Introduction

Obesity is becoming more and more prevalent in the world and has many recognized impacts on different body systems. Chronic obstructive pulmonary disease (COPD) is also very common and affects different systems but mainly the respiratory system. Of particular interest to us is the impact of obesity on respiratory function in general and more specifically in COPD patients.

The objectives of the chapter are to: 1) explore the different impacts of obesity on respiratory function in healthy and COPD patients; 2) to try to explain the impact of obesity on exercise tolerance and exercise dyspnea; and 3) the study the impact of obesity on the outcomes of a pulmonary rehabilitation program for COPD patients.

2. Definition of obesity

The definition of obesity is based on body mass index (BMI) which is the ratio of body mass in kilograms to the square of the height in meters. A person is overweight if BMI is between 25 and 30 kg/m^2 and obese if BMI is over 30 kg/m^2 [5]. This definition, although being simple and easily applicable to everyday clinical contexts, is somewhat simplistic in the sense that it does not take into account either body mass distribution or fat vs. fat free mass. These variables have important impact on the respiratory physiology and on the chronic obstructive pulmonary disease (COPD).

3. Epidemiology

Overweight and obesity are very prevalent in western countries. For instance, in Canada, it is estimated that, in 2004, 23.1 % of adults were obese and 36.1 % were overweight, up from 13.8 and 28.5 % respectively compared to 1979 [6]. This has led the scientific community to talk about this phenomenon in terms of "obesity epidemic", since the condition has recently been recognized as a disease [7].

4. Effects of obesity on respiratory physiology at rest

Obesity has many different effects on respiratory physiology at rest. These effects will be explained in more detail in the following text and are summarized in table 1.

At rest	Lung volumes	Reduced functional residual capacity and expiratory reserve volume exponentially with increases in BMI. Total lung capacity and residual volume within normal limits.
	Respiratory system compliance	Reduced compliance mainly due to extra upper body weight (abdomen and thorax) and breathing at lower volumes.
	Expiratory flows	Airways narrowed and more reactive but no consistent influence of BMI on either FEV1 or FEV1/FVC ratio.
	Oxygenation	Alveoar collapsing at the lung bases causing V/Q mismatch leading to chronic hypoxia. Worse during sleep.
During exercise	Oxygen comsuption and ventilation	VO2, VCO2, and VE higher for any given workload due to higher metabolic cost of moving a heavier body mass and increased work of breathing.
	Lung volumes	Dynamic hyperinflation that raises lung volumes to a more compliant zone.
	Dyspnea	Dyspnea is increased at any given workload but is proportional to the increase of VE.

Table 1. Summary of the effects of obesity on respiratory physiology at rest and during exercise.

4.1 Lung volumes and respiratory mechanics

The best described effect of obesity is the reduction of the end-expiratory lung volume and functional residual capacity [2,8]. End-expiratory lung volume is the volume left in the lung at the end of a normal expiration and under most circumstances. functional residual capacity is the resting respiratory system volume determined by the equilibrium of two opposing forces [9]; the elastic recoil of the lung which exerts a deflating effect and the elastic properties of the chest wall that tends to expand because its resting volume is higher than the functional residual capacity in healthy individuals [9]. In the obese subject, reduction of the resting respiratory system volume at functional residual capacity is caused by the extra weight of the thoracic wall and the abdomen which reduces significantly the respiratory system compliance [10]. There is an exponential relationship between BMI and both functional residual capacity and end-expiratory lung volume [2]. Total lung capacity and residual volume are relatively unaffected by obesity [11]. So, with a preserved total lung capacity and residual volume, decreased functional residual capacity has two physiologic corollaries: 1) decreased expiratory reserve volume and, 2) increased inspiratory capacity [1].

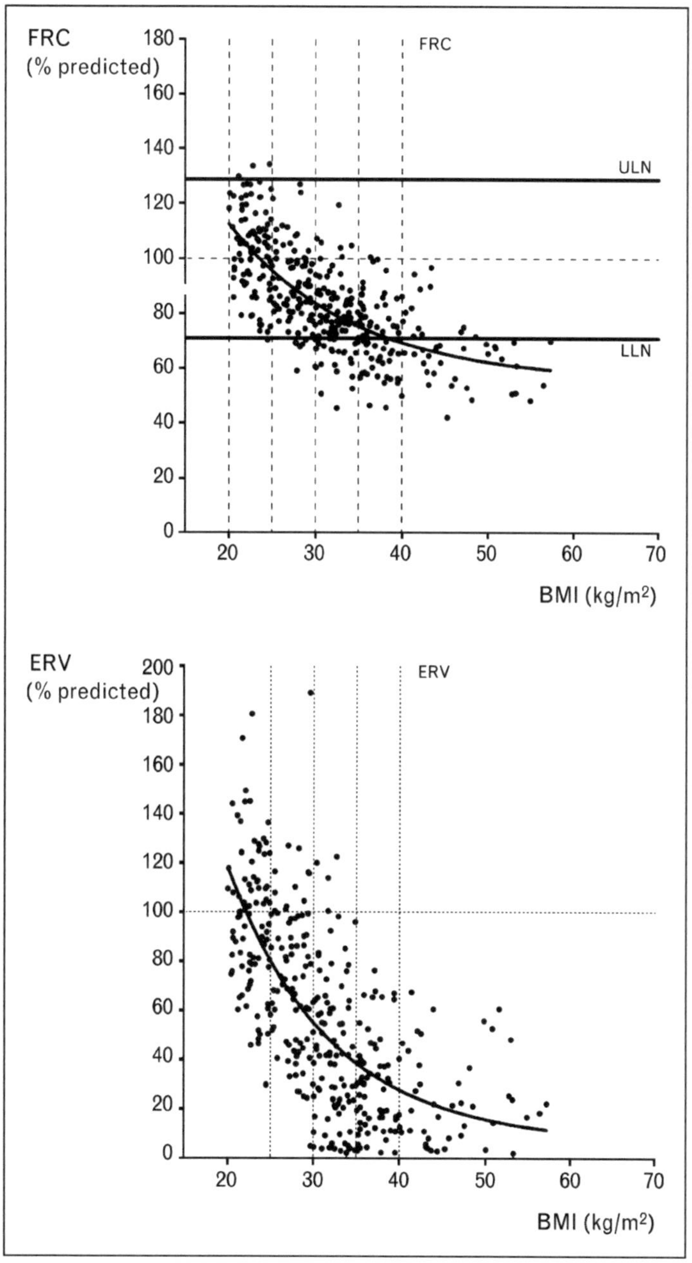

Fig. 1. Exponential relation between BMI and both functional residual capacity (FRC) and expiratory reserve volume (ERV). Shown on the functional residual capacity graph are the upper and lower limits of normal. Adapted from [2].

Although airways are narrower and more reactive than normal weight subjects, both maximal ventilatory capacity and expiratory volumes are preserved in the obese subject. There is no consistent evidence of BMI influencing forced expiratory volume in 1 second (FEV1) or FEV1/forced vital capacity [12,13].

4.2 Oxygenation

As functional residual capacity gets lower, it draws near the residual volume so much that, in some subjects, each tidal volume breath results in alveolar collapsing at the lung bases. This creates ventilation perfusion mismatch and can lead to chronic hypoxemia [14]. This phenomenon is exacerbated during sleep but can also be observed during daytime [15].

4.3 Importance of body mass distribution

Fat mass distribution is of paramount importance when considering the effects of obesity on respiratory physiology. Waist size and waist-to-hip ratio is more closely related to the previously described changes than BMI alone [16,17]. Studies using dual X-ray absorptiometry (DEXA) allowed establishing that upper body fat, as opposed to lower body fat, is linked to reductions of functional residual capacity and expiratory reserve volume [18]. This association was observed for thoracic as well as abdominal fat. It thus seems that upper body mass is the main determinant of the lower lung volumes observed in the obese subject and that, because of the interdependence of the thoracic and abdominal cavity in terms of volume and pressure, the location of fat mass within the upper body is not an important determinant of lung volumes.

5. Effects of obesity on respiratory physiology during exercise

5.1 Oxygen consumption

Both oxygen consumption (VO_2) and carbon dioxide production (VCO_2) are increased for a given workload in the obese individual [3]. This higher metabolic expenditure is due to the higher energy demand caused by the extra body mass that obese subjects have to carry around. Also, decreased respiratory system compliance increases significantly the work of breathing [19]. Maximal exercise capacity in terms of VO_2 is not affected and is even increased [20,21]. Actually, absolute VO_2 tends to be higher with increasing BMI, but specific VO_2 expressed as VO_2/kg tends to be lower with increasing BMI. This effect of obesity on VO_2 is particularly evident in weight baring activities.

5.2 Lung volumes during exercise

As already mentioned, obese patients' tidal volume is very close to their residual volume at rest. During exercise however, functional residual capacity increases to normal levels allowing the expansion in tidal volume to accommodate the increasing ventilatory demand in a fashion that is similar to healthy subject. In contrast to patients with obstructive lung disease, the increase in functional residual capacity is not deleterious in obese individuals as it serves to restore normal physiology and places the respiratory system in a more compliant position [22].

5.3 Ventilation and dyspnea relationship

For a given workload, obese subjects feel more dyspnea than non-obese subjects. However, the relationship between ventilation and dyspnea is unchanged [3]. Because of the increased metabolic cost associated with obesity, ventilation is higher for a given workload [3]. It thus seems that the higher perception of dyspnea in obese subjects is only a normal response to higher minute ventilation and that changes in respiratory mechanics and physiology do not really impact on subjective sensations.

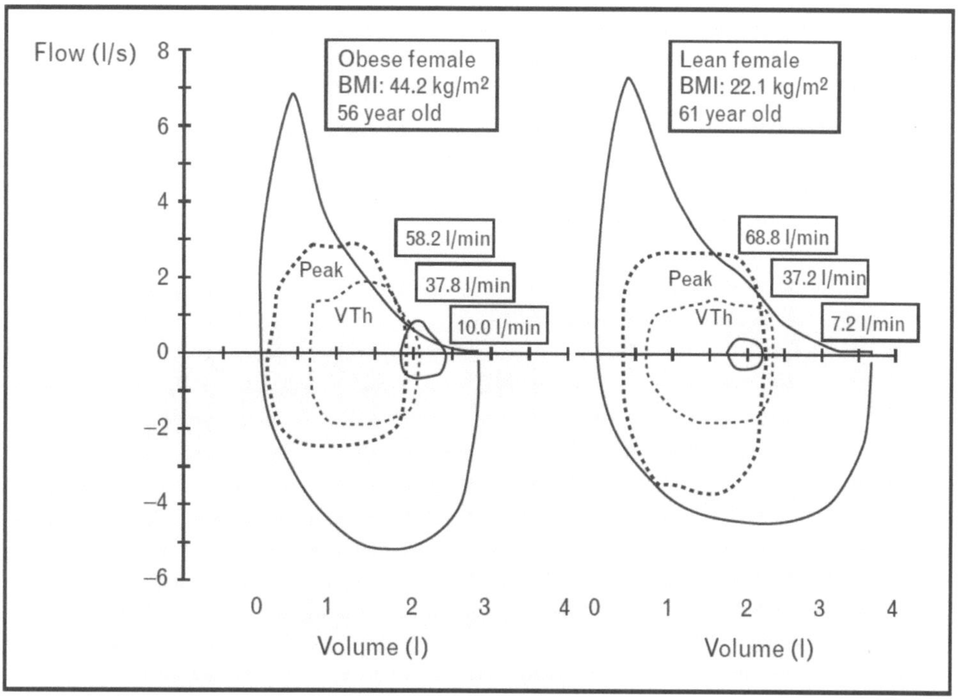

Fig. 2. Expiratory flow volume curve of an obese woman compared to a lean one. At rest, respiration is performed at lower lung volumes but with increasing ventilation, expiratory patterns tend to be closer. Adapted [3].

6. Effects of obesity on COPD

6.1 How frequently obesity and COPD coexist in the same subject

It was traditionally thought that COPD patients were less likely to be obese. The rationale was that systemic inflammation in the more advanced stages of disease would lead to cachexia [23] rather than overweight. However, in the most recent studies looking at the association of high BMI and COPD, approximately two thirds is overweight or obese [24].

6.2 Impact of obesity on survival

A BMI below 21 kg/m^2 was shown to be a negative prognosis marker [25] while obesity appears to convey a survival advantage in COPD, as it is the case in other chronic disease [26]. However, data relating to this so called "obesity paradox", whereby obesity seems beneficial on survival, is often biased because more obese patients tend to have less severe or less advanced disease.

6.3 The main physiologic changes in COPD

The main characteristics of COPD are limitation of expiratory flow and hyperinflation. At rest, FEV1 and the ratio of FEV1 to forced vital capacity are decreased while functional residual capacity, end-expiratory lung volume, total lung capacity and residual volume are elevated. The main consequence of lower expiratory flows is a limitation in maximal ventilatory capacity [27]. The consequence of higher functional residual capacity and residual volume is reduction in the respiratory capacity (IC). The main pathophysiological reasons for these reduction in flows and elevated lung volumes are an increased airway resistance due to inflammation and mucus production and an increased lung compliance due to parenchymal destruction [28,29].

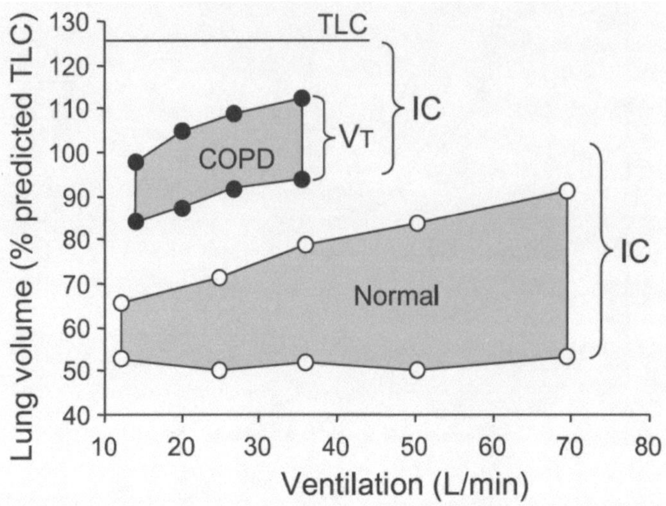

Fig. 3. Schematic representation of dynamic hyperinflation in a COPD subject. During exercise, rising lung volumes lead to a decreased inspiratory capacity and respiration occurs at higher lung volumes [4].

During exercise, the lower inspiratory capacity constraints the expansion in tidal volume in such a way that the increased ventilatory demand is more dependent upon the progression of the respiratory rate. This breathing pattern characterized by a rapid and shallow breathing shortens expiration, preventing full expiration to occur [4]. The increased airway resistance also contributes to this phenomenon leading to gas retention and dynamic hyperinflation [30]. Because of dynamic hyperinflation, COPD subjects breathe at higher lung volumes during exercise (closer to total lung capacity), in a less compliant portion of the volume-pressure relationship of the respiratory system. Work of breathing is increased in this situation and the resulting tidal volume for a given respiratory effort is decreased, a phenomenon being referred to as neuro-mechanical uncoupling. The final results of these physiological abnormalities for the patients is increased dyspnea perception [31].

Another important systemic consequence of COPD is limb muscle atrophy which is observed especially in the more advanced stages of the disease [23,32]. Total as well as lower limb muscle mass is decreased leading to fatigue during exercise [33]. In fact, some COPD subjects are not primarily limited by dyspnea but by leg fatigue during exercise [34]. This symptom also contributes significantly to exercise intolerance in COPD [35].

6.4 Effect of obesity on COPD at rest

Obesity and COPD have various influences on respiratory physiology, some are similar and some are opposite.

The relationship between BMI and either functional residual capacity or expiratory reserve volume are not affected by the presence of airflow obstruction [1]. However, obese COPD patients are less hyperinflated compared to their lean counterparts [1]. Moreover, for a given

FEV1, IC is higher in obese subjects [2]. These changes seem beneficial to COPD subjects, counteracting some of the deleterious effects of the disease. However, as previously mentioned, oxygen consumption is higher for a given workload for obese subjects, leading to higher ventilatory demand. This increased in ventilatory requirement further stresses the respiratory system whose capacity is already reduced by the presence of airflow limitation [35].

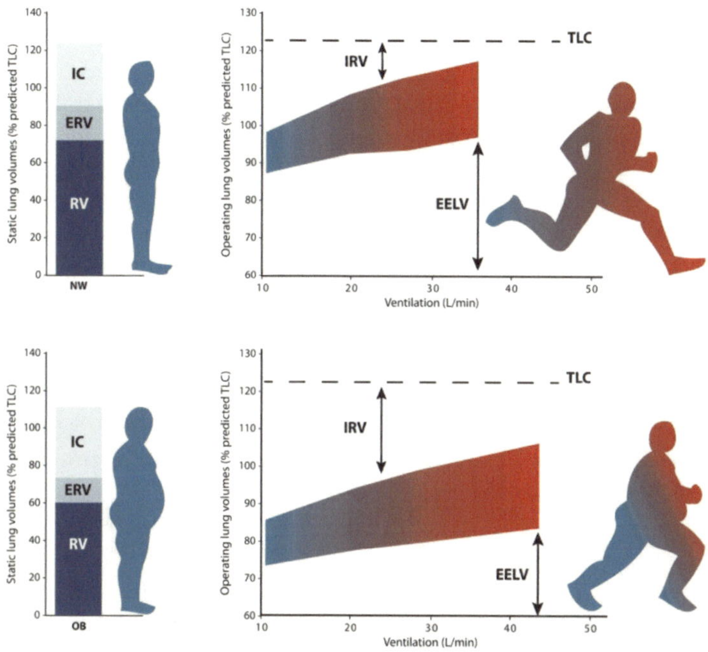

Fig. 4. Lung volumes of an obese and a non-obese COPD subject. A : At rest, lung volumes are reduced in the obese subject. B : During exercise, dynamic hyperinflation is reduced in the obese subject although still present. Adapted from [1].

6.5 Exercise tolerance of the obese patients with COPD

The effects of obesity on exercise tolerance in patients with COPD have not been studied extensively. In one study, obese patients with COPD had higher exercise capacity and were less dyspneic for a given ventilation during cycling exercise [1]. These effects were felt to be related to lower operating lung volumes and reduced dynamic hyperinflation [3]. Other studies have reported marked decreases in exercise tolerance during a 6-minutes walking test [36] but not during a cycling endurance test [37] in obese patients with COPD. It thus appears that obese patients with COPD perform better when cycling than in weight bearing activities such as walking [35].

7. Effects of obesity of pulmonary rehabilitation

7.1 Rehabilitation as a therapeutic intervention in COPD

Pulmonary rehabilitation is a multidisciplinary intervention focusing on exercise training and patient education and self-management [38]. The exercise component is essential if the goal of rehabilitation is to improve exercise tolerance and reduce dyspnea [39]. It is recommended for patients experiencing persisting symptoms despite maximal pharmacologic therapy [38]. Rehabilitation can be provided in an outpatient setting or at home, with comparable benefits on exercise tolerance, dyspnea, quality of life and exacerbations [40]. It is considered the most effective therapy to improve symptoms and quality of life in COPD [41,42].

7.2 Specific exercise limitations

Obese patients with COPD entering a rehabilitation program typically have a reduced exercise tolerance. [24]. In one study, their cycling capacity was comparable to lean patients with COPD while their walking capacity was reduced. Walking is more representative of daily activities, so it is felt that patients with COPD subjects that are also obese are more limited than their non-obese counterparts. Obese patients with COPD usually show similar improvements in exercise capacity than non-obese although they are less likely to achieve clinically significant improvements during walking [24]. These observations are important because identifying obese patients as having specific exercise limitations can help tailoring the rehabilitation program to their specific needs. Although obesity is associated with more functional impairment, quality of life of obese COPD subjects is not different than their non obese counterparts and improves to a similar extent with rehabilitation [24]. The fact that obesity does not seems to alter quality of life may be related to the subjective nature of the quality of life measures and to chronic adaptation to obesity with the progressive avoidance of certain tasks that are more challenging to obese individuals.

7.3 Good opportunity to adopt healthier lifestyles

The fact that upon entering pulmonary rehabilitation, obese COPD patients have a reduced walking capacity suggests that weight loss could be beneficial to improve their functional status. Although never formally tested, this is a legitimate assumption. Pulmonary rehabilitation could be an ideal setting to help patients with COPD adopting a healthier lifestyle that will eventually lead to long lasting weight loss [38].

8. References

[1] Ora J, Laveneziana P, Ofir D, Deesomchok A, Webb KA, O'Donnell DE: Combined effects of obesity and chronic obstructive pulmonary disease on dyspnea and exercise tolerance. *Am J Respir Crit Care Med* 2009, 180: 964-971.

[2] Jones RL, Nzekwu MM: The effects of body mass index on lung volumes. *Chest* 2006, 130: 827-833.

[3] Ofir D, Laveneziana P, Webb KA, O'Donnell DE: Ventilatory and perceptual responses to cycle exercise in obese women. *J Appl Physiol* 2007, 102: 2217-2226.

[4] O'Donnell DE, Bertley JC, Chau LK, Webb KA: Qualitative aspects of exertional breathlessness in chronic airflow limitation: pathophysiologic mechanisms. *Am J Respir Crit Care Med* 1997, 155: 109-115.

[5] Clinical Guidelines on the Identification, Evaluation, and Treatment of Overweight and Obesity in Adults--The Evidence Report. National Institutes of Health. *Obes Res* 1998, 6 Suppl 2: 51S-209S.

[6] Tjepkema M: Nutrition: Findings from the Canadian Community Health Survey. *Statistics Canada Catalog* 2005.

[7] Allison DB, Downey M, Atkinson RL, Billington CJ, Bray GA, Eckel RH, Finkelstein EA, Jensen MD, Tremblay A: Obesity as a disease: a white paper on evidence and arguments commissioned by the Council of the Obesity Society. *Obesity (Silver Spring)* 2008, 16: 1161-1177.
[8] Pelosi P, Croci M, Ravagnan I, Vicardi P, Gattinoni L: Total respiratory system, lung, and chest wall mechanics in sedated-paralyzed postoperative morbidly obese patients. *Chest* 1996, 109: 144-151.
[9] West J: *Respiratory Physiology*, 8 edn. Philadelphia: Lippincott Williams Wilkins; 2008.
[10] Sharp JT, Henry JP, Sweany SK, Meadows WR, Pietras RJ: Effects of Mass Loading the Respiratory System in Man. *J Appl Physiol* 1964, 19: 959-966.
[11] Collins LC, Hoberty PD, Walker JF, Fletcher EC, Peiris AN: The effect of body fat distribution on pulmonary function tests. *Chest* 1995, 107: 1298-1302.
[12] Schachter LM, Salome CM, Peat JK, Woolcock AJ: Obesity is a risk for asthma and wheeze but not airway hyperresponsiveness. *Thorax* 2001, 56: 4-8.
[13] Zerah F, Harf A, Perlemuter L, Lorino H, Lorino AM, Atlan G: Effects of obesity on respiratory resistance. *Chest* 1993, 103: 1470-1476.
[14] Hedenstierna G, Santesson J, Norlander O: Airway closure and distribution of inspired gas in the extremely obese, breathing spontaneously and during anaesthesia with intermittent positive pressure ventilation. *Acta Anaesthesiol Scand* 1976, 20: 334-342.
[15] Farebrother MJ, McHardy GJ, Munro JF: Relation between pulmonary gas exchange and closing volume before and after substantial weight loss in obese subjects. *Br Med J* 1974, 3: 391-393.
[16] Canoy D, Luben R, Welch A, Bingham S, Wareham N, Day N, Khaw KT: Abdominal obesity and respiratory function in men and women in the EPIC-Norfolk Study, United Kingdom. *Am J Epidemiol* 2004, 159: 1140-1149.
[17] Chen Y, Rennie D, Cormier YF, Dosman J: Waist circumference is associated with pulmonary function in normal-weight, overweight, and obese subjects. *Am J Clin Nutr* 2007, 85: 35-39.
[18] Sutherland TJ, Goulding A, Grant AM, Cowan JO, Williamson A, Williams SM, Skinner MA, Taylor DR: The effect of adiposity measured by dual-energy X-ray absorptiometry on lung function. *Eur Respir J* 2008, 32: 85-91.
[19] Dempsey JA, Reddan W, Balke B, Rankin J: Work capacity determinants and physiologic cost of weight-supported work in obesity. *J Appl Physiol* 1966, 21: 1815-1820.
[20] Babb TG, Ranasinghe KG, Comeau LA, Semon TL, Schwartz B: Dyspnea on exertion in obese women: association with an increased oxygen cost of breathing. *Am J Respir Crit Care Med* 2008, 178: 116-123.
[21] Babb TG, DeLorey DS, Wyrick BL, Gardner PP: Mild obesity does not limit change in end-expiratory lung volume during cycling in young women. *J Appl Physiol* 2002, 92: 2483-2490.
[22] Babb TG, Buskirk ER, Hodgson JL: Exercise end-expiratory lung volumes in lean and moderately obese women. *Int J Obes* 1989, 13: 11-19.
[23] Decramer M, De BF, Del PA, Marinari S: Systemic effects of COPD. *Respir Med* 2005, 99 Suppl B: S3-10.
[24] Sava F, Laviolette L, Bernard S, Breton MJ, Bourbeau J, Maltais F: The impact of obesity on walking and cycling performance and response to pulmonary rehabilitation in COPD. *BMC Pulm Med* 2010, 10: 55.
[25] Cote CG, Celli BR: BODE index: a new tool to stage and monitor progression of chronic obstructive pulmonary disease. *Pneumonol Alergol Pol* 2009, 77: 305-313.

[26] Schols AM, Slangen J, Volovics L, Wouters EF: Weight loss is a reversible factor in the prognosis of chronic obstructive pulmonary disease. *Am J Respir Crit Care Med* 1998, 157: 1791-1797.

[27] Hogg JC, Chu F, Utokaparch S, Woods R, Elliott WM, Buzatu L, Cherniack RM, Rogers RM, Sciurba FC, Coxson HO, Pare PD: The nature of small-airway obstruction in chronic obstructive pulmonary disease. *N Engl J Med* 2004, 350: 2645-2653.

[28] Leopold JG, Gough J: The centrilobular form of hypertrophic emphysema and its relation to chronic bronchitis. *Thorax* 1957, 12: 219-235.

[29] McLean KH: The pathogenesis of pulmonary emphysema. *Am J Med* 1958, 25: 62-74.

[30] O'Donnell DE, Revill SM, Webb KA: Dynamic hyperinflation and exercise intolerance in chronic obstructive pulmonary disease. *Am J Respir Crit Care Med* 2001, 164: 770-777.

[31] O'Donnell DE, Webb KA: Exertional breathlessness in patients with chronic airflow limitation. The role of lung hyperinflation. *Am Rev Respir Dis* 1993, 148: 1351-1357.

[32] Skeletal muscle dysfunction in chronic obstructive pulmonary disease. A statement of the American Thoracic Society and European Respiratory Society. *Am J Respir Crit Care Med* 1999, 159: S1-40.

[33] Casaburi R, Patessio A, Ioli F, Zanaboni S, Donner CF, Wasserman K: Reductions in exercise lactic acidosis and ventilation as a result of exercise training in patients with obstructive lung disease. *Am Rev Respir Dis* 1991, 143: 9-18.

[34] Killian KJ, LeBlanc P, Martin DH, Summers E, Jones NL, Campbell EJ: Exercise capacity and ventilatory, circulatory, and symptom limitation in patients with chronic airflow limitation. *Am Rev Respir Dis* 1992, 146: 935-940.

[35] Pepin V, Saey D, Laviolette L, Maltais F: Exercise capacity in chronic obstructive pulmonary disease: mechanisms of limitation. *COPD* 2007, 4: 195-204.

[36] Ramachandran K, McCusker C, Connors M, Zuwallack R, Lahiri B: The influence of obesity on pulmonary rehabilitation outcomes in patients with COPD. *Chron Respir Dis* 2008, 5: 205-209.

[37] Laviolette L, Sava F, O'Donnell DE, Webb KA, Hamilton AL, Kesten S, Maltais F: Effect of obesity on constant workrate exercise in hyperinflated men with COPD. *BMC Pulm Med* 2010, 10: 33.

[38] O'Donnell DE, Aaron S, Bourbeau J, Hernandez P, Marciniuk DD, Balter M, Ford G, Gervais A, Goldstein R, Hodder R, Kaplan A, Keenan S, Lacasse Y, Maltais F, Road J, Rocker G, Sin D, Sinuff T, Voduc N: Canadian Thoracic Society recommendations for management of chronic obstructive pulmonary disease - 2007 update. *Can Respir J* 2007, 14 Suppl B: 5B-32B.

[39] Ries AL, Kaplan RM, Limberg TM, Prewitt LM: Effects of pulmonary rehabilitation on physiologic and psychosocial outcomes in patients with chronic obstructive pulmonary disease. *Ann Intern Med* 1995, 122: 823-832.

[40] Maltais F, Bourbeau J, Shapiro S, Lacasse Y, Perrault H, Baltzan M, Hernandez P, Rouleau M, Julien M, Parenteau S, Paradis B, Levy RD, Camp P, Lecours R, Audet R, Hutton B, Penrod JR, Picard D, Bernard S: Effects of home-based pulmonary rehabilitation in patients with chronic obstructive pulmonary disease: a randomized trial. *Ann Intern Med* 2008, 149: 869-878.

[41] Lacasse Y, Wong E, Guyatt GH, King D, Cook DJ, Goldstein RS: Meta-analysis of respiratory rehabilitation in chronic obstructive pulmonary disease. *Lancet* 1996, 348: 1115-1119.

[42] Lacasse Y, Martin S, Lasserson TJ, Goldstein RS: Meta-analysis of respiratory rehabilitation in chronic obstructive pulmonary disease. A Cochrane systematic review. *Eura Medicophys* 2007, 43: 475-485.

2

The Importance of Chronic Bronchitis in Chronic Obstructive Pulmonary Disease

Elizabeth Sapey and Robert A Stockley
University of Birmingham
United Kingdom

1. Introduction

Chronic obstructive pulmonary disease (COPD) is a common and important group of conditions characterised by airflow obstruction with related symptoms including cough, shortness of breath, expectoration and wheeze. The widely accepted Global Initiative for Chronic Obstructive Lung Disease (GOLD) has classified COPD as "a disease state characterised by airflow limitation that is not fully reversible. The airflow limitation is usually both progressive and associated with an abnormal inflammatory response of the lungs to noxious particles or gases" (1). The current GOLD definition for airflow limitation is a forced expiratory volume in 1 second (FEV_1) / forced vital capacity (FVC) ratio of < 70% and disease severity is classified into four physiological stages: stage 1 ($FEV_1 \geq 80\%$ predicted); stage 2 ($FEV_1 \geq 50$ to < 80% predicted); stage 3 ($FEV_1 \geq 30$ to < 50% predicted); stage 4 ($FEV_1 < 30$ or < 50% predicted in the presence of chronic respiratory failure) (2).

COPD is one of the foremost causes of chronic morbidity and mortality worldwide. Globally, it affected 44 million people in 1990 (3) and recent estimates suggest that COPD affects approximately 210 million people (4) or 10% of all adults (5) with the prevalence continuing to rise. In 2007, COPD accounted for 5% of all deaths (4) but the WHO predicts an increase in COPD-related deaths of more than 30% in the next 10 years, emphasising the continued impact this disease will have internationally (6).

Cigarette smoking remains the most important risk factor for the development of COPD (7) although only approximately 20% of smokers develop clinically significant disease (8). This suggests that a combination of genetic and environmental factors interact to cause COPD, and there has been much research aiming to identify candidate genes that may confer genetic susceptibility. To date, however, only deficiency alleles on the α1AT gene have been robustly identified as predisposing to disease (9).

Pathologically, COPD is characterised by widespread inflammation of the peripheral and central airways with destruction of the lung parenchyma. Oedema, fibrosis, smooth muscle hypertrophy and loss of elastic recoil lead to bronchial wall thickening, which affects airflow (10).

COPD, while primarily a lung disease, is associated with increased co-morbidity including cardiovascular disease, type 2 diabetes, osteoporosis and systemic pathology such as muscle wasting and dysfunction. It has been hypothesised that persistent low-grade inflammation may drive the co-morbidity and the systemic effects noted with this disease (11). The systemic manifestations of COPD are important, as they are not only associated with

increased morbidity, but are also predictive of disease outcome, especially Body Mass Index (BMI) which forms part of the BODE index (Body Mass, airflow obstruction, dyspnoea and exercise capacity) and is used to classify the impact of the disease (12).
There is great heterogeneity in COPD, and disease presentation and the underlying pathology seen varies between individuals. Although COPD is defined by airflow obstruction, disease phenotypes include emphysema (defined pathologically as the destruction of alveolar walls and the permanent enlargement of the airspaces distal to the terminal bronchioles); bronchiectasis (defined pathologically as localised, permanently dilated bronchi and characterised by excess mucus production and reduction of mucociliary clearance), bronchiolitis (inflammation of the bronchioles) and chronic bronchitis. Chronic bronchitis is defined clinically as the presence of chronic productive cough for at least 3 months in each of 2 successive years in patients in whom other causes of chronic cough such as tuberculosis, heart failure and carcinoma of the lung, have been excluded (13). It is a feature of approximately 50% of people who smoke (14) and 30% of patients with COPD (15), although air pollution, the inhalation of toxic gases and upper gastrointestinal pathology such as reflux disease have also been associated with the condition (16).
Chronic Bronchitis is thought to be of special significance in COPD, as it is associated with increased inflammation and poorer patient outcomes. This chapter will review the pathology of chronic bronchitis, its' inflammatory basis, associated morbidity and mortality and potential treatments.

2. Background

Chronic bronchitis is common, affecting approximately 6 to 12% of adults, over 20 years of age. Cigarette smoke -exposure remains the most important aetiological risk factor for development of both chronic bronchitis and COPD (17-19). There is a six-fold rise in prevalence from 6.3% in non-smokers to 40% in heavy smokers (20), with a linear relationship between cigarette smoke exposure and chronic bronchitis(19). Other risk factors associated independently with chronic bronchitis include poor socioeconomic background, recurrent or severe childhood respiratory illness and exposure to dusty/polluted environments (18, 21).
There is great heterogeneity between patients, and both time of presentation and disease course vary. In a proportion of patients, sputum expectoration occurs without airflow obstruction, while in others, airflow obstruction precedes sputum expectoration (22). There is some debate whether chronic bronchitis is solely a recognised phenotype of COPD, or whether it is an entirely independent disease process. Certainly, while often present in unison, chronic expectoration and airflow obstruction behave largely as independent variables (23). This is perhaps unsurprising as bronchial gland hypertrophy (seen in chronic bronchitis) occurs predominantly in larger bronchioles (24), whereas the dominant site of irreversible airflow obstruction occurs in more peripheral and smaller airways(25).
Often, chronic bronchitis is preceded by recurrent episodes of acute bronchitis (26), and the frequency and severity of these acute episodes influences the rate of decline in lung function, patients quality of life and the risk of death (27) (see later).
Symptoms can be restricted to chronic sputum expectoration, or include those related to airflow obstruction, including breathlessness and wheeze. Sputum expectoration varies between and within individuals and in individual patients, in terms of the frequency of cough, the volume and tenacity of sputum produced (which can alter the patients ability to

clear secretions effectively) and sputum purulence. The majority of patients initially describe low-volume, mucoid sputum (clear to grey in colour), but as many as 30% of patients have airways which are colonised with potentially pathogenic bacteria, and this is more likely to be associated with the expectoration of purulent (green) sputum (28). See Figure 1

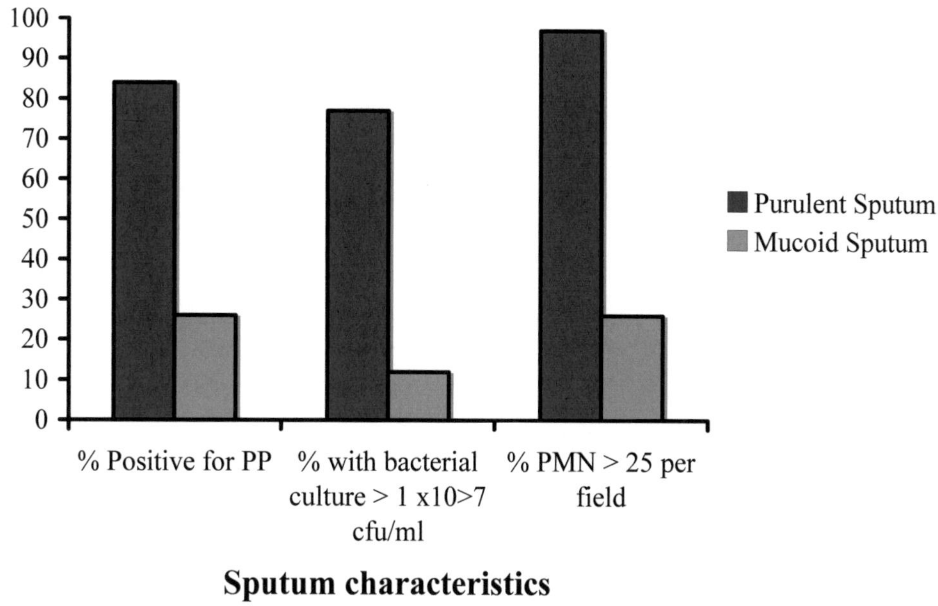

Fig. 1. The characteristics of sputum collected from patients with Chronic Bronchitis with either purulent or mucoid sputum.

Legend. Sputum samples were collected from clinically stable patients with chronic bronchitis. 87 had purulent sputum and 36 had mucoid sputum. Samples were studied for the presence or absence of putative pathogenic bacteria (PP), bacteria were quantified in colony forming units/ml of sample, and classified as being above or below 1 x 10^7 cfu/ml, and neutrophils (PMN) were counted in a random viewing field on light phase microscopy. Purulent sputum was consistently and significantly associated with the presence of putative pathogens, a higher number of bacterial colonies, and more neutrophils than mucoid sample.

Modified from (29) and (30).

Although standard definitions of chronic bronchitis only include chronic sputum expectoration, early descriptive series of patients found that 70% of patients had bronchospasm, 88% had either sporadic or constant breathlessness and "spells of sickness for several weeks or a few months" with infection thought to be causal in all cases (31). The disease is characterised with periods of stability, interspersed with episodes of worsening symptoms (exacerbations). These will be described later.

Physical examination can be normal, but it can reveal signs consistent with COPD and emphysema (including evidence of hyper-inflated lung fields, peripheral and central cyanosis, cor-pulmonale and hyper-capnia). Radiographic signs in pure chronic bronchitis are poorly documented, as the most frequently quoted studies (for example (32, 33)) did not exclude patients with emphysema. However, it is likely that chest radiographs in the majority of patients with chronic bronchitis are normal (34), as the bronchial wall thickening which is characteristic of chronic bronchitis is approximately 0.1 - 0.5mm (24, 35) and therefore too small to be noticeable in plain x-rays. Bronchial wall thickening can be seen on high resolution computer tomography scans of the thorax (36). See figure 2.

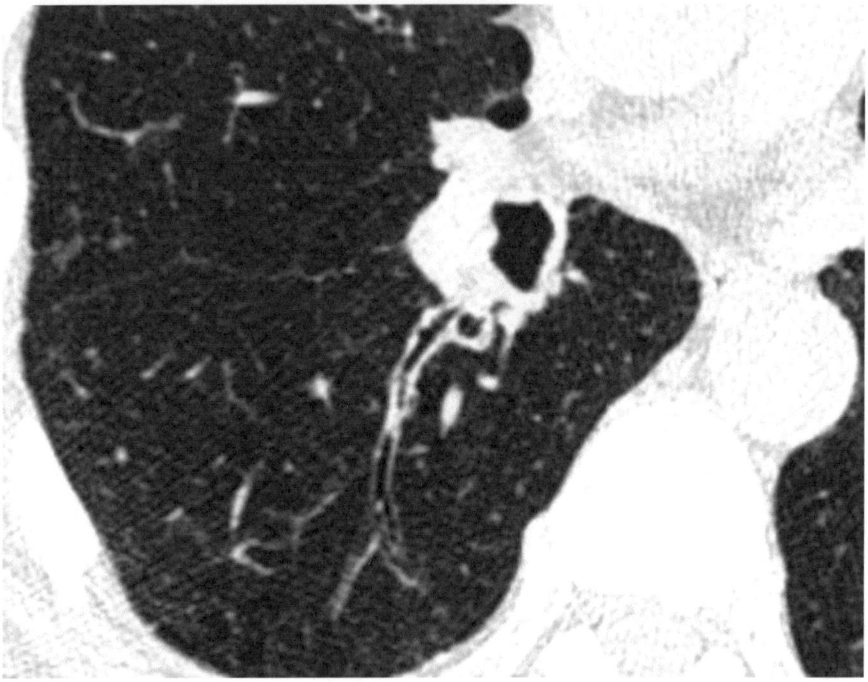

Fig. 2. High resolution CT image showing moderate bronchial wall thickening and mild bronchial dilatation in a patient with chronic bronchitis.
Used with permission from Hochhegger et al, Imaging, 2008; 20 (37).

There is a robust series of studies demonstrating that Chronic Bronchitis is associated with increased morbidity and mortality. It is an independent risk factor for all cause mortality both in COPD (38), and in subjects with normal lung function, even when smoking has been accounted for (38-40). The overall ten year mortality following a diagnosis of chronic bronchitis is 50%, with respiratory failure following an acute exacerbation being the most frequent terminal event (41).

Currently there are no clearly identified genetic risk factors for Chronic Bronchitis, however, twin studies have suggested that the heritability estimate for this condition is 40%, with only 14% of genetic influences shared with those related to smoking habits (42). Studies of polymorphisms of the TNFα gene (which reside in the promoter region of the gene, are associated with increased secretion of TNFα in the lung, and an increase in neutrophilic inflammation (43)) have shown a strong association with a chronic bronchitis phenotype in COPD (43, 44). However, this polymorphism has a minor allele frequency of 4 - 6% (43), and hence, other susceptibility factors must exist. There is currently an interest in genome wide association studies, and perhaps these will identify more potential candidate genes (45).

3. The pathology of chronic bronchitis

3.1 An overview of the histological changes seen in chronic bronchitis

Chronic bronchitis is characterised pathologically by mucus hyper-secretion with bronchial mucous gland hypertrophy and chronic inflammation of the bronchi and bronchioles, with a subsequent inflammatory cell infiltrate. Inflammation of the bronchial epithelium can produce squamous metaplasia, with a loss of ciliated cells. The metaplastic squamous epithelium can become dysplastic from persistent injury by smoking, and may become malignant (squamous cell carcinoma of the bronchus). Typical changes seen histologically with chronic bronchits are shown in Figure 3.

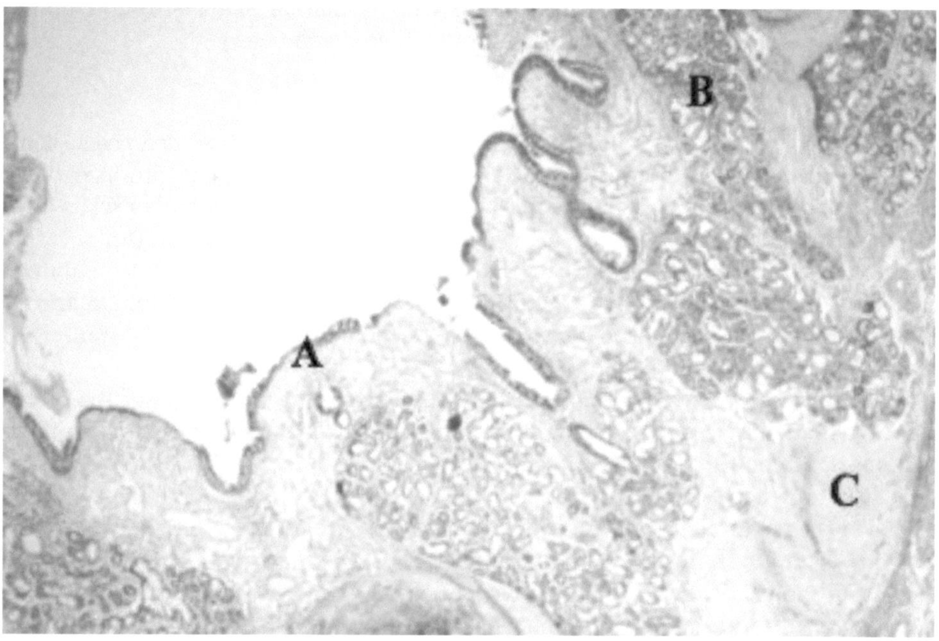

Fig. 3. Histology of Chronic Bronchitis

Legend. This figure demonstrates epithelial thickening (A), mucous gland hypertrophy and metaplasia (B) and prominence of airway smooth musculature (C), all of which are typical features in chronic bronchitis.

The earliest abnormality in chronic bronchitis is thought to be a respiratory bronchiolitis, affecting airways of less than 2mm in diameter, in response to chronic cigarette smoke or toxin exposure. Destruction of the airway wall and surrounding parenchymal elastin can lead to mural weakness and this coupled with mucus hyper-secretion predisposes towards bronchiolar obstruction.

The bronchioles are so numerous, that bronchiolar obstruction must be widespread and extensive to give clinical symptoms and studies confirm that pathological changes are seen before the clinical manifestations of disease (46). Squamous metaplasia and increased epithelial thickening is also seen prior to symptomatology and without airflow obstruction, although there is a relationship between epithelial layer thickness and COPD severity (25). However, all of these changes vary between patients, even in those with a similar degree of airflow obstruction (47).

Mucous gland hypertrophy and metaplasia occurs in response to inflammatory signals present in the airways of patients with chronic obstructive pulmonary disease (48) and contribute to airflow obstruction (49). Cigarette smoke-induced chronic airway inflammation also causes constriction and hypertrophy of airway smooth muscle cells (49) which become more prominent in biopsies taken from subjects with chronic bronchitis. In keeping with this observation, some studies have described an increase in airway smooth muscle mass in COPD (50) and have associated this with increases in airway wall thickness, greater luminal narrowing, and increased airflow resistance with poorer clearance of pulmonary secretions (51).

The inflammatory changes seen in chronic bronchitis occur in the mucosa, gland ducts and glands of both the intermediate sized bronchi (with an internal diameter of 2 - 4mm) and smaller bronchi and bronchioles (less than 2mm in internal diameter).

3.2 Pulmonary secretions

Airways secretions form an important component of the primary host defence system. In the trachea, there are approximately 4000 submucosal glands which produce both the mucus (52), and important proteins such as antibacterial proteins (including lysozyme (53) and lactoferrin (54)), secretory component necessary for immunoglobulin (Ig) A transport (55), and the antiproteinase, secretory leukoprotease inhibitor (SLPI) (56). Submucosal glands are composed of a central acinus consisting of serous cells, and a tubule lined with mucous cells. Plasma cells (responsible for the production of IgA) are also found in the submucosal glands (57).

The serous and mucous cells of the bronchial glands secrete the majority of the bronchial secretions, although goblet cells, and both the serous and clara cells of the airway epithelium make important contributions. Secretions are further diluted by alveoli surfactant and plasma fluid transudate (58). Bronchial mucus is composed of a continuous watery sol layer which overlays the bronchial epithelium and in which the cilia beat; and a more viscous gel layer, which lies on the tips of the cilia. The sol layer is 5 - 10μm deep, and is derived from the clara cells in the airway epithelium at the bronchiolar level with some contribution from fluid transudation. The sol layer enables the cilia to propel the gel layer over its surface, and is fundamental to mucociliary clearance. The mucus gel layer is derived from several sources including goblet and serous cells in the airway epithelium, clara cells at the bronchiolar level (59) and the submucosal glands (60). The sol phase contains soluble bronchial proteins and serum proteins, whilst the gel phase contains the mucinous glycoproteins, other serum proteins and also proteins bound to mucins (61). Bronchial mucus has many functions. It reduces evaporative loss from the respiratory tract, provides a protective barrier over the bronchial epithelium and removes trapped inhaled particles via ciliary action. The mucus also provides a medium for immunoglobulins and other protective proteins.

In healthy individuals, airway secretions are moved up to the mouth by ciliary action in the mucociliary escalator. Ciliated cells are found primarily in the tracheo-bronchial epithelium, although they are also present in the bronchioles (60, 62). There are approximately 200 – 300 cilia per cell; each is 4 – 6 μm long and 0.1 – 0.2 μm in diameter. The cilia beat 1000 times per minute, and in health the action of the cilia is co-ordinated, both within a single cell and between adjacent cells (63). The ciliary beat cycle has two components. The first is movement towards the larynx; this is the effective stroke, and is followed by a recovery stroke in the opposite direction where the cilia bend and disengage from the mucus (64).

Microvili project between the cilia and are believed to regulate the depth of the periciliary fluid level.

The clearance of mucus depends on ciliary action (65), cough, mucus volume, and the viscoelasticity and adhesiveness of the mucus to the airway epithelium. Mucus transportation has two phases, a fast phase related to ciliary clearance and cough, which is completed after a few hours in healthy individuals, and a slower phase which represents alveolar clearance and occurs over weeks or months (66, 67).

Mucocilary clearance is impaired in chronic bronchitis. There are many reasons for the impairment, including inhibition of ciliary activity by proteinases such as neutrophil elastase (NE) released from neutrophils recruited to the lungs (68), the presence of bacterial products (69) and epithelial damage. In chronic bronchitis, the inflammatory exudate overwhelms the normal clearance mechanisms, and the excess and accumulated secretions are expectorated in the form of sputum, which is a mixture of bronchial secretions, cells, cellular debris, cleared organisms and saliva, resulting in the chronic productive cough that characterises chronic bronchitis.

Mucinous glycoproteins are synthesised in mucus and goblet cells. Activated transcription factors upregulate expression of *MUC* genes in the nucleus of these cells. New MUC transcripts are translated to MUC proteins on ribosomes and cotranslationally inserted into the endoplasmic reticulum (ER). Glycosylation of the MUC protein backbone is initiated post-translationally in the *cis*-Golgi. Mature (fully glycosylated), mucins are packaged and stored in secretory granules until a mucin secretagogue triggers mucin secretion at the apical surface of the cell (70).

Airway mucins are overproduced by patients with chronic airway diseases like chronic bronchitis/COPD. This sustained mucin secretion, requires increased biosynthesis of mucins to replenish secretory granules, which in turn necessitates upregulation of *MUC* genes. Eight *MUC* genes (*MUC1, MUC2, MUC4, MUC5AC, MUC5B, MUC7, MUC8* and *MUC13)* are expressed in normal respiratory tract tissues (70), and although they are basally active in order to maintain mucin release to promote muco-ciliary clearance, protein transcription can be up-regulated dramatically in inflammation and infection.

In Chronic Bronchitis, a number of factors have been shown to up-regulate *MUC* genes, including neutrophil elastase, a proteolytic enzyme stored within neutrophil granules (see later). Inflammatory mediators have also been implicated, including IL-8 (71) and LTB4 (72) and oxidative stress (73). It is hypothesized that the on-going inflammation, intermittent infection and viral and bacterial colonization that is present in some patients with chronic bronchitis leads to excessive *MUC* gene activation, mucin production and goblet cell hypertrophy. If these genes were amenable to modulation, they would be a potential therapeutic target in the treatment of this disease.

3.3 Immunology and inflammation in chronic bronchitis

The inflammatory response seen in the lungs of patients with chronic bronchitis is complex, involves the innate and acquired immune system and serves as a self-perpetuating stimulus for further immune activation. Cigarette smoke exposure is the most important risk factor for developing chronic bronchitis, but the symptoms, the inflammation and the decline in lung function parameters continue, even after smoking cessation (74, 75).

Chronic Bronchitis is associated with the recruitment of leucocytes into lung tissue, the production of inflammatory mediators and the release of destructive proteins into the milieu, including proteinases. Bronchial biopsies taken from patient with chronic bronchitis show an increase in inflammatory cells compared with non-smokers and smokers with no symptoms of chronic mucus production (10). The cellular composition varies between individuals, but typically includes neutrophils, macrophages and CD8+ T cells. There are also smaller numbers of CD4+ T cells, but these may be monoclonal (76), and limited to pulmonary follicles (77).

Consistently, research has highlighted the importance of the neutrophil in the pathogenesis of COPD and chronic bronchitis. Patients with chronic bronchitis and COPD have increased numbers of neutrophils in proximal airway secretions (78, 79) and broncheoalveolar lavage fluid (BALF) (80) compared with asymptomatic smokers, and numbers increase with increasing disease (81, 82). Airway neutrophil numbers are also raised in patients with chronic bronchitis without COPD, although less so than when airflow obstruction is present (83). Sputum neutrophilia is associated with a faster decline in FEV_1 compared with those with lower neutrophil counts, losing approximately 1% more than predicted each year (84) and neutrophil counts decline with smoking cessation (85), consistent with the benefits of this intervention.

The neutrophil is the most abundant circulating leukocyte. The average peripheral blood neutrophil count is 2.5 - 7.5 x 10^6 /ml and when inactive, its' circulating half life is only 6 - 8 hours, which means that the bone marrow is required to produce and release more than 5 - 10 x 10^{10} neutrophils daily, with the capacity to increase production further if needed. Exposure to cigarette smoke appears to stimulate neutrophil differentiation and maturation, causing a peripheral leucocytosis (86, 87) which has been found to correlate with the severity of airflow obstruction (88). Fully mature neutrophils leave the bone marrow in a non-activated state and have a half life of 4 to 8 hours before marginating and entering tissue pools (89). Once in tissue, neutrophils are usually removed by apoptosis leading to their recognition and phagocytosis by macrophages in the main and by other neutrophils when the macrophage clearance system is overwhelmed (90). This mechanism prevents cell necrosis and the release of the remaining cellular content of proteinase and other mediators.

Neutrophils migrate into the lung in response to soluble pro-migratory stimuli, which include non-chemotactic cytokines (such as TNFα and IL-1β), chemotactic cytokines (chemokines including Interleukin 8) or chemoattractants (such as Leukotriene B4, (LTB4) and Complement factor C5a). Neutrophils are present at both the bronchial and alveolar level in chronic bronchitis and COPD, and therefore it is likely that neutrophil migration occurs from both the bronchial and pulmonary circulation.

In the bronchial circulation, neutrophils appear to migrate from vessel to tissue in a step-like process, dictated by the sequential activation of adhesive proteins and their ligands on neutrophils and endothelial cells. Migration begins with the capture of neutrophils from flowing blood, causing the cell to roll along the endothelial surface. Tethering and rolling of the neutrophil along the vessel wall is a normal feature of circulating neutrophils and is due to reversible binding of transmembrane glycoprotein adhesive molecules called "selectins", which are found both on neutrophils and endothelial cells (91). The next step in neutrophil migration is the transition from reversible rolling to firm adhesion with the endothelium. This is achieved by the sequential activation of neutrophil receptors called Integrins (92, 93). The final step of neutrophil recruitment from the bronchial circulation to the lungs is transendothelial migration. This is believed to occur preferentially at tricellular junctions (94), requiring the activation of Platelet endothelial cell adhesion molecule (PECAM1) (95) which is distributed evenly around the neutrophil and at intercellular junctions of endothelial cells. Once through the endothelial cell layer, leukocytes bind to matrix components such as collagen and laminin via ß1 integrins, with VLA-6 and 9 being perhaps the most important in allowing neutrophils to move through venule basement membrane and lung tissue (96-98). See figure 4. After this step, the neutrophil may come in close contact with the sub-mucosal glands and mucus containing epithelial cells. This is associated with mucus emptying from cellular tissues via a proteinase/ epidermal growth factor axis (73).

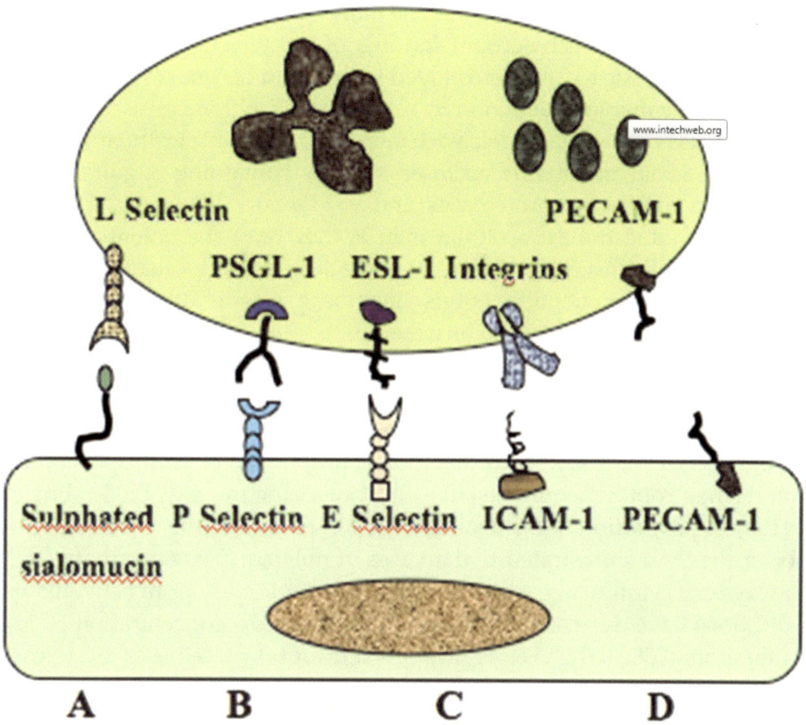

Fig. 4. Schematic summary of Neutrophil and Endothelial Cell Adhesion Molecules and their ligands in neutrophil transendothelial migration.

Legend. A: Early but short lived binding between L-Selectin and it's ligand initiates transient rolling on the endothelium surface. **B**. Interactions betweem P selectin and PSGL-1 and E-selctin and ESL-1 slows neutrophil rolling and allows transient tethering. **C**. Firm adhesion occurs through integrins and ICAM-1 associations. **D**. PECAM-1 interactions allow homing to intracellular junctions and diapedis via β1 Integrins.

Neutrophils are capable of sensing and migrating to sites of inflammation by sensing chemotactic gradients formed by pro-inflammatory stimuli. Neutrophils migrating within the lung encounter multiple chemoattractants signals in complex spatial and temporal patterns as endothelial, epithelial cells and immune cells respond to infection or injury, releasing a cocktail of cytokines and chemokines. *In vitro* models have demonstrated that neutrophils can migrate up and down chemical gradients, responding to one signal, migrating to its concentration peak and then migrating up a novel, more distant chemoattractant gradient, from endothelium to tissue (99). Thus the size and source of the gradient will influence any affect of neutrophils on mucus production.

Once neutrophils have migrated to the source of inflamed and infected tissue, their role is to kill and remove micro-organisms. The neutrophil achieves this by a process of phagocytosis, the respiratory burst and the release of cytotoxic peptides and proteins. These proteins include proteinases, which are bactericidal. Neutrophil elastase (the most well-studied of the proteinases) can break down the Outer membrane protein A (OmpA) of *E. coli* and other Gram-negative bacteria, and break down Shigella virulence factors, by cleaving peptide bonds in target proteins including small, hydrophobic amino acids such as glycine, alanine, and valine (100). Other cytotoxic peptides include the human neutrophil peptides 1 - 4 (collectively known as "the defensins") which account for 50% of the total protein content of azurophil granules and are highly toxic to fungi, enveloped viruses and bacteria (89).
Defensins also enhance mucin production by activating *MUC* gene transciption (101).
Neutrophil proteinases are usually released in a controlled intracellular environment, by fusing phagasomes (lipid membrane enclosed vesicles containing engulfed bacteria) with lysosymes (vesicles containing proteinases and oxidants). However, if proteinases are released from the cell into the extracellular matrix, they have the potential to be extremely destructive. Neutrophil elastase is capable of degrading all components of the extracellular matrix (ECM) by cleaving peptide bonds, including elastin, fibronectin and collagen, causing structural damage to tissue and airways (102).
Neutrophil elastase release is thought to be an important driver of disease pathogenesis in chronic bronchitis (28), and occurs during neutrophil migration, phagocytosis and cell death. Indeed, elastase is the most potent secretogogue studied to date. When neutrophils migrate through the ECM, it is known that a high proportion of neutrophil proteinases are expressed on the neutrophil membrane (103-105), polarising towards the leading edge of the neutrophil (106). A proportion of the proteinase is left behind as the cell moves on (106, 107) and it has been clearly demonstrated that an area of obligate elastase activity (or "collateral damage") always exists following the secretion of free proteinase from activated neutrophils until concentrations have decreased by diffusion to match the concentration of surrounding proteinase inhibitors (108, 109). See Figure 5. Neutrophil proteinases are released during degranulation, and phagocytosis ("sloppy eating"), especially during "frustrated phagocytosis", when cells attempt to ingest large particles (110). In contrast with apoptotic cells, proteinases are released during cell necrosis (111) and finally, proteinases can be released from activated macrophages, which scavenge the proteinases from apoptotic neutrophils via endocytosis and subsequently release them during the first 24 hours of their own inflammatory response (112).
As well as degrading lung tissue, neutrophil proteinases have many other effects in chronic bronchitis and COPD. When released from neutrophils, they damages the respiratory epithelium, reducing ciliary beating (68, 113) and triggering a state of oxidative stress in cells (114). Proteinases can induce apoptosis of epithelial cells (115) and detachment of bronchial epithelial cells from the extra cellular matrix (116), which is thought to be important in COPD and chronic bronchitis (117). Proteinases stimulate the release of other pro-inflammatory signals such as LTB4 by macrophages (118) and IL-8 from bronchial epithelial cells which enhances more neutrophil migration into the lung. Proteinases also decrease the function of immunoglobulins and activate components of the complement cascade (119, 120) and may also effect wound healing, by effecting transforming growth factor β and the epithelins (121). The inflammatory consequences of neutrophil proteinases on lung tissue and cells relevant to the development of chronic bronchitis and COPD are summarised in table 1.

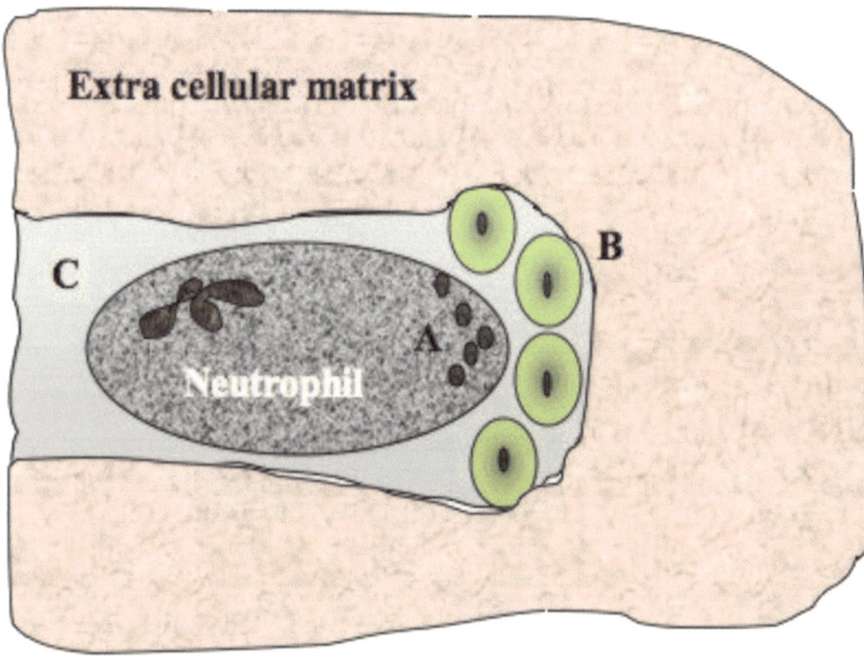

Fig. 5. The potential mechanism for tissue damage during extracellular proteinase release from neutrophils

Legend. As neutrophils migrate towards a source of inflammation, granules containing proteinases including neutrophil elastase (NE) are mobilised towards the leading edge of the cell (**A**). These proteinases are thought to be released during migration through complex media (such as the extracellular matrix (ECM)) to allow a path to be made for the neutrophil. Upon exocytosis, NE has a concentration of 5mM. Alpha-1 anti-trypsin (A1AT) (an anti-proteinase and inhibitor of NE) is thought to be present in the interstitium at concentrations which are 200 times lower than NE when it is first released from a granule, and since the inhibitor inactivates NE on a one molecule to one molecule basis, the proteinase remains active. NE concentrations decrease by diffusion (represented by the dark green to pale green graduated circles) and it is only when concentrations have reduced to approximately 24uM that NE can be fully inhibited by A1AT (**B**). This leads an obligate area of proteolysis around the leading edge of the cell, theoretically aiding the cell's transmigration, and potentially leaving damaged ECM behind the cell (**C**).

Although neutrophils are clearly associated with chronic bronchitis, it is likely that many immune cell populations are involved in the pathogenesis of this disease. Interestingly, there are few differences in the cellular content of bronchial biopsies taken from patients with COPD with and without chronic bronchitis (122) although one study has suggested a predominance of eosinophils in airway secretions when chronic bronchitis is present (123), however this observation has not been replicated. The numbers of CD8+ lymphocytes in bronchial tissue relate inversely with FEV_1 (122) and have been shown capable of causing lung tissue damage both by their own cytotoxicity and by recruiting macrophages by secreting IFN-γ. Macrophages are the most abundant cell recovered in bronchoalveolar lavage in patients with chronic bronchitis and COPD, and numbers also correlate with disease severity (124, 125). These cells are believed to participate in tissue damage by the release of their own proteinases, such as MMP-12 (although they are less potent than neutrophil elastase) and reactive oxygen species. Whether macrophage proteinases stimulate mucus production and release is unknown. Certainly, more studies are needed to fully understand and identify pivotal inflammatory signals or biomarkers which could differentiate those smokers who are at most risk of chronic bronchitis and COPD, those who are most likely to experience frequent exacerbations of their symptoms and those at risk of bacterial colonisation of their airways, as these disease features are related to worsening clinical outcomes.

Bacterial Killing	Intra-cellular : bactericidal following engulfment of organisms in phagosome Extra cellular: Targeting and cleaving bacterial virulence factors in released granule proteins
Induces Inflammatory Cell migration	NE/alpha 1 antitrypsin complexes are chemotactic for neutrophils Modification of ICAM1 expression enhancing adhesion
Degradation by proteolysis	Degrades all components of Extracellular Matrix Degrades Cystatin C Degrades inhibitors of proteinases Cleaves T Lymphocyte surface antigen
Activation of proteinases by post-transcriptional modifications	Activates proteinases including MMP-2, MMP-3, MMP-9, and Cathepsin B
Modification of inflammatory mediators, enhancing inflammation	Enhances epithelial secretion of IL8 Enhances macrophage secretion of LTB4 Inhibits cellular response to inhibitors of inflammatory mediators, for example, TNFsR1 Prolongs the half life of inflammatory mediators including TNFα Increases alpha1-AT expression by monocytes and alveolar macrophages
Enhances Cell Apoptosis	Increases epithelial and endothelial cell apoptosis
Alteration of Cell function	Disruption and detachment of epithelial cells Reduces ciliary beating of columnar epithelium Enhances oxidative stress Increases mucin production Increases bacterial adherence and colonisation on the epithelium

Table 1. An overview of the inflammatory consequences of neutrophil proteinases thought relevant to the development and progression of Chronic Bronchitis and COPD.

Legend. References are included in the text.

4. Bacterial colonisation in chronic bronchitis

Approximately 25% of patients with chronic bronchitis have pulmonary secretions from which potentially pathogenic bacteria are cultured, even when they are clinically stable. These patients are deemed to have airways that are colonised with bacteria (126). The most common bacteria cultured in clinically stable patients are *Haemophilus influenzae, Streptococcus viridans* and *Streptococcus pneumoniae* (127) although *Neisseria* species and *Proteus mirabilis* have also been isolated. Interestingly, these bacteria have been cultured in lower airway secretions despite the presence of antibodies in serum and sputum against the bacterium (128) and despite courses of appropriate oral antibiotics (129), which suggests that when established, colonisation is difficult to eradicate.

Identified risk factors for colonisation include behavioural factors such as current smoking (127, 130), and repeated bacterial infections in the form of exacerbations (see later). Cigarette smoke exposure is known to effect lower airway mucociliary clearance by reducing ciliary beat frequency (131) and the neutrophilic inflammation present in chronic bronchitis has been shown to be conducive to bacterial colonisation (132). Colonisation is associated with increased sputum concentrations of inflammatory mediators including IL-8, LTB4 as well as neutrophil elastase (30). Lower airway bacterial colonisation in the stable state appears to increase the frequency and alter the character of COPD exacerbations (with patients with Chronic Bronchitis experiencing more exacerbations) (133). Exacerbation frequency relates to subsequent decline in lung function (134) and health status (135); suggesting that colonisation may be important in disease progression, although it does not directly relate to decline in FEV_1 (127).

The numbers of bacteria present may also alter immune cellular responses which could impact on subsequent inflammation, as patients with sputum bacterial loads of > 10^6 cfu/ml have been shown to have a more robust inflammatory response than those with bacterial loads that are lower (30). In animal models, bacterial loads of less than 10^5 organisms can be eradicated by macrophages and other components of the innate host defence without inducing much inflammation. In patients with chronic bronchitis, a load of this magnitude can co-exist without secondary inflammation perhaps because a balance between bacterial killing and replication controls the situation. However, greater bacterial loads require neutrophil recruitment and the involvement of the secondary acquired immune response (136). Macrophages and dendritic cells facilitate bacterial clearance in a variety of ways. They are able to migrate to the bronchial lymph nodes, particularly to the T cell paracortical areas (137) where the antigen they carry is available for primary stimulation of the T cell clones. T cell derived cytokines then amplify the effector function of macrophages by enhancing their phagocytic and anti-microbial capacity (138).

5. Exacerbations of chronic bronchitis

Chronic Bronchitis is characterised by periods of disease stability punctuated by exacerbations. Several different definitions of exacerbations exist (for example (139, 140)) but a common definition is a subjective increase from baseline of one or more chronic symptoms including cough frequency, sputum production or sputum purulence and breathlessness (27). The episodes can be defined by severity or aetiology (bacterial, viral, environmental or unknown). Approximately 30% of exacerbations are thought to be caused by viral infections (141) with 30% of these being caused by influenza, 25% by parainfluenza, 20% by rhinovirus and 15% by coronovirus (27). In exacerbations requiring ventilatory support, only 15% of cases were associated with positive identification of a viral pathogen, and half of these were also associated with a concomitant bacterial infection, suggesting that viruses are less important in more severe exacerbations (142).

Pathogenic bacterial organisms are found in 50 - 80% of patients during exacerbations (143, 144), with the most common organisms being *Streptococcus pneumoniae*, nontypable *Haemophilus influenzae* and *Moraxella catarrhalis* (19, 145). Less frequently, gram negative organisms are isolated, including *pseudomonas aeruginosa* (146). Previously there was controversy as to whether bacteria isolated from sputum during exacerbation were truly causative, or whether they represented colonization. However, recent studies have demonstrated that mean bacteria colony forming units per ml of sample (counted during quantitative sputum culture) are at least a log higher in exacerbations compared with those seen in the stable state (27). Further more, bacterial exacerbations such as these are characterized by a significant increase in pulmonary inflammation including neutrophil recruitment and can be identified by the presence of purulent sputum (147) which resolves with resolution of symptoms (148).

Examination of sputum purulence is a simple and accurate way to differentiate between bacterial and non-bacterial exacerbations of chronic bronchitis (29), and can be used to rationalize antibiotic therapy to target those patients likely to benefit, and to protect others from unnecessary antibiotic exposure and potential side effects.

Exacerbation frequency appears to increase with decreasing FEV_1 and the presence of chronic bronchitis, but in patients with moderate to severe disease, the median exacerbation frequency is 2 -3 per annum and patients with more frequent exacerbations experience a faster decline in FEV_1 (134). There is also a correlation with the degree of airflow obstruction and the type of bacteria isolated from sputum during acute exacerbations of Chronic Bronchitis and COPD, with Pseudomonas species and Enterobacteriaceae being predominant in patients with an $FEV_1 \leq 35\%$ of the predicted value (149) although it is difficult to ascertain whether the bacteria are the cause or a consequence of reduced lung function.

Exacerbations are a significant cause of morbidity and mortality, with increasing exacerbation frequency being related to worsening patient outcomes, reduced exercise capacity and a reduced quality of life (150). Exacerbations remain the commonest precipitant of death and even after an exacerbation resolves, respiratory, physical, social and emotional impairment may persist for prolonged time (150). The decline in health status is thought to be the result of prolonged periods of heightened pulmonary inflammation, with more immune cell recruitment to the lungs, more proteinase release, and more tissue damage (151). Preventing exacerbations and treating them expeditiously is a priority in order to slow disease progression.

6. Established and emerging therapies in chronic bronchitis

Treatments for chronic bronchitis have focused upon improving or reducing sputum clearance and treating airflow obstruction, when present. Airflow obstruction is treated in accordance with guidelines for the treatment of COPD, and these will not be covered here.

6.1 The treatment of exacerbations of chronic bronchitis

During clinical exacerbations of chronic bronchitis and COPD, studies have demonstrated that oral prednisolone (continued for 10 days) is efficacious, improving dyspnoea, increasing improvements in FEV_1 and increasing the time until the next exacerbation (152).

Results from trials of antibiotic treatment during exacerbations have been more confusing, as they have often not proved clinically effective (for example, (153, 154)). However, these trials have often been limited in their design, as they have not differentiated between bacterial exacerbations (where one would expect an improvement in clinical outcomes following appropriate treatment) and non-bacterial exacerbations (where antibiotics should not effect outcomes). Antibiotics are an appropriate therapy for suspected bacterial exacerbations, and should be reserved for patients with symptoms and signs consistent with infection, in the presence of purulent sputum (30, 147). Given the bacteria isolated from sputum during exacerbations (see earlier), an appropriate choice of antibiotic includes broad spectrum penicillins such as amoxicillin (155), tetracyclines such as doxycyline (156) and quinolones and macrolides where allergies and bacterial resistance are important determinants of anti-bacterial choice . International guidelines for treatment choice have not altered in the past ten years and the majority of guidelines suggest that an initial sputum culture is only required prior to treatment initiation when resistance is suspected.

Salbutamol and ipratropium have been shown to improve symptoms of breathlessness and wheeze during exacerbations of chronic bronchitis and COPD, and increase FEV_1 (157), and these therapies are routinely used where these symptoms predominate. Both appear equally efficacious and while only a select group of patients benefit from both therapies in unison, side effects are minimal, supporting their use (158). Delivery device (nebulised or via an inhaler) does not effect outcome (159). It is less clear if they are beneficial in the absence of chronic airflow obstruction, as studies have shown mixed results (160). There are currently no published studies which support the use of long acting $Beta_2$ agonists or anti-muscurinic medicants during acute exacerbations of chronic bronchitis.

A meta-analysis of 23 trials suggested that mucolytics also reduce symptom scores, days of illness and increase time until next exacerbation in chronic bronchitis (161) supporting their use in patients with frequent exacerbations.

Not all patients respond to therapy, and a poorer response (with increased risk of death) is more commonly seen in patients aged over 65 years, those with significant co-morbidities, significant airflow obstruction ($FEV_1 < 50\%$ predicted) and more than 4 exacerbations per year (139). Patients fulfilling these criteria should be assessed carefully to ensure that treatment, where needed, is started promptly. In order to facilitate this, many patients are now being managed in the community with prophylactic antibiotics and oral corticosteroids, as it has been shown that early intervention is associated with better clinical outcomes (162).

6.2 Treatments for stable disease

Most studies of potential treatments used in chronic bronchitis have not differentiated between chronic bronchitis and COPD, and therefore results should be interpreted with caution. Certainly, patients with mild symptoms and infrequent exacerbations may not necessitate regular pharmacotherapy and no treatments (apart from smoking cessation) have been shown to reduce symptoms and alter progression or the development of airflow obstruction. In light of this, all patients should be encouraged and supported with appropriate pharmacotherapy to stop smoking, as this has clear health benefits and has been shown to reduce disease progression.

Inhaled corticosteroids are a common treatment in COPD, and recommended for patients with a FEV_1 less than 50% predicted or in patients who experience frequent exacerbations. Studies of inhaled corticosteroids in chronic bronchitis without airflow obstruction are limited, and contradictory. Llewellyn-Jones et al, saw a reduction in the chemotactic activity of lung secretions with reduced neutrophil activity in sputum from patients with chronic bronchitis and emphysema (163), however, other authors have not shown a similar response in short term trials (164). Furthermore, a three year trial of inhaled budesonide in mild and moderate COPD did not show any benefit in lung function decline, symptom scores or exacerbation rates, questioning the role for inhaled steroids in the absence of severe airflow obstruction (165). Similarly, there is no clinical evidence to support the use of bronchodilators in chronic bronchitis in the absence of airflow obstruction, however, long acting β2 agonists have been shown to increase ciliary beat frequency, which could enhance sputum clearance (166).

Phosphodiesterase 4 (PDE4) inhibitors are effective anti-inflammatory agents in animal models and have been shown to reduce inflammation in COPD and chronic bronchitis (167). PDE4 hydrolyzes cyclic adenosine monophosphate (cAMP) to inactive adenosine monophosphate (AMP). Inhibition of PDE4 blocks hydrolysis of cAMP thereby increasing levels of cAMP within cells. Increases in the intracellular levels of cyclic AMP can reduce the activation of a wide range of inflammatory and lung resident cells (168).

There have been trials of PDE4 inhibitors in COPD (169-171), that have confirmed a modest but significant improvement in spirometry in COPD, and quality of life scores and a reduction in the number of exacerbations experienced. There is evidence that Roflumilast may be particularly beneficial in patients with COPD and chronic bronchitis (172), but it is unclear if this drug is effective in chronic bronchitis without airflow obstruction, and further trials are awaited. PDE4 inhibitors appear to reduce the number of neutrophils recruited to the airways, with a reduction of between 30 – 50%, which could explain their clinical efficacy (168).

N-acetylcysteine is both a mucolytic and an anti-inflammatory and antioxidant drug (173, 174). It is widely prescribed for the treatment of chronic bronchitis in mainland Europe (175) and studies have confirmed that it is effective in reducing the risk of exacerbations and improves symptoms of chronic bronchitis (reducing sputum volume) (176). The use of other mucolytics including carbocysteine, have been reviewed in a recent Cochrane publication (177) of 28 trials. This review surmised that regular use of mucolytics reduced exacerbation frequency and days of disability during exacerbations in patients with chronic bronchitis, however, this benefit was not seen in patients taking regular inhaled corticosteroids. The authors suggest that oral mucolytics are a potentially useful treatment in patients with frequent exacerbations who are not on inhaled corticosteroids(177).

Prophylactic antibiotics have been used in patients with stable chronic bronchitis in an attempt to treat bacterial colonisation, and reduce associated inflammation. There have been few trials examining the efficacy of this, however a meta-analysis of 9 trials suggested that antibiotics reduced the days of illness experienced due to exacerbations of chronic bronchitis, without reducing actual exacerbation frequency (178). Erythromycin has been shown to reduce exacerbation frequency in patients with chronic bronchitis and COPD (179) and clarithromycin has been shown to reduce the development of emphysema in smoke-exposed mice (180). These actions are thought to be mediated via the macrolides effect on matrix metalloproteinase 9 secretion (a proteinase) and are separate from the anti-microbial properties of the drugs (181). Further trials are needed to assess the longterm impact of macrolide therapy in chronic bronchitis.

If chronic bronchitis is caused and perpetuated by neutrophilic inflammation, one would expect that therapies which decrease the inflammatory response would improve clinical outcomes. Unfortunately, neutrophilic inflammation (as seen in COPD and chronic bronchitis) is, in the main, resistant to the generic inflammatory treatments employed in other respiratory conditions, such as asthma and new therapeutic strategies are urgently required. It may be that there is no single treatment that is effective in all patients with chronic bronchitis, and perhaps as more is learned about its genetic and environmental drivers, more specific treatments for subsets of patients will be developed (practicing pharmacogenetics). Until that point, there are no clear therapeutic options for patients with stable disease without airflow obstruction, and no treatments that prevent the decline in FEV_1 in patients with airflow obstruction. Current best practice includes the prompt treatment of exacerbations, coupled with smoking cessation support.

7. Conclusion

Chronic bronchitis is a common and debilitating feature of COPD, which effects between 8 and 12 % of adults globally and despite improvements in air quality in developed countries, it's prevalence has not fallen. The main risk factor for developing chronic bronchitis is now chronic cigarette smoke exposure, but environmental air quality remains an important contributing factor in the developing world.

Chronic bronchitis is associated with bronchial inflammation, and although the neutrophil and its products have been shown to cause all of the pathological features of disease *in vitro*, many other cell types have been implicated in its pathogenesis.

In COPD, the presence of chronic sputum expectoration is associated with worse clinical outcomes than those without. The inflammatory burden is higher in patients with chronic bronchitis compared with matched patients without (182) and chronic mucus hyper-secretion is consistently associated with both an excess FEV_1 decline, an increased risk of subsequent hospitalization (183) and death from respiratory infections (184).

Despite it's importance in terms of prevalence, morbidity and mortality, chronic bronchitis remains under-investigated and poorly treated. No medicants have been shown to robustly improve symptoms, decline in FEV_1 or exacerbation frequency. The mainstay of treatment remains smoking cessation and prompt treatment of exacerbations. New therapeutic strategies are urgently required.

8. References

[1] Pauwels RA, Buist AS, Calverley PM, Jenkins CR, Hurd SS, Committee GS. Global strategy for the diagnosis, management and prevention of chronic obstructive pulmonary disease. Nhlbi/who global initiative for chronic obstructive lung disease (gold) workshop summary. *Am J Respir Crit Care Med* 2001;163:1256 - 1276.

[2] Global Initiative for chronic obstructive lung disease. Guidelines and resources. *wwwgoldcopdcom/index* 2007.

[3] Lomas DA. Chronic obstructive pulmonary disease. Introduction. *Thorax* 2002;57:735

[4] World Health Organization. Chronic obstructive pulmonary disease (copd). Fact sheet 315. *wwwwhoint/mediacentre/factsheet/fs315* 2007.

[5] Buist AS, McBurnie MA, Vollmer WM, Gillespie S, Burney P, Mannino DM, Menzes AM, Sullivan SD, Lee TA, Weiss KB, et al. International variation in the prevalence of copd (the bold study): A population-based prevalene study. *Lancet* 2007;370:741 - 750.

[6] Mannino DM, Holguin F. Epidemiology and global impact of obstructive pulmonary disease. *Respir Med* 2006;1:114 - 120.

[7] Doll R, Peto R, Wheatley K, Gray R, Sutherland I. Mortality in relation to smoking: 40 years' observations on male british doctors. *BMJ* 1994;309:901 - 911.

[8] Tashkin DP, Clark VA, Coulson AH, Simmons M, Bourque LB, Reems C, Detels R, Sayre JW, Rokaw SN. The ucla population studies of chronic obstructive respiratory disease. Viii. Effects of smoking cessation on lung function; a prospective study of a free-living population. *Am Rev Respir Dis* 1984;130:707 - 715.

[9] Sanford AJ, Silverman EK. Chronic obstructive pulmonary disease.1: Susceptibility factors for copd the genotype-environment interaction. *Thorax* 2002;57:736 - 741.

[10] Saetta M, Turato G, Maestrelli P, Ciaccia A, Fabbri LM. Cellular and structural basis of chronic obstructive pulmonary disease. *Am J Respir Crit Care Med* 2001;163:1304 - 1309.

[11] Sin DD, Anthonisen NR, Soriano JB, Agusti AG. Mortality on copd. Role of co-morbidities. *Eur Respir J* 2006;28:1245 - 1257.

[12] Celli BR, Cote CG, Martin JM, Caanova C, Montes de Oca M, Mendez RA, Pinto-Plara V, Cabral HJ. The body mass index, airflow obstruction, dyspnoea and exercise capacity index in chronic obstructive pulmonary disease. *N Engl J Med* 2004;350:1005 - 1012.

[13] Medical Research Council. Definition and classification of chronic bronchitis for clinical and epidemiological purposes. A report to the medical research council by their committee on the aetiology of chronic bronchitis. *Lancet* 1965;1:775 - 779.

[14] Redline S. Epidemiology of copd. In n. Cherniack editor. *Chronic Obstructive Pulmonary Disease* 1991;1st Edition. Philadelphia: Saunders.

[15] Sapey E, Stockley RA. The neutrophil and its special role in chronic obstructive pulmonary disease. . *In Asthma and COPD: Basic Mechanisms and clinical management* 2008;Editor: P J Barnes.

[16] Caruso G, Catalano D, Scalisi N, Terrnova S, Virgilio C, Mazzone O. Association of chronic obstructive bronchitis and upper digestive pathology. *Recenti Prog Med* 1991;82:585 - 587.

[17] Dalphin JC, Bildstein F, Pernet D, Dubiez A, Depierre A. Prevalance of chronic bronchitis and respiratory function in a group of diary farmers in the french doubs province. *Chest* 1989;95:1244 - 1247.

[18] Menezes AMB, Victora CG, Rigatto M. Prevalance and risk factors for chronic bronchitis in pelotas, rs, brazil: A population-based study. *Thorax* 1994;49:1217 - 1221.

[19] Tager IB, Speizer FE. Risk estmates for chronic bronchitis in smokers: A study of male to female differences. *Am Rev Respir Dis* 1976;113:619 - 625.

[20] Thurlbeck WM. Chronic airflow obstruction in lung disease. *In Bennington JL, ed Major problems in pathology Vol %* 1976;Philadelphia, 1976:WB Saunders.

[21] Barker DJP, Godfrey KM, Fall C, Osmond C, Winter PD, Shaheen SO. Relation of birth weight and childhood respiratory infections to adult lung function and death from chronic obstructive lung disease. *BMJ* 1991;303:671 - 675.

[22] Demoly P, Simony-Lafontaine J, Chanez P, Pujol JL, Lequeux N, Michel FB. Cell proliferation in the bronchial mucosa of asthmatics and chronic bronchitis. *Am J Respir Crit Care Med* 1994;150:214 - 217.

[23] Jamel K, Cooney TP, Fleetham JA. Chronic bronchitis, correlation of morphological findings to sputum production and flow rates. *Am Rev Respir Dis* 1984;129:719 - 722.
[24] Reid L. Measurement of the bronchial mucous gland layer; a diagnostic yardstick in chronic bronchitis. *Thorax* 1960;15:132 - 141.
[25] Hogg JC, Chu F, Utokaparch S, Woods R, Elliott WM, Buzatu L, Cherniack RM, Rogers RM, Sciurba FC, Coxon OR, et al. The nature of small airway obstruction in chronic obstructive pulmonary disease. *N Engl J Med* 2004;350:2645 - 2653.
[26] Graham NWH. The epidemiology of acute respiratoy infection in children and adults: A global perspective. *Epidemiol Rev* 1990;12:149 - 178.
[27] Sethi S. Infectious etiology of acute exacerbations of chronic bronchitis. *Chest* 2000;117:380s - 385s.
[28] Hill AT, Bayley D, Stockley RA. The interrelationship of sputum inflammatory markers in patients with chronic bronchitis. *Am J Respir Crit Care Med* 1999;160:893 - 898.
[29] Stockley RA, O'Brien CO, Pye A, Hill SL. Relationship of sputum color to nature and outpatient management of acute exacerbations of copd. *Chest* 2000;117:1638 - 1645.
[30] Hill AT, Campbell EJ, Hill SL, Bayley D, Stockley RA. Association between airway bacterial load and markers of airways inflammation in patients with stable chronic bronchitis. *Am J Med* 2000;109:288 - 295.
[31] Oswald NC, Harold TJ, Martin WJ. Clinical pattern of chronic bronchitis. *Lancet* 1953;2:639 - 643.
[32] Bates DV, Gordon CA, Paul GI. Chronic bronchitis: Report on the third and fourth stages of the co-ordinated study of chronic bronchitis in the department of veterans affairs, canada. *Med Serv J Can* 1966;22:1 - 59.
[33] Simon G. Chronic bronchitis and emphysema; a symposium. Iii. Pathological findings and radiological changes in chronic bronchitis and empysema. B. Radiological changes in chronic bronchitis. *Br J Radiol* 1959;32:292 - 294.
[34] Gamsu G, Nadel JA. The roentgenologic manifestations of emphysema and chronic bronchitis. *Med Clin North Am* 1973;57:719 - 733.
[35] Thurlbeck WM, Angus AE. A distribution curve for chronic bronchitis. *Thorax* 1964;19:436 - 442.
[36] Hartman TE, Tazelaar HD, Swensen SJ, Muller NL. Cigarette smoking: Ct and patholgic findings of associated pulmonary disease. *Radiographics* 1997;17:377 - 390.
[37] Hochhegger B, Dixon S, Screaton N, Cardinal Da Silva V, Marchiori E, Binukrishnn S, Holemans JA, Gosney JR, McCann C. Emphysema and smoking related lung disease. *Imaging* 2008;20:219 - 235.
[38] Stavem K, Sandvik L, Erikssen J. Breathlessness, phelgm and mortality: 26 years of follow-up in healthy middle aged norwegian men. *J Intern Med* 2006;260:332 - 343.
[39] Ebi-Kryston KL, Hawthorne VM, Rose G, Shipley MJ, Gillis CR, Hole D, Carmen W, Eshleman S, Higgins MW. Breathlessness, chronic bronchitis and reduced pulmonary function as predictors of cardiovascular disease mortality amoung men in england, scotland and the united states. *Int J Epidemiol* 1989;18:84 - 88.
[40] Frostad A, Soyseth V, Anderson A, Gulsvik A. Respiratory symptoms as predictors of all cause mortality in an urban community. *J Intern Med* 2006;259:520 - 529.

[41] Turato G, Di Stefano A, Maestrelli P, Mapp CE, Ruggieri MP, Roggeri A, Fabbri LM, Saetta M. Effect of smoking cessation on airway inflammation in chronic bronchitis. *Am J Respir Crit Care Med* 1995;152:1262 - 1267.

[42] Hallberg J, Dominicus A, Eriksson UK, Gerhardsson de Verdier M, Pedersen NL, Dahlback M, HNihlen U, Higenbottam T, Svartengren M. Interaction between smokng and genetic factors in the development of chronic bronchitis. *Am J Respir Crit Care Med* 2007;177:486 - 490.

[43] Sapey E, Wood AM, Ahmad A, Stockley RA. Tnf alpha rs361525 polymorphism is associated with increased local production and downstream inflammation in copd. *Am J Respir Crit Care Med* 2010;180:192 - 199.

[44] Huang S.L., Chern-Huey S, Shi-Chuan C. Tumor necrosis factor alpha gene polymorphism in chronic bronchitis. *Am J Respir Crit Care Med* 1997;156:1436 - 1439.

[45] Dijkstra A. Genetic susceptibilities for chronic bronchitis: A genome-wide association study. *Am J Respir Crit Care Med* 2010;181:A3834 (Abstract).

[46] Niewoeher DE, Kleinerman J, Rice DB. Pathologic changes in the periheral airways of young cigarette smokers. *N Engl J Med* 1974;291:755 - 758.

[47] Kim V, Criner GJ, Abdallah HY, Graughan JP, Furukawa S, Solomides CC. Small airways morphometry and improvement in pulmonary function after lung volume reduction surgery. *Am J Respir Crit Care Med* 2005;171:40 - 47.

[48] Williams OW, Sharafkhaneh A, Kim V, Dickey BF, Evans CM. Airway mucus, from production to secretion. *Am J Respir Cell Mol Biol* 2006;34:527 - 536.

[49] Baraldo S, saetta M, Cosio MG. Pathophysology of small airways *Semin Respir Crit Care Med* 2003;24:465 - 472.

[50] Nagai A, West WW, Thurlbeck WM, The National Institute of Health Intermittent Positive-Pressure breathing trial: pathological studies : II. Correlation between morphologic findings, clinical findings and evidence of expiratory airflow obstruction. *Am Rev Respir Dis* 1985;132:946 - 953.

[51] Lambert RK, Wiggs BR, Kuwano K, Hogg JC, Pare PD. Functional significance of increased airflow smooth muscle in asthma and copd. *J Appl Physiol* 1993;74:2771 - 2781.

[52] Tos M. Mucus glands of the trachea in children. Quantitative studies. *Anat Anz* 1970;126:146 - 160.

[53] Bowes D, Corrin B. Ultrastructural immunocytochemical localisation of lysozyme in human bronchial glands. *Thorax* 1977;32:163 - 170.

[54] Bowes D, Clark AE, Corrin B. Ultrastructural localisation of lactoferrin and glycoprotein in human bronchial glands. *Thorax* 1981;36:108 - 115.

[55] Brandtzaeg P. Mucosal and glandular distribution of immunoglobulin components. Immunohistochemistry with a cold ethanol-fixation technique. *Immunology* 1974;26:1101 - 1114.

[56] Kramps JA, Franken C, Meijer CJ, Dijkman JH. Localisation of low molecular weight protease inhibitor in serous secretory cells of the respiratory tract. *J Histochem Cytochem* 1981;29:712 - 719.

[57] Soutar CA. Distribution of plasma cells and other cells containing immunoglobulin in the respiratory tract of normal man and class of immunoglobulins contained therein. *Thorax* 1976;31:158 - 166.

[58] Puchelle E, Girod de Bentzmann S, Higenbottam T. Airway secretions and lung liquids. In brewis, r.A.L., editor. *Respiratory Medicine* 1995;W.B.Saunders. London:97 - 111.
[59] Widdicombe Jg, Pack RJ. The clara cell. *Eur J Respir Dis* 1982;63:202 - 220.
[60] Shimura S, Takishima T. Airway submucosal gland secretion. In shimura, s., editor. *Airway secretion, physiological basis for the control of mucous hypersecretion* 1994;Marcel Decker. New York:23 - 35.
[61] Kim WD. Lung mucus: A clinician's view. *Eur Respir J* 1997;10:1914 - 1917.
[62] Widdicombe JH, Widdicombe JG. Regulation of human airway surface liquid. *Respir Physiol* 1995;99:3 - 12.
[63] Sanderson MJ, Sleigh MA. Ciliary activity of cultured rabbit tracheal epithelium: Beat pattern and metachrony. *J Cell Sci* 1981;47:331 - 347.
[64] Sleigh MA, Blake JR, Liron N. The propulsion of mucus by cilia. *Am Rev Respir Dis* 1988;137:726 - 741.
[65] Puchelle E, Zahm JM, Girard F, Bertrand A, Polu JM, Aug F, Sdoul P. Mucociliary transport in vivo and in vitro. Relations to sputum properties in chronic bronchitis. *Eur J Respir Dis* 1980;61:254 - 264.
[66] Hasania A, Pavia D. Cough as a clearance mechanism. In braga, p.C., editor. *Cough* 1989;Raven Press. New York.
[67] Pavia D. Lung mucociliary clearance. In clarke, s.W., editor. *Aerosols and the lung* 1984;Butterworths. Boston.
[68] Smallman LA, Hill SL, Stockley RA. Reduction of ciliary beat frequency in vitro by sputum from patients with bronchiectasis: A serine proteinase effect. *Thorax* 1984;39:663 - 667.
[69] Wilson R, Pitt T, Taylor G, Watson D, MacDermot J, Sykes D, Roberts D, Cole P. Pyocyanin and 1-hydroxyphenazine produced by pseudomonas aeruginosa inhibit the beating of human respiratory cilia in vitro. *J Clin Invest* 1987;79:221 - 229.
[70] Callaghan Rose M, Voynow JA. Respiratory tract mucin genes and mucin glycoproteins in health and disease. *Physiological Review* 2006;88:245 - 278.
[71] Bautista M, Chen Y, Ivanova VS, Rahimi MK, Watson AM, Rose MC. Il-8 regulates mucin gene expression at the post-transcriptional level in lung epithelial cells. *J Immunol* 2009;13:2159 - 2166.
[72] Miyahara N, Takeda K, Miyahara S, Matsubara S, Koya T, Joetham A, Krishnan E, KDakhama A, Haribabu B, Gelfand EW. Requirement for leukotrine b4 receptor 1 in allergen-induced airway hyperresponsiveness. *Am J Respir Crit Care Med* 2005;175:161 - 167.
[73] Takeyama K, Dabbagh K, Jeong-Shim J, Dao-Pick T, Ueki IF, Nadel JA. Oxidative stress causes mucin synthesis via transactivation of epidermal growth factor receptor: Role of neutrophils. *J Immunol* 2000;164:1546 - 1552.
[74] Retamales I, Elliot MW, Meshi B, Coxon HO, Pare PD, Sciurba FC, Rogers RM, Hayashi S, Hogg JC. Amplification of inflammation in emphysema and its association with latent adenoviral infection. 2001;Am J Respir Crit Care Med:469 - 473.
[75] Rutgers SR, Postma DS, ten Hecken NH, Kauffman HF, van der Mark TW, Koeter GH, Timens W. Ongoing airway inflammation in patients with copd who do not smoke. *Thorax* 2000;55:12 - 18.

[76] Sullivan AK, Simonian PL, Falta MT, et al. Oligoclonal cd4+ t cells in the lungs of patients with severe emphysema. *Am J Respir Crit Care Med* 2005;172:590 - 596.

[77] van der Strate BW, Postma DS, Brandsma CA, Melgert BN, Luinge MA, Geerlings M, Hylkema MN, van den DA, Timens W, Kerstjens HA, . Cigarette smoke induced emphysema: A role for the b cell? *Am J Respir Crit Care Med* 2006;173:751 - 758.

[78] Rutgers SR, Timens W, Kaufmann HF, van der Mark TW, Koeter GH, Postma DS. Comparison of induced sputum with bronchial wash, bronchoalveolar lavage and bronchial biopsies in copd. *Eur Respir J* 2000;15:109 - 115.

[79] Stansecu D, Sanna A, Veriter C, Kostinev S, Calcagni PG, Fabbri LM. Airways obstruction, chronic expectoration and rapid decline in fev1 in smokers are associated with increased levels of sputum neutropils. *Thorax* 1996;51:267 - 271.

[80] Martin TR, Raghu G, Maunder RJ, Springmeyer SC. The effects of chronic bronchitis and chronic airflow obstruction on lung cell populations recovered by bronchoalveolar lavage. *Am Rev Respir Dis* 1985;132:260.

[81] Thompson AB, Daughton D, Robbins RA, Ghafouri MA, Ohlerking M, Rennard SI. Intraluminal airway inflammation in chronic bronchitis. Chracterization and correlation with clinical parameters. *Am Rev Respir Dis* 1989;140:1527 - 1537.

[82] Lacoste JY, Bousquet J, Chanez P, Van Vyve T, Simony-Lafontaine J, Lequeu N, Vic P, Enander I, Godard P, Miche FB. Eosinophilic and neutrophilic inflammation in asthma, chronic bronchitis and chronic obstructive pulmonary disease. *J Allergy Clin Immunol* 1993;92:537 - 548.

[83] O'Shaughnessy T, Ansari TW, Barnes NC, Jeffery PK. Inflammatory cells in the airway surface epithelium of bronchitis smokers with and without airflow obstruction. *Eur Respir J* 1996;9:14s (Abstract).

[84] Donaldson GC, Seemungal TA, Patal IS, Bhowmik A, Wilkinson TM, Hurst JR, MacCallum PK, Wedzicha JA. Airway and systemic inflammation and decline in lung function in patients with copd. *Chest* 2005;128:1995 - 2004.

[85] Rennard SI, Daughton DM, Fujita J, Oehlerking MB, Dobson JR, Stahl MG, Robbins RA, Thompson AB. Short-term smoking reduction is associated with reduction in measures of lower respiratory tract inflammation in heavy smokers. *Eur Respir J* 1990;3:752 - 759.

[86] Corre F, Lellouch J, Schwartz D. Smoking and leucocyte counts: Results of an epidemiological study. *Lancet* 1971;2:632 - 634.

[87] Van Eeden SF, Hogg JC. The response of human bone marrow to chronic cigarette smoking. *Eur Respir J* 2000;15:915 - 921.

[88] Yeung MC, Buncio AD. Leukocyte count, smoking and lung function. *Am J Med* 1984;76:383 - 386.

[89] Burnett D. Neutrophils and the pathogenesis of copd in stockley, r.A., editor. *Pulmonary defences* 1997;WileyEurope. Chichester.:113 - 126.

[90] Rydell-Tormanen K, Uller L, Erjefalt JS. Neutrophil cannibalism - a back up when the macrophage clearance system is insufficient. . *Respir Res* 2006;14:143 - 149.

[91] Wagner JG, Roth RA. Neutrophil migration mechanisms with an emphasis on pulmonary vasculature. *Pharmacological Review* 2000;52:349 - 374.

[92] Crockett-Torabi A, Fantone JC. The selectins. Insights into selectin induced intra-cellular signaling in leukocytes. *Immunol Res* 1995;14:237 - 251.

[93] Williams MA, Solomkin JS. Integrin mediated signaling in human neutrophil functioning. *J Leuk Biol* 1999;65:725 - 736.
[94] Burns MJ, Walker DC, Brown ES, Thurmon LT, Bowden RA, Keese CR. Neutrophil transendothelial migration is independent of tight junctions and occurs preferentially at tricellular corners. *J Immunol* 1997;159:2893 - 2903.
[95] Newman PJ. The biology of pecam-1. *J Clin Invest* 1997;99:3 - 7.
[96] Yadav R, Larbi KY, Young RE, Nourshargh S. Migration of leukocytes through the vessel wall and beyond. *Thromb Haemost* 2002;90:598 - 606.
[97] Shang XZ, Issekutz AC. Beta-2 (cd18) and beta-1 (cd29) integrin mechanisms in migration of human polymorphonuclear leucocytes and monocytes through lung fibroblast barriers. Shared and distinct mechanisms. *Immunol* 1997;92:527 - 535.
[98] Shang XZ, Yednock T, Issekutz AC. Alpha-9 beta-1 integrin is expressed on human neutrophils and contributes to neutrophil migration through human lung and synovial fibroblast barriers. *J Leuk Biol* 1999;66:809 - 816.
[99] Foxman EF, Kundel EJ, Butcher EC. Integrating conflicting chemotactic signals; the role of memory in leukocyte navigation. *J Cell Biol* 1999;147:577 - 587.
[100] Belaaouaj A. Neutrophil elastase-mediated killing of bacteria: Lessons from targeted mutagenesis. *Microbes and Infection* 2002;4:1259 - 1264.
[101] Aarbiou J, Verhoosel RM, Van Wetering S, De Boer WI, Van Krieken JH, Litinov SV, Rabe KF, Hiemstra PS. Neutrophil defensins enhance lung epithelial wound closure and mucin gene expression in vitro. *Am J Resp Cell Mol Biol* 2004;30:193 - 201.
[102] Cepinskas G, Sandig M, Kvietys PR. Paf induced elastase dependent neutrophil transendothelial migration is associated with the mobilisation of elastase to the neutrophil surface and localised to the migrating front. *J Cell Sci* 1999;112:1937 - 1945.
[103] Owen CA, Campbell MA, Sannes PL, Boukedes SS, Campbell EJ. Cell surface bound elastase and cathepsin g on human neutrophils; a novel, non-oxidative mechanism by which neutrophils focus and preserve catalytic activity of serine proteinases. *J Cell Biol* 1995;131:775 - 789.
[104] Campbell EJ, Campbell MA, Owen CA. Bioactive proteinase three on the cell surface of human neutrophils; quantification, catalytic activity and susceptibility to inhibition. *J Immunol* 2000;165:3366 - 3374.
[105] Owen CA, Campbell MA, Boukedes SS, Campbell EJ. Cytokines regulate membrane-bound leucocytes elastase on neutrophils, a novel mechanism for effector activity. *Am J Physiol Lung Cell Mol Physiol* 1997;272:L385 - L393.
[106] Cepinskas G, Sandig M, Kvietys PR. Paf induced elastase dependent neutrophil transendothelial migration is associated with mobilisation of elastase to the neutrophil surface and localised to the migrating front. *J Cell Sci* 1999;112:1937 - 1945.
[107] Clayton A, Evans RA, Pettit E, Hallett M, Williams JD, Steadman R. Cellular activation through the ligation of intracellular adhesion molecule 1. *J Cell Sci* 1998;111:443 - 453.
[108] Liou TG, Campbell EJ. Quantum proteolysis resulting from release of single granules by human neutrophils; a novel, non oxidative mechanism of extra cellular proteolytic activity. *J Immunol* 1996;157:2624 - 2631.

[109] Campbell EJ, Campbell MA, Boukedes SS, Owen CA. Quantum proteolysis by neutrophils; implications for pulmonary emphysema in alpha 1 anti-trypsin deficiency. *J Clin Invest* 1999;104:337 - 344.
[110] Ohlsson K, Linder C, Lundberg E, Axelsson L. Release of cytokines and proteases from human peripheral blood mononuclear and polymorphonuclear cells following phagocytosis and lps stimulation. *Scand J Clin Lab Invest* 1996;56:461-470.
[111] Fadok VA, Bratton DL, Guthrie L, Henson PM. Differential effects of apoptotic versus lysed cells on macrophage production of cytokines: Role of proteases. *J Immunol* 2001;166:6847-6854.
[112] Weitz JI, Huang AJ, Landman SL, Nicholson SC, Silverstein SC. Elastase-mediated fibrinogenolysis by chemoattractant-stimulated neutrophils occurs in the presence of physiologic concentrations of antiproteinases. *J Exp Med* 1987;166:1836-1850.
[113] Amitani R, Wilson R, Rutman A, Read R, Ward C, Burnett D, Stockley RA, Cole PJ. Effects of human neutrophil elastase and pseudomonas aeruginosa proteinases on human respiratory epithelium. *Am J Respir Cell Mol Biol* 1991;4:26 - 32.
[114] Aoshiba K, Yasuda K, Yasui S, Tamaoki J, Nagai A. Serine proteinases increase oxidative stress in lung cells. *Am J Physiol Lung Cell Mol Physiol* 2001;281:L556 - L564.
[115] Nakajoh M, Fukushima T, Suzuki K, Yamaya M, Nakayama K, Sekizawa K, Sasaki H. Retinoic acid inhibits elastase-induced injury in human lung epithelial cells. *Am J Respir Cell Mol Biol* 2002;28:296 - 304.
[116] Rickard K, Rennard S. Neutrophil elastase causes detachment of bronhial epithelial cells from extracellular matrix. *Am Rev Respir Dis* 1989;139:406.
[117] Tuder RM, Zhen L, Cho CY, Taraseviciene-Stewart L, Kasahara Y, Salvemini D, Voelkel NF, Flores SC. Oxidative stress and apoptosis interact and cause emphysema due to vascular endothelial growth factor receptor blockade. *Am J Respir Cell Mol Biol* 2003;29:88-97.
[118] Hubbard RC, Fells G, Gadek J, Pacholok S, Humes J, Crystal RG. Neutrophil accumulation in the lung in alpha 1-antitrypsin deficiency. Spontaneous release of leukotriene b4 by alveolar macrophages. *J Clin Invest* 1991;88:891-897.
[119] Niederman MS, Merrill WW, Polomski LM, Reynolds HY, Gee JB. Influence of iga and elastase on trachea cell bacterial adherence. *Am Rev Respir Dis* 1986;133:255 - 260.
[120] Vogt W. Cleavage of the fifth component of complement and generation of a functionally active c5b6-like complex by human leukocyte elastase. *Immunobiology* 2000;201:470 - 477.
[121] Ashcroft GS, Lei K, Jin W, Longenecker G, Kulkarni AB, Greenwell-Wild T, Hale-Donze H, McGrady G, Song XY, Wahl SM. Secretory leukocyte protease inhibitor mediates non-redundant functions necessary for normal wound healing. *Nat Med* 2000;6:1147 - 1153.
[122] O'Shaughnessy TC, Ansari TW, Barnes NC, Jeffery PK. Inflammation in bronchial biopsies of subjects with chronic bronchitis: Inverse relationship of cd8+ t lymphocytes with fev1. *Am J Respir Crit Care Med* 1997;155:852-857.
[123] Snoeck-Strobard JB, Lapperre TS, Gosman MM, Boezen HM, Timens W, ten Hacken NH, Sont JK, Sterk P, Hiemstra PS. Chronic bronchitis sub-phenotype within copd; inflammation in sputum and biopsies. *Eur Respir J* 2008;31:70 - 77.

[124] MacNee W. Pathogenesis of chronic obstructive pulmonary disease. *Proc Am Thorac Soc* 2005;2:258 - 266.
[125] Jeffery PK. Structural and inflammatory changes in copd: A comparison with asthma. *Thorax* 1998;53:129-136.
[126] Monso E, Ruiz J, Rosell A, et al. Bacterial infection in chronic obstructive pulmonary disease. *Am J Respir Crit Care Med* 1995;152:1316 - 1320.
[127] Monso E, Rosell A, Bonet G, Manterola J, Cardona PJ, Ruiz J, Morera J. Risk factors for lower airways bacterial colonisation in stable chronic bronchitis. *Eur Respir J* 1999;13:338 - 342.
[128] Groeneveld K, Eijk PP, Van Alpen L, Jansen HM, Zanen HC. Haemophilus influenzae infections in patients with chronic obtructive pulmonary disease despite specific antibodies in serum and sputum. *Am Rev Respir Dis* 1990;141:1316 - 1321.
[129] Groeneveld K, Van Alphen L, Eijk PP, Visschers G, Jansen HM, Zanen HC. Endogenous and exogenous reinfections by haemophilus influenzae in pateints with chronic obstructive pulmonary disease: The effect of antibiotis treatment on persistence. *J Infect Dis* 1990;161:512 - 517.
[130] Irwin RS, Erickson AD, Pratter MR. Prediction of tracheobronchial colonisation in current cigarette smokers with chronic obstructive bronchitis. *J Infect Dis* 1982;145:34 - 241.
[131] Del Donno M, Pavia D, Agnew JE, Lopez-Vidriero MT, Clarke SW. Variability and reproducibility in the measurement of tracheobronchial clearance in healthy subjects and patients with different obstructive lung diseases. *Eur Respir J* 1988;1:613 - 620.
[132] Riise GC, Ahlstedt S, Larsson S. Bronchial inflammation in chronic bronchitis assessed by measurement of cell products in bronchealveolar lavage fluid. *Thorax* 1995;50:360 - 365.
[133] Patel IS, Seemungal TAR, Wilks M, Lloyd-Owen SJ, Donaldson GC, Wedzicha JA. Relationship between bacterial colonisation and the frequency, character and severity of copd exacerbations. *Thorax* 2002;57:759 - 764.
[134] Donaldson GC, Seemungal TA, Bhowmik A, Wedzicha JA. Relationship between exacerbation frequency and lung function decline in chronic obstructiv pulmonary disease. *Thorax* 2002;57:847 - 852.
[135] Seemungal TAR, Donaldson GC, Paul EA, Bestall JC, Jeffries DJ, Wedzicha JA. Effect of exacerbation on quality of life in patients with chronic obstructive pulmonary disease. *Am J Respir Crit Care Med* 1998;157:1418 - 1422.
[136] Onofrio JM, Toews GB, Lipscomb MF, Pierce AK. Granulocyte-alveolar-macrophage interaction in the pulmonary clearance of staphlococcus aureus. . *Am Rev Respir Dis* 1983;127:335 - 341.
[137] Thepen T, Claassen E, Hoeban K, Breve J, Kraal G. Migration of alveolar macrophages from alveolar space to paracortical t area of draining lymph node. *Adv Exp Med Biol* 1993;329:305 - 310.
[138] Skerrett SJ, Martin TR. Intratracheal interferon gamma augments pulmonary defenses in experimental legionellosis. *Am J Respir Crit Care Med* 1994;149:50 - 58.
[139] Anthonisen NR, Manfreda J, Warren CP, Hershfield ES, Harding GK, Nelson NA. Antibiotic therapy in exacerbations of chronic obstructive pulmonary disease. *Ann Intern Med* 1987;106:196 - 204.

[140] Burge S, Wedzicha JA. Copd exacerbations: Definitions and classification. *Eur Respir J* 2003;21:46s - 53s.
[141] Guasti L, Marino F, Cosentino M, Maio RC, Rasini E, Ferrari M, Castiglioni L, Klersy C, Gaudio G, Grandi AM, et al. Prolonged statin-associated reduction in neutrophil rective oxygen species and angiotensin ii type 1 receptor expression: 1 year follow up. *Eur Heart J* 2008;29:1118 - 1126.
[142] Sparrow D, Glynn RJ, Cohen M. The relationship of the peripheral leukocyte count and cigarette smoking to pulmonary function among adult men. *Chest* 1984;86:383 - 386.
[143] Muzio M, Chinnaiyan AM, Kischkel FC, O'Rourke K, Shevchenko A, Ni J, Scaffidi C, Bretz JD, Zhang M, Gentz R, et al. Flice, a novel fadd-homologous ice/ced-3-like protease, is recruited to the cd95 (fas/apo-1) death-inducing signalling complex. *Cell* 1996;85:817 - 827.
[144] Morrison HM, Kramps JA, Burnett D, stockley RA. Lung lavage fluid from patients with alpha 1 proteinase inhibitor deficiency or chronic obstructive bronchitis; anti-elastase function and cell profile. *Clin Sci (Colch)* 1987;72:373 - 381.
[145] Muller WA. The role of pecam-1 in leukocyte emigration. Studies in vitro and in vivo. *J Leuk Biol* 1995;66:698 - 704.
[146] Soler N, Torres A, Ewig S, et al. Bronchial microbial patterns in sever exacerbations of copd requiring mechanical ventilation. *Am J Respir Crit Care Med* 1998;157:1498 - 1505.
[147] Gompertz S, O'Brien C, Bayley D, Hill SL, Stockley RA. Changes in bronchial inflammation during acute exacerbations of chronic bronchitis. *Eur Respir J* 2001;17:1112 - 1119.
[148] Gompertz S, Bayley D, Hill SL, Stockley RA. Relationship between airway inflammation and the frequency of exacerbations in patients with smoking related copd. . *Thorax* 2001;56:36 - 41.
[149] Eller J, Ede A, Schaberg T, Niederman MS, Mauch H, Lode H. Infective exacerbations of chronic bronchitis. Relation between bacteriologic etiology and lung function. *Chest* 1998;113:1542 - 1548.
[150] Anzueto A. Impact of exacerbations on copd. *Eur Respir Rev* 2010;19:113 - 118.
[151] Sapey E, Stockley RA. Copd exacerbations: Aetiology. *Thorax* 2006;61:250 - 258.
[152] Aaron SD, Vandemheen KL, Hebert P, Dales R, Stiell IG, Ahuja J, Dickinson G, Brison R, Rowe BH, Dreyer J, et al. Outpatient oral prednisolone after emergency treatment of chronic obstructive pulmonary disease. *New Engl J Med* 2003;348:26 18 - 2625.
[153] Tager I, Speizer TE. The role of infection in chronic bronchitis. *New Engl J Med* 1975;292:563 - 571.
[154] Saint S, Bent S, Vittinghoff E, Grady D. Antibiotics in chronic obstructive pulmonary disease exacerbations. *JAMA* 1995;273:957 - 960.
[155] Mackay, A.D.,. Amoxycillin versus ampicillin in treatment of exacerbations of chronic bronchitis. *Br J Dis Chest* 1980;74:379 - 384.
[156] Ball P. Infective pathogenesis and outcomes in chronic bronchitis. *Curr Opin Pulm Med* 1996;2:181 - 185.
[157] Petrie GR, Palmer KNV. Comparison of aerosol ipratropium bromide and salbutamol in chronic bronchitis and asthma. *BMJ* 1975;1:430 - 432.

[158] Balter MS, La Forge J, Low DE, Mandell L, Grossman RF. Canadian guidelines for the management of acute exacerbations of chronic bronchitis. *Can Respir J* 2003;10:248 = 258.
[159] Turner M, Patel A, Ginsberg S, Fitzgerald J. Bronchodilator delivery in acute airflow obstruction. A meta-analysis. *Arch Intern Med* 1997;157:1736 - 1744.
[160] Smucny J, Flynn C, Becker L, Glazier R. Beta2 agonists for acute bronchitis. *Cochrane Database of Systematic Reviews* 2004;CD001726-CD001726.
[161] Poole PJ, Black PN. Oral mucolytic drugs for exacerbations of chornic obstructive pulmonary disease: Systemic review. *BMJ* 2001;322:1 - 6.
[162] Wilkinson TMA, Donaldson GC, Hurst JR, Seemungal TAR, Wedzicha JA. Early therapy improves outcomes of exacerbations of chronic obstructive pulmonary disease. *Am J Respir Crit Care Med* 2004;169:1298 - 1303.
[163] Llewellyn-Jones CG, Harris TA, Stockley RA. Effect of fluticasone propionate on sputum of patients with chronic bronchitis and emphysema. *Am J Respir Crit Care Med* 1996;153:616 - 621.
[164] Loppow D, Schleiss MB, Kanniess F, Taube C, Jores RA, Magnussen H. In patients with chronic bronchitis, a four week trial with inhaled steroids does not attenuate airway inflammation. *Respir Med* 2000;95:115 - 121.
[165] Vestbo J, Soorensen T, Lange P, Brix A, Torre P, Viskum K. Long term effect of inhaled budesonide in mild and moderate chronic obstructive pulmonary disease: A randomised controlled trial. *The Lancet* 1999;353:1819 - 1823.
[166] Piatti G, Ambrosetti U, Santus P, Allegra L. Effects of salmeterol on cilia and mucus in copd and pneumonia patients *Pharmacological Research* 2005;51:165 - 168.
[167] Gamble E, Grootendorst DC, Brightling CE, Troy S, Qiu Y, Zhu J, Parker D, Matin D, Majumdar S, Vignola AM, et al. Antiinflammatory effects of the phosphodiesterase-4 inhibitor cilomilast (arifo) in chronic obstructive pulmonary disease. *Am J Respir Crit Care Med* 2003;168:976 - 982.
[168] Spina D. Pde4 inhibitors: Current status. *British Journal of Pharmacology* 2008;155:308 - 315.
[169] Calverley PA, Sanchez-Toril F, McIvor A, Teichmann P, Bredenbroeker D, Fabbri LM. Effect of 1 year treatment with roflumilast in severe chronic obstructive pulmonary disease. *Am J Respir Crit Care Med* 2007;176:154 - 161.
[170] Rennard SI, Schachter N, Strek M, Rickard K, Amit O. Cilomilast for copd: Results of a six month, placebo controlled study of a potent, selective inhibitor of phosphodiesterase 4. *Chest* 2006;129:56 - 66.
[171] Rabe KF, Bateman ED, O'Donnell D, et al. Roflumilast - an oral anti-inflammatory treatment for copd; a randomised control trial. *The Lancet* 2005;9485:563 - 571.
[172] Rennard SI, Calverley PA, Goethring UM, Martinez FJ. Reduction of exacerbations by the pde4 inhibitor roflumilast - the importance of defining different subsets of patients with copd. *Respiratory Research* 2011;12:doi:10.1186/1465-9921-1112-1118.
[173] Larson M. Clinical recognition of n-acetylcysteine in chronic bronchits. *Eur Respir Rev* 1992;2:5 - 8.
[174] Tunek A. Possible mechanisms behind the anti-inflammatory effects of n-acetylcysteine: Is metabolism essential? *Eur Respir Rev* 1992;2:35 - 38.
[175] Leuenberger P, Anderhub PJ, Brandli O, et al. Management of chronic obstructive pulmonary disease. *Schwei Med Wochens* 1997;127:766 - 782.

[176] Stey C, Steurer J, Bachmann S, Medici TC, Tramer MR. The effect of oral n-acetylcycteine in chronic bronchitis; a quantitative systemic review. *Eur Respir J* 2000;16:253 - 262.

[177] Poole P., Black PN. Mucolytic agents for chronic bronchitis or chronic obstructive pulmonary disease. . *Cochrane Database of Systematic Reviews* 2010;2:Art No: CD001287. DOI 001210.001002/14651858.CD14001287.pub14651853.

[178] Staykova T, Black PN, Chacko EE, Poole P. Prophylactic antibiotic therapy for chronic bronchitis. *Cochrane Database of Systematic Reviews* 2003;1:Art No> CD004105. DOI:004110.001002/14651858.CD14004105.

[179] Kunisaki KD, Niewoeher DE. Antibiotic prophylaxis for chronic on=bstructive pulmonary disease. Resurrecting an old idea. *Am J Respir Crit Care Med* 2008;178:1098 - 1099.

[180] Nakanishi Y, Kobayashi D, Asano Y, Sakurai T, Kashimura M, Okuyama S, Yoneda Y, Shapiro SD, Takayama K. Clarithromycin prevents smoke induced emphysema in mice. *Am J Respir Crit Care Med* 2009;179:271 - 278.

[181] Hashimoto N, Kawabe T, Hara T, Imaizumi K, Wakayama H, Saito H, Shimokata K, Hasegawa Y. Effect of erythromycin on matrix metalloproteinase-9 and cell migration. *The Journal of Laboratory and Clinical Medicine* 2001;137:176 - 183.

[182] Gompertz S, Hill AT, Bayley D, Stockley RA. Effect of expectoration on inflammation in induced sputum in alpha-1-antitrypsin deficiency. *Respir Med* 2006;100:1094 - 1099.

[183] Vestbo J, Prescott E, Lange P. Association of chronic mucus hypersecretion with fev1 decline and chronic obstructive pulmonary disease morbidity. Copenhagen city heart study group. . *Am J Respir Crit Care Med* 1996;153:1530 - 1535.

[184] Prescott E, Lange P, Vestbo J. Chronic mucus hypersecretion in copd and death from pulmonary infection. *Eur Respir J* 1995;8:1333 - 1338.

3

In Vitro Models of Chronic Obstructive Pulmonary Disease (COPD)

Jason Adamson, Linsey E Haswell,
Gary Phillips and Marianna D Gaça
*British American Tobacco, GR&D Centre,
Regents Park Road, Southampton,
United Kingdom*

1. Introduction

1.1 The lung

The lungs are situated at the air-blood interface and are a crucial boundary between the organism and the environment, protecting the host from a battery of potential insults such as inhaled particles, pollutants, carcinogens and infectious agents that deposit on airway surfaces during normal tidal breathing. The upper or conducting airways (tracheo-bronchial region) are covered with a columnar epithelium composed of ciliated cells and mucus producing goblet cells (Figure 1A). The apical surface of the epithelium is covered by a surface liquid which is comprised of two distinct layers. The outer mucus layer provides a physical barrier that traps inhaled particles. The underlying periciliary fluid is a low viscosity liquid which allows cilia to beat and continually move the mucus layer towards the pharynx. Thus inhaled particles trapped in the mucus are cleared from the airways. Under normal conditions mucus protects the lung airway epithelium; however abnormalities in mucus hypersecretion or clearance can lead to respiratory disease (Rogers 2007). In the lower bronchioles, the epithelium is simple columnar, containing secretary Clara cells and has progressively fewer ciliated cells. The alveolar epithelium is composed primarily (95%) of flattened alveolar type I (AT-I) cells that form a thin barrier for gas exchange. These cells are interspersed with rounded alveolar type II (AT-II) cells that secrete pulmonary surfactant to decrease the surface tension within the alveoli and prevent alveolar collapse during expiration (Figure 1B).

1.2 Chronic obstructive pulmonary disease (COPD)

COPD is an umbrella term that is used to describe chronic lung disease and includes the familiar terms of chronic bronchitis, small airways disease and emphysema. A more specific definition of COPD is; 'a preventable and treatable disease with some significant extrapulmonary effects that may contribute to the severity in individual patients. Its pulmonary component is characterised by airflow limitation that is not fully reversible. The airflow limitation is usually progressive and associated with an abnormal inflammatory response of the lung to noxious particles or gases' (Global Initiative for Chronic Obstructive Lung Disease, 2009).

Pathologically the small bronchi (structures 2-4mm in diameter), small airways (<2mm in diameter) and the lower airway lung parenchyma are the main sites in which chronic bronchitis, small airways disease and emphysema develop. To monitor airflow and the changes in lung function that occur as a consequence of COPD, the volume of air forcibly expelled from the lungs in one second (forced expiratory volume in one second [FEV_1]) is measured. Lung function alters due to changes in the distensibility (compliance) of the lung and in the obstruction of the small airways. Increased compliance (emphysema) and/or decreased airflow (small airways disease), results in prolonged emptying of the lung and thus reduced FEV_1. The classic description of the changes in FEV_1 in smokers and those smokers that develop COPD is summarized in the study conducted by Fletcher & Peto in 1977.

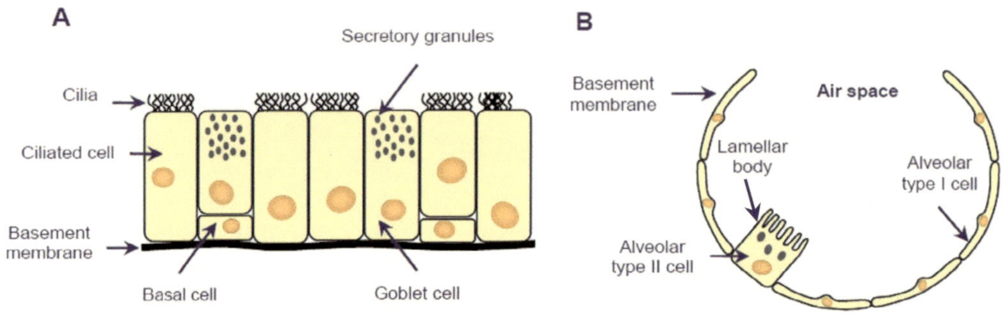

Fig. 1. A. Schematic representing the tracheal bronchial epithelium. The epithelium consists of ciliated, goblet and basal cells situated on top of the basement membrane. B. Schematic representing the alveolar epithelium. The epithelium consists of alveolar type I and type II cells situated on top of the basement membrane.

Inhalation of cigarette smoke, occupational and environmental pollutants are the main causes of COPD (Driscoll et al., 2005; Sethi et al., 2000) and affect all major compartments of the lung, including the central and peripheral airways, the parenchyma and the pulmonary vasculature. Smoking is known to be the most important risk factor for this disease (Oswald et al., 1955) but although some 80-90% of all COPD cases can be attributed to this activity (Sethi et al., 2000) considerable variation in the response to smoke is observed. It has been estimated that only 15% of the variation in lung function is explained by smoking (Beck et al., 1981) thus implicating a genetic predisposition to the disease.

Smoke exposure can directly injure the lung through the action of toxicants found within smoke but also through the attraction, activation and the release of pro-inflammatory mediators from cells of the immune system. These mediators, which can act locally to damage tissue, can also perpetuate the inflammatory response through the attraction of further inflammatory cells to the site of injury. In addition, smoke exposure also contributes to injury through an imbalance in the oxidant–antioxidant profile within the lungs of smokers. If the exogenous (cigarette smoke) and endogenous (inflammatory cells) oxidants outweigh the lung's antioxidant capacity, this can lead to injury and further inflammation. Thus oxidative stress and direct toxicant induced tissue injury drives inflammation and in susceptible individuals drives the disease process and the subsequent development of COPD. To fully understand the causes and elucidate the mechanisms associated with the pathogenesis of this disease and to develop appropriate therapeutic regimes, *in vivo* and *in vitro* studies are and have been vital.

2. *In vivo* models of COPD

Studying COPD using *in vivo* models is not ideal as there is no one model that encompasses all aspects of the clinical disease pathology. Instead there are a number of models that represent individual disease mechanisms or endpoints (MacNee 2005; Pauwels et al., 2001). Animal studies also possess the disadvantage of species variation including differences in respiratory anatomy, breathing patterns and lung protein expression profiles. The most common animal species used to date have been the mouse, rat and guinea pig; the mouse offering the unique opportunity for genetic manipulation, which have and will continue to help unravel key mechanisms underlying the development of cigarette smoke-induced COPD, including emphysema, small airway disease and chronic bronchitis.

2.1 Emphysema

Cigarette smoke-induced emphysema has been the one pathology of COPD that has attracted the most interest over the years and the use of animals to elucidate the mechanisms involved in this destructive process has been previously reviewed (Wright & Churg 2010; Yoshida et al., 2007). Studies conducted in mice, rats and guinea pigs demonstrate that prolonged cigarette smoke exposure results in the development of emphysematous like lesions. However, these lesions form primarily in the alveolar ducts, regions distinct from those seen in humans where the focus is mainly around the respiratory bronchioles. The degree of emphysema, even in the most chronically exposed animals is fairly mild compared to that seen in humans. This not only represents the intrinsic differences in the susceptibility of animals to cigarette smoke exposure but also to the fact that emphysema develops over many years of chronic smoke exposure, an exposure period that may not be fully captured *in vivo*.

Destruction of the connective tissue framework is the primary mechanism of alveolar destruction in emphysema which is brought about by an imbalance in the protease-antiprotease profile within the lung (Gross et al., 1964). In the Pallid mouse, a strain of mice with reduced alpha 1-proteinase inhibitor levels, cigarette smoke exposure leads to the development of emphysema (Takubo et al., 2002). Furthermore, neutrophil elastase null mice are protected against chronic cigarette smoke-induced emphysema and treatment with a neutrophil elastase inhibitor has been shown to decrease the airspace enlargement observed in control mice following cigarette smoke exposure (Wright et al., 2002). Hautamaki et al., 1997, demonstrated that matrix matelloproteinase 12 (MMP-12) null mice are also protected from the development of cigarette smoke-induced emphysema. The role for other MMPs in the development of emphysema is still under study, although early transgenic studies with MMP-1 indicated that this proteinase may also be involved in the development of emphysema (D'Armiento et al., 1992).

The important role that antioxidants play in protecting the lungs from smoke-induced emphysema has also been shown by the use of transgenic animal models. Nrf2, the key transcription factor involved in upregulating intracellular antioxidants is key in protecting the lungs against smoke-induced emphysema (Sussen et al, 2009). In rats, administration of antioxidants in smoke-exposed or elastase-treated animals decreases inflammation and ameliorates the emphysematous lesions that develop (Smith et al., 2002). These observations have been mirrored in chronically smoke-exposed transgenic CuZnSOD animals that are 100% protected (Foronjy et al., 2006). The use of antiproteases and anti-inflammatory compounds have been considered in the treatment regime of patients with emphysema and have been proved effective in animal models (Roh et al., 2010). However, few human trials of compounds based on predictions from animal studies have been successful (Barnes, 2007). This discrepancy between human and animal data and the efficacy of anti-inflammatory and anti-oxidant therapy needs to be resolved.

2.2 Small airway disease

Small airway disease is an important cause of airflow limitation in smokers with COPD (Pare et al., 1991). Although little attention has been paid to the use of animal models of small airways disease many studies now show that small airways disease manifests in animals as an increase in airway wall collagen after smoke exposure. Studies conducted in mice (Churg et al., 2006) and guinea pigs (Churg et al., 2007) demonstrate that smoke exposure increases airway thickness and correlates with reduced expiratory flow and increased airway resistance (Wright et al., 2007).

Both B and T lymphocytes are increased in the small airway walls of humans with COPD (Cosio et al., 2002; Hogg et al., 2004). The interaction between inflammation and small airway remodeling has been addressed in rodent models (Lee et al., 2002). Interleukin (IL) 10 over expression causes mucus cell metaplasia, B and T cell inflammation and the sub-epithelial fibrosis of the airways. Fibrosis of the peribronchial region was also seen in mice over expressing IL-1β (Lappalainen et al., 2005) indicating that many of the mechanisms involved in the features of small airways disease are mediated by multiple mechanisms.

2.3 Chronic bronchitis

Chronic bronchitis is associated with an inflammatory response involving the small bronchi, leading to abnormal remodelling, chronic cough and the accumulation of excessive mucus in the airway lumen due to goblet cell metaplasia and/or hypersecretion. The use of animal models to explore the mechanisms associated with chronic bronchitis has not been extensive, but has been previously reviewed (Nikula et al., 2000). In the guinea pig cigarette smoke induces secretary cell metaplasia (Wright et al., 1992) which is analogous to that seen in humans. In contrast, cigarette smoke exposure has little effect in the mouse (Bartalesi et al., 2005) with only a few secretory cells appearing in the small airways. In the larger airways cigarette smoke-exposed rats (Rogers et al., 1986) and guinea pigs (Komori et al., 2001) exhibit significant goblet cell metaplasia which can be attenuated with treatment with anti-inflammatory agents and antioxidants.

2.4 Transgenic and gene targeted models and COPD

Gene depletion and over expression in mice is a way of identifying the function and role of distinct genes in disease. An early application of this approach was the over expression of collagenase 1 which resulted in airspace enlargement in the mouse (D'Armiento et al., 1992). This challenged the elastase-antielastase hypothesis and identified collagen as a potential player in the development of emphysema. However, mice do not express collagenase 1 but rather two other similar proteases, collagenase 2 and 3 and thus limited the interpretation of this study. Another transgenic mouse model that may prove useful in future COPD related research is the Marlboro mouse (Shapiro, 2000). These animals carry the null gene for macrophage elastase (MMP-12), which in man is expressed in the macrophages of cigarette smokers and in patients with emphysema. In chronically smoke-exposed MMP-12 null mice, macrophages are not recruited to the lung and nor do these animals develop emphysema. Over expression of IL-13 has been shown to lead to emphysema in adult mice (Zheng et al., 2000). The resultant inflammation and lung destruction is metallo- and cysteine proteinase dependent. These mice exhibit airway remodeling with goblet cell hypertrophy, driven in part by the MMP-9 mediated activation of transforming growth factor-beta (TGF-β). A similar proteinase dependent pathway has also been established for emphysema through the effects of over expressed interferon- gamma (IFN-γ) (Wang et al., 2000). This also results in inflammation and suggests a potential Th1 pathway involvement in the development of emphysema.

Prior to the advent of gene targeting technology, several natural mutants were known to develop airspace enlargement and included the tight skin (Tsk) (Green et al., 1976), Pallid (de Santi et al., 1995), Blotchy (McCartney et al., 1988)) and Beige (Barbosa et al., 1996) mice. Tsk mice have a mutation in fibrillin-1, a matrix protein that is an important component of elastic fibres (Kielty et al., 1998), whilst the Blotchy mouse has a deficiency in copper metabolism that results in reduced lysyl oxidase activity, a key collagen and elastin cross linking enzyme. These naturally occurring mutations can help to uncover key pathways in lung development but also in the development of tissue injury and remodeling following cigarette smoke exposure. These gene targeting techniques are useful tools to examine potential molecular mechanisms underlying human COPD. In combination with cigarette smoke exposure new transgenic and gene-targeted models will help further elucidate the role of key inflammatory and immuno-regulatory molecules in the development of COPD.

Currently available animal models are restricted to investigating a limited number of the varied and extensive characteristic features of COPD. Although in future combined models of inhalation exposure, gene targeting techniques and naturally occurring mutations may provide more appropriate models of COPD, these may not necessarily be better. There is still concern with *in vivo* systems as to their utility in predicting the pathophysiology and pathogenesis of COPD. There are clear structural, biochemical and physiological differences between animal and human lungs that make translation of animal data to man difficult. However, in conjunction with other experimental approaches, such as the use of *in vitro* models utilising tissue derived from smokers, non smokers and individuals with COPD, a clearer understanding of the molecular and biochemical process involved in the development of COPD will be established.

3. *In vitro* models of COPD

In vitro tests are often used prior to or in place of *in vivo* and subsequent clinical studies. *In vitro* tests are designed to generate rapid, initial data that will give general insight into disease mechanisms and the biological effect of test compounds and materials. There is a general shift in employing human cells and tissues to ensure as many of the physiological parameters are maintained in the *in vitro* test systems. Typical *in vitro* systems modelling an organ such as the lung can include the use of established continuous cell lines, primary cells and tissues (such as organ slices). Primary cell cultures are explanted directly from either a healthy or diseased donor organism and can keep their functional differentiated state for a short period (days to weeks). These cells have a limited life span. However maintenance of the differentiated properties has been improved slightly with the addition of additives to the culture medium, the use of biological scaffoldings using components of the extracellular matrix or by different forms of co-culture. Permanent, continuous cell cultures have acquired the ability to proliferate indefinitely either through a natural or introduced mutation. Most continuous cell lines have originated from embryos, tumors or transformed cells. There are countless well established cell lines representative of different cell types, for example NCI-H292 that are specific for human lung epithelial cells. The disadvantages of continuous cell lines are that they do not retain many features of the original tissue; they may not accurately represent the *in vivo* situation as the phenotype of immortalised cells often differs from that of the normal tissue. A major advantage of using immortalised cell lines is that they are readily available, stable, easy to handle and convenient. Cell lines are homogenous populations therefore reducing donor to donor variability.

In comparison to *in vivo, in vitro* studies offer a number of advantages including:

- more flexibility
- generation of reproducible data as *in vitro* studies can be better controlled
- avoidance of animal species variation and animal/human extrapolation due to the availability of human tissue
- direct access and investigation to cellular components and biomolecules
- easier and quicker to perform
- more economical
- reduction in the number of animals used in research.

Each *in vitro* system has advantages and disadvantages, but it is generally accepted that the closer the system is to the whole organ (as it functions naturally and with endogenous cell types), the more accurate the predictive results will be.

COPD is a multifaceted disease and one *in vitro* model would not be able to replicate the entire disease pathogenesis. Consequently informative *in vitro* models of COPD must utilise the different cell types involved in disease pathogenesis and model endpoints with clinical relevance such as pro-inflammatory mediator release, goblet cell hyperplasia, cilia dysfunction, squamous cell metaplasia and emphysema. The development of pulmonary *in vitro* models began in the 1990's (Sporty et al., 2008) and despite the large number of pulmonary *in vitro* models described in the literature, currently there are no validated *in vitro* models of COPD. To demonstrate their utility, we will describe a number of *in vitro* models of the respiratory tract commonly used by researchers to investigate the mechanisms of COPD and some developed in our laboratories investigating the effect of cigarette smoke. We will focus predominately on *in vitro* models utilising human tissue.

3.1 Modelling the tracheo-bronchial airways

3.1.1 Primary cell cultures

Publications documenting the differentiation of primary lung cells into a mucociliary epithelium found in the tracheo-bronchial airways have been reported as early as 1984 (Lee et al., 1984). Initial studies described primary epithelial cells cultured on plastic and submerged in medium, however, more recent protocols describe the culture of cells at an air-liquid interface (ALI) (Gray et al., 1996). Primary human bronchial epithelial cells (HBECs) obtained directly from surgical tissue or low passage primary cells are available from several commercial sources. Cells are seeded on collagen coated surfaces in hormone and growth factor supplemented medium. Initially cells proliferate quickly to form a monolayer of undifferentiated cells. Proliferation then decreases and, after placing cells at an ALI, cells undergo differentiation in 2-3 weeks, producing a columnar epithelium containing goblet, ciliated and basal cells (Figure 2). Well-differentiated tracheo–bronchial cultures have been described for a variety of species including mouse (Davidson et al., 2004), rat (Ostrowski et al., 1995) horse (Schwab et al., 2010) hamster (Lee et al., 1984), ferret, pig (Liu et al., 2007) and human (Gray et al., 1996; Haswell et al., 2010).

Commercial 'ready-to-use' fully differentiated HBEC cultures are now readily available and include EpiAirway® by MatTek (http://www.mattek.com/pages/products/epiairway) and

MucilAir™ by Epithelix (http://www.epithelix.com/content/view/4/4/lang,en/).The MucilAir™ product has a unique advantage over both in-house derived HBEC cultures and the commercially available EpiAirway® model: the cultures are able to remain fully functionally differentiated for more than one year. This provides the potential for long-term or repeat exposure studies which could help model clinically relevant COPD pathologies that require chronic exposure to agents such as cigarette smoke.

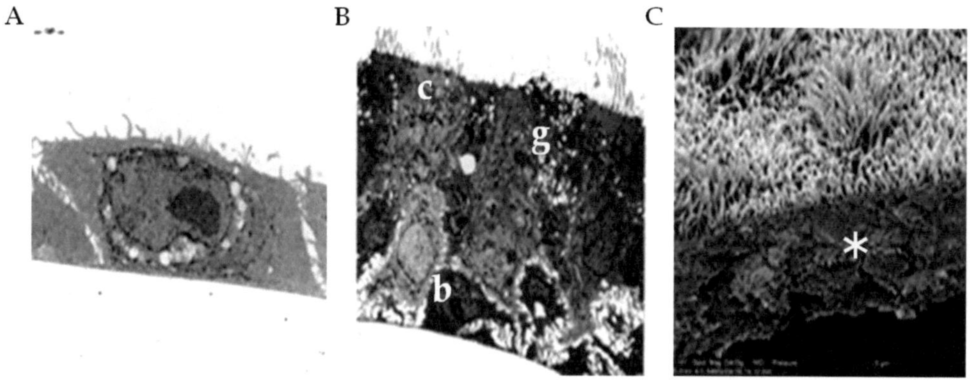

Fig. 2. Transmission (A and B) and scanning (C) electron micrographs of human bronchial epithelial cell air-liquid interface cultures at day 1 (A) and day 28 (B and C). At day 28 cultures had developed into a columnar epithelium containing basal cells (b), mucus containing goblet cells (g) and ciliated cells (c). The fractured culture edge of a culture is indicated by * in the scanning electron micrograph. (Haswell et al., 2010).

The use of highly differentiated models of the conducting airways allows for the investigation of inhaled agents to specific cell types and the simultaneous interaction between different cell types in response to exposure. Moreover, culturing cells at an ALI supports the direct exposure of cultures to aerosols and gases thus better modelling an *in vivo* exposure. Despite these clear physiological advantages for using primary differentiated cells, HBEC cultures have several limitations including, tissue availability, limited number of cells harvested from each isolation, a limited replicative lifespan, donor to donor variation and relatively high cost. Regardless of these constraints, primary differentiated cell cultures have been used in a large number of studies to investigate the effects of cigarette smoke on the conducting airways.

Goblet cell hyperplasia is a characteristic feature of the lung epithelium in patients with COPD contributing to the overproduction of airway mucus, including the mucin MUC5AC (Rogers, 2007). Chronic inhalation of mainstream cigarette smoke has been shown to increase the number of goblet cells, up-regulate MUC5AC at the gene level in the airways of smokers (Cosio et al., 1980; Innes et al., 2006; Saetta et al., 2000) and at the protein level in patients with COPD (Ma et al., 2005). We recently reported a study using primary HBECs as an *in vitro* model of differentiated lung epithelium, investigating the morphological and cellular changes in response to non-cytotoxic doses of cigarette smoke particulate matter (PM) and three mainstream cigarette smoke constituents: acrolein, formaldehyde and acetaldehyde (Haswell et al., 2010). HBECs from three different donors were exposed basally to cigarette smoke PM and the constituents for 28 days during the differentiation period. Using both flow cytometry and immunocytochemical techniques for identification of MUC5AC positive cells, cigarette smoke PM treatment induced an increase in MUC5AC positive cells when compared to untreated control cultures. Treatment with acrolein also increased the percentage of MUC5AC positive cells in the HBEC cultures. However, formaldehyde and acetaldehyde (maximum dose 1μM) had little effect. This study demonstrated for the first time that cigarette smoke and acrolein, known lung toxicants, induce an increase in the percentage of goblet cells in an *in vitro* model of human lung epithelium. This response reflects, to an extent, the goblet cell hyperplasia observed in animal inhalation models, smokers and patients with COPD.

Another frequent observation in the tracheo-bronchial mucosa of cigarette smokers who develop COPD is squamous cell metaplasia (SCM) (Jeffery, 2000). SCM is the replacement of the normal mucociliary epithelium with a stratified squamous epithelium. SCM is considered to be an adaptive response, protecting the lumen from the effects of inhaled agents. However, the assessment of cigarette smoke on SCM induction often relies on human epidemiological data or *in vivo* animal inhalation studies. HBECs cultured using medium without retinoic acid became squamous, mucin secretion decreases and expression of the squamous cell markers transglutaminase-1 (Gray et al., 2007) and involucrin (BAT unpublished data) are elevated. Although culturing HBECs without retinoic acid has not been fully developed and characterised as an *in vitro* model of SCM it could potentially provide a method to allow the assessment of cigarette smoke and its constituents on SCM induction.

Mucociliary dysfunction is caused by mucus hypersecretion coupled with a decrease in mucus transport, and represents an important pathophysiological component of COPD. Effective mucociliary clearance requires both the appropriate amount of mucus and the co-ordinated cilia beating to clear mucus and remove inhaled agents from the lung. Smoking has been reported to adversely affect the function of cilia (Elliott et al., 2006; Simet et al., 2010; Sisson et al., 1991;Verra et al., 1995). Differentiated HBEC cultures are highly ciliated (Figure 2C) therefore the investigation of cilia beat frequency (CBF) following exposure to cigarette smoke could provide important information on mucociliary dysfunction. CBF is a measurable and tightly regulated function of the ciliated epithelium. CBF can be determined by high speed video microscopy; this requires specialised equipment, trained personnel and is highly time consuming. However, the development of the SAVA system, a high-speed all-digital video imaging system to measure CBF could shorten the analysis time and negate the need for expensive microscopy equipment (Sisson et al., 2003).

Primary HBEC cultures have also been used to investigate the effects of cigarette smoke on cell signalling and function. In a study by Maunders et al., 2007, HBECs from three different donors were exposed to air or non-cytotoxic doses of whole mainstream cigarette smoke for 1 hour and gene expression profiles were then determined post-exposure using whole genome Affymetrix microarrays. Many direct effects of cigarette smoke found in this study were consistent with previous reports of *in vivo* and *in vitro* cigarette smoke toxicity studies, such as increased epithelial permeability, activation of antioxidant responses, and cell signaling pathways (Boucher et al., 1980; Hackett et al., 2003; Mossman et al., 2006), thus demonstrating HBEC cultures are able to model key features of cigarette smoke-exposed conducting airways.

Many cigarette smoke toxicants are biologically inactive until transformed by metabolic enzymes into reactive intermediates. For example, the cigarette smoke constituent benzo(a)pyrene, when activated generates reactive forms capable of binding to DNA (Castell et al., 2005). Therefore the metabolic capacity of *in vitro* models of COPD is important. In a recent study Newland et al., 2001, characterised the expression and activity of relevant cytochrome P450 (CYP) metabolizing enzymes, CYP1A1/1B1, and CYP2A6/2A13, in primary ALI HBEC cultures. HBEC CYP activity and inducibility was conserved over the 28 day culture period (Newland et al., 2011).

3.1.2 Cell lines

Immortal or continuous cell lines are commonly used to model COPD *in vitro.* NCI-H292 is a bronchial epithelial cell line derived from a mucoepidermoid carcinoma (Carney, 1985). Several studies have reported the responses of NCI-H292 cells to cigarette smoke are similar to that of primary HBECs and the airway epithelium *in vivo* (Baginski et al., 2006; Newland & Richter 2008; Phillips et al., 2005; Shao et al., 2004). In a study by Phillips et al., 2005, NCI-H292 cells were cultured on inserts and exposed at the ALI to whole smoke for 30 minutes. Low doses of smoke were shown to induce COPD associated markers including the up-regulation of MUC5AC mRNA and the production of the inflammatory mediators IL-6, IL-8 and MMP-1. NCI-H292 cells have also been shown to respond to a variety of agents associated with inhalation toxicity including cigarette smoke PM via various endpoints linked to inflammation (IL-6 and IL-8), airway remodelling (MMP-1, GM-CSF), and mucin overproduction (MUC5AC) (Newland & Richter 2008). Although NCI-H292 cells have been extensively used as a lung model for toxicological assessment, they lack critical metabolic activation capability, in particular they did not show CYP2A6/2A13 activity (Newland et al., 2011).

There are several other cells lines that have been used to model the tracheo-bronchial airways. 16HBE14σ cells originate from a normal human bronchial epithelial cell line that has been transformed by the SV40 large T-antigen. These cells retain differentiated epithelial morphology and functions, forming polarised monolayers with functional tight junctions (Cozens et al., 1994). The cell line BEAS-2B is another normal human bronchial epithelial cell line and was transformed using the adenovirus 12-simian virus 40 hybrid virus. Although continuous cell lines have been around for a while there is no general agreement as to which is the most appropriate.

3.2 Modelling the alveolar region

3.2.1 Primary cells

Currently there are no available or reported cell lines that possess significant functional properties of alveolar epithelial cells (Forbes & Ehrhardt, 2005). The primary culture of alveolar epithelial cells is therefore used for most *in vitro* studies of the alveolar epithelium. Human alveolar epithelial cells are isolated from human patients undergoing lung resection. These cells, when plated on permeable supports or plastic exhibit AT-II cell characteristics that include lamellar bodies, apical microvilli, tight junctions, and expressed surfactant (Witherden, 2004). After approximately eight days of culture AT-II cells can acquire the AT-I cell-like morphology (Elbert et al., 1999; Fuchs et al., 2003). As with primary HBECs, primary alveolar cells have the same limitations including a limited replicative lifespan, the limited number cells obtained from each isolation, tissue availability and donor variation.

3.2.2 Cell lines

The adenocarcinoma cell line A549 is the most widely used alveolar cell line, however, due the lack of tight junction formation, a key feature of the alveolar epithelium, the cell line potentially has limited value (Forbes & Ehrhardt 2005). In addition A549s have low levels of

P450 activities, a limited number of phase I enzymes (Castell et al., 2005) and they do not retain significant metabolic activity, having reduced CYP1A1/1B1 or CYP2A6/2A13 activity (Newland et al., 2011). Moreover studies have shown A549s are not as sensitive to cigarette smoke exposure as primary cultures (Kode et al., 2006; Newland & Richter 2008).

3.3 Airway epithelium co-cultures

COPD involves the interplay of several systems including the respiratory, immune and cardiovascular systems. Therefore to model more complex endpoints and to investigate the underlying mechanisms by which cigarette smoke and other agents cause disease requires more complex culture systems that model the interactions between different cell types. Co-cultures contain either primary or continuous cell lines of epithelial origin in culture with either primary or continuous cell lines from a variety of different sources including the endothelial cells, fibroblasts and immune cells (Table 1). The co-culture of different cell types can be achieved in different ways. The simplest is the culture of two different cell types in the same medium e.g., a collagen gel, but more commonly inserts are used to separate the cell types. The cells can be seeded both on the insert or either side of the semi-permeable membrane, thus creating a bi-layer or co-culture system, as in Figure 3. The establishment of co-cultures is not easy as the differing culture requirements of each cell type creates a technical challenge. The development of co-cultures has allowed the cell-to-cell communication and interactions of differing cell types to be modelled *in vitro*, which is not possible using mono-cultured cells.

Airway cell	Other cell type	Interaction being modelled	Reference
16HBE14σ	Human umbilical vein endothelial cells	Epithelial-endothelial	(Chowdhury et al. 2010)
A549 or NCI-H441	Human pulmonary microvascular endothelial cells	Epithelial-endothelial	(Hermanns et al. 2004)
NCI-H441	ISO-HAS-1	Epithelial-endothelial	(Papritz et al. 2010)
NCI-H441	Human pulmonary microvascular endothelial cells	Epithelial-endothelial	(Hermanns et al., 2009)
Calu-3 or A549	Peripheral blood mononuclear cells	Epithelial-immune	(Korpi-Steiner et al. 2010; Torvinen, Campwala, & Kilty 2007)
HBECs	Monocytes	Epithelial-immune	(Korpi-Steiner et al., 2010)
16HBE14σ or A549 or primary human AT-I	Human monocyte-derived macrophages and dendritic cells	Epithelial-immune	(Blank et al. 2011; Lehmann et al. 2011; Rothen-Rutishauser, Kiama, & Gehr 2005)
16HBE14σ or A549	Human monocyte-derived macrophages or dendritic cells	Epithelial-immune	(Blank, Rothen-Rutishauser, & Gehr 2007)
A549	Fibroblasts	Epithelial-mesenchymal	(Noguchi et al. 2007)
HBECs	Fibroblasts	Epithelial-mesenchymal	(Araya et al. 2007)
A549	Fibroblasts	Epithelial-mesenchymal	(Liu, Gao, & Zhang 2010)
HBECs	Fibroblast cell line Wi-38	Epithelial-mesenchymal	(Pohl et al. 2009)
Primary human AT-II	Human pulmonary microvascular endothelial cells	Epithelial-endothelial	(Hermanns et al. 2009)

Table 1. A summary of various *in vitro* co-culture COPD systems described in the literature.

To date only two studies have reported exposing airway co-cultures to cigarette smoke. Both studies were co-culture models of A549 cells with fibroblasts. Fibrosis of the small airways and respiratory bronchioles has been found to cause increased airway wall thickness in smokers compared with nonsmokers (Kim et al., 2008) and it is thought that epithelial cells and fibroblasts are involved in matrix deposition at the sites of lung injury. In one study human foetal lung fibroblasts and A549 cells were cultured in a collagen gel and exposed to cigarette smoke extract (Noguchi et al., 2007). The authors found these co-cultures prevented the inhibition of fibroblast-mediated collagen gel contraction induced by cigarette smoke and suggest that the epithelial cells protected the fibroblasts from cigarette smoke induced injury. The effect of cigarette smoke extract on the interaction of the alveolar epithelial cells and fibroblasts was also investigated by Liu et al., 2010. Human lung fibroblasts were cultured below an insert containing A549 cells and differing responses between both mono-cultured cells and co-cultured cells were observed. Low concentrations of cigarette smoke extract produced epithelial-mesenchymal transition in co-cultured A549 cells but not in mono-cultured A549 cells. This co-culture system may resemble the *in vivo* situation more closely than in mono-cultured cell systems by allowing cell-to-cell interactions important in disease pathogenesis to be modelled.

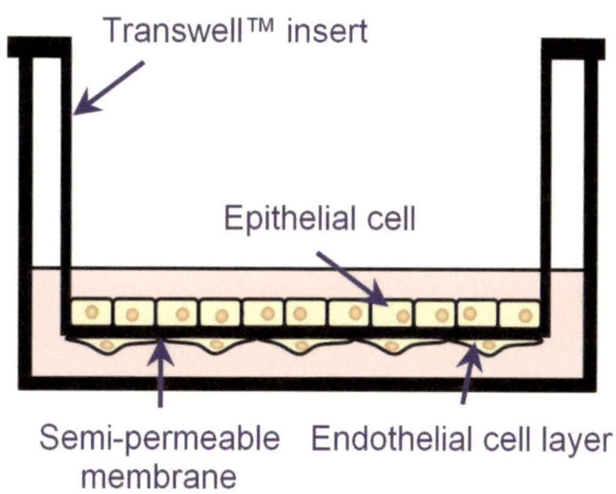

Fig. 3. Schematic of a bi-layer co-culture model. Lung epithelial cells and endothelial cells are grown either side of a semi permeable membrane.

Several other co-culture systems have been reported that model endpoints key in the development of COPD. The co-culture of HBECs with airway fibroblasts, to model human airway-mesenchymal interactions, has allowed the investigation of mechanisms by which SCM induces a fibrotic response in the adjacent airway fibroblasts (Araya et al., 2007). HBECs and human monocytic cell co-cultures have modelled interactions between the airway epithelium and the immune system during human rhinovirus infection, which is a major cause of exacerbations in patients with COPD (Korpi-Steiner et al., 2010). In addition co-culture of HBECs with fibroblasts have indicated that co-culturing these cell types extends the culture life of HBECs. HBECs grown in a bi-layer model with the fibroblast cell line Wi-38 were shown to differentiate and maintain a mucociliary phenotype for at least 3 months (Pohl et al., 2009). This type of culture system could permit the investigation of epithelial-mesenchymal interactions in a chronic or repeated exposure situation.

Recently a bi-layer system with primary human AT-II cells with human pulmonary microvascular endothelial cells has been described (Hermanns et al., 2009). In this system AT-II cells partly differentiated into AT-I like cells establishing a bi-layer model that reflects the cellular composition of the alveolar epithelium *in vivo*. This complex co-culture system could provide a suitable *in vitro* model to investigate the effects of cigarette smoke on the structural and functional behaviour of the alveolar epithelium using primary tissue. Studies using co-culture systems have not been limited to just two cell types. The cell lines 16HBE14σ and A549 and human primary AT-I cells have all been co-cultured with macrophages and dendritic cells (Blank et al., 2007; Lehmann et al., 2010; Rothen-Rutishauser et al., 2005). Co-cultures are becoming increasingly more complex and enable the study of the interactions between the immune system and cells of the human airway barrier.

3.4 Lung slices

Organ slices have been used for a wide range of biochemical studies for several decades (Parrish et al., 1995). Organ-slice cultures can be particularly beneficial for modelling the pathological processes and the underlying mechanisms of a complex disease such as COPD for several reasons. Organ-slice cultures maintained *in vitro* have the potential to preserve all cell types present in the original tissue in the correct spatial configuration. Data derived from organ slices maintained *in vitro* could provide an important link between studies on isolated cells and *in vivo* models. Unlike many continuous cell lines, lung slices retain the composite metabolic activity of the lung parenchyma and can be used in studies requiring bioactivation (Freeman & O'Neil 1984). Relatively large numbers of slices, up to 30 from one resection, can be generated from each donor (Wohlsen et al., 2003). However, large variation exists between sequential slices and also from donor to donor. One major disadvantage of lung slices is their limited life span, approximately one week *in vitro* (Parrish et al., 1995). Therefore their utility is currently restricted to short term studies. Lung slices for *in vitro* culture have been produced from a variety of species including rats, hamsters, guinea pigs, rabbits, horses and humans.

In the literature there are many different methods available that have not been standardised with respect to slice preparation, thickness, stabilisation and culture media. Organ slices can be prepared by either tissue slicers or mechanical slicers, the latter are often referred to as precision cut lung slices. An important consideration when deciding upon slice thickness is that cut surfaces will contain damaged cells (Freeman & O'Neil 1984). As the slice thickness increases the percentage of damaged cells will decrease. However, as slice thickness increases diffusion pathways are extended, potentially leading to inadequate gas diffusion and substrate delivery. Optimal lung slice thickness has been described as between 500-700µm, this is relatively thick when compared to 200-350µm for slices of the liver, kidneys and heart (Parrish, et al 1995). Stabilisation of the organ slices prior to exposure can reduce the impact of slicing induced cell damage. A large number of different culture media have been used to maintain the lung slices *in vitro* but as yet there is no consensus on which is the best approach.

To date there have been very few studies that have utilised lung slices to model cigarette smoke exposure. In a recent study precision-cut lung slices from guinea pigs exposed to cigarette smoke were used to detect endothelial dysfunction in pulmonary arteries (Wright & Churg 2008). Several studies have also used lung slices to examine the effects of cigarette smoke constituents including acrolein (Fisher et al., 1994), benzo(a)pyrene (Harrigan et al., 2004) and cadmium (Lin et al., 2010).

4. Exposure systems

Appropriate exposure of *in vitro* models to cigarette smoke, diesel emissions and other aerosols and particles implicated in the development of COPD is crucial. How aerosols and particles are collected and presented to the *in vitro* model system needs careful consideration. In the field of cigarette smoke toxicity and biological testing many studies have attempted to develop relevant and appropriate cigarette smoke test substances and systems. The impotance and intricacies of these systems will be discussed.

4.1 What is cigarette smoke?

Cigarette smoke is a concentrated, complex and dynamic aerosol consisting of several thousands of chemicals (Rodgman & Perfetti, 2008). The smoke aerosol is divided into two phases: a particulate and a gas/vapour phase. The particulate phase is the minority fraction and constitutes 4-9%of the total smoke by weight; the gas phase is the majority fraction and comprises the remaining 91-96% by weight (Clunes, 2008). The combination of the particulate and gas phase is termed 'whole smoke', capturing any interactions or synergies between the two. The exact number of chemicals in cigarette smoke is unknown, and this is due to the technical challenges in identifying and quantifying the chemical constituents present in smoke. Some researches have speculated that as many as 100,000 chemicals are present (Wakeham, 1972, as cited in Liu et al., 2011), however a more conservative estimate would put the number at 5,300 identified compounds (Rodgman & Perfetti, 2008). Examples of chemicals in the gas phase include formaldehyde, acrolein, and hydrogen cyanide (associated with COPD); examples of chemicals in the particulate phase include polycyclic aromatic hydrocarbons and tobacco specific nitrosamines (TSNAs) (associated with cancer) (Hoffmann et al., 1997). The leading smoke toxicants identified as relating to disease are largely products of combustion and are found in the gas phase rather than in the particulate phase (Laugesen & Fowles, 2005), hence the importance of performing biological assessment using whole smoke rather than any individual phase alone.

4.2 Generating smoke for *in vitro* testing

For *in vitro* testing cigarette smoke can be generated on smoking machines, of which there are many commercially available and will be described later. There are several methods to trap either or both of the particulate and gas phases of the smoke for exposure to cell and tissue cultures. The three main types of 'smoke' generated for *in vitro* tests described here are PM, aqueous extracts of smoke also termed cigarette smoke extract (CSE), and direct whole smoke exposures in an exposure chamber.

PM is trapped on a Cambridge filter pad (CFP) when inserted directly in-line of the smoke generation. The pad efficiently traps 99.9% of all particles >0.1μm (Johnson et al., 2009) which can later be eluted using a solvent such as dimethyl sulphoxide (DMSO) and diluted in cell culture medium prior to exposure to submerged cell culture systems (Figure. 4A). This is a relatively simple, quick and robust method for the biological assessment of cigarette smoke exposure (Haswell et al., 2010; Newland & Richter 2008) but crucially it only captures <5% of whole smoke (Clunes, 2008) and will not contain volatile compounds (Johnson et al., 2009). Solvents used to extract PM from filters can also affect the way in which cells respond, for example DMSO is a known antioxidant. Furthermore, these cell cultures are submerged and this type of exposure method lacks in physiological relevance to the human lung where epithelial cells are exposed to air.

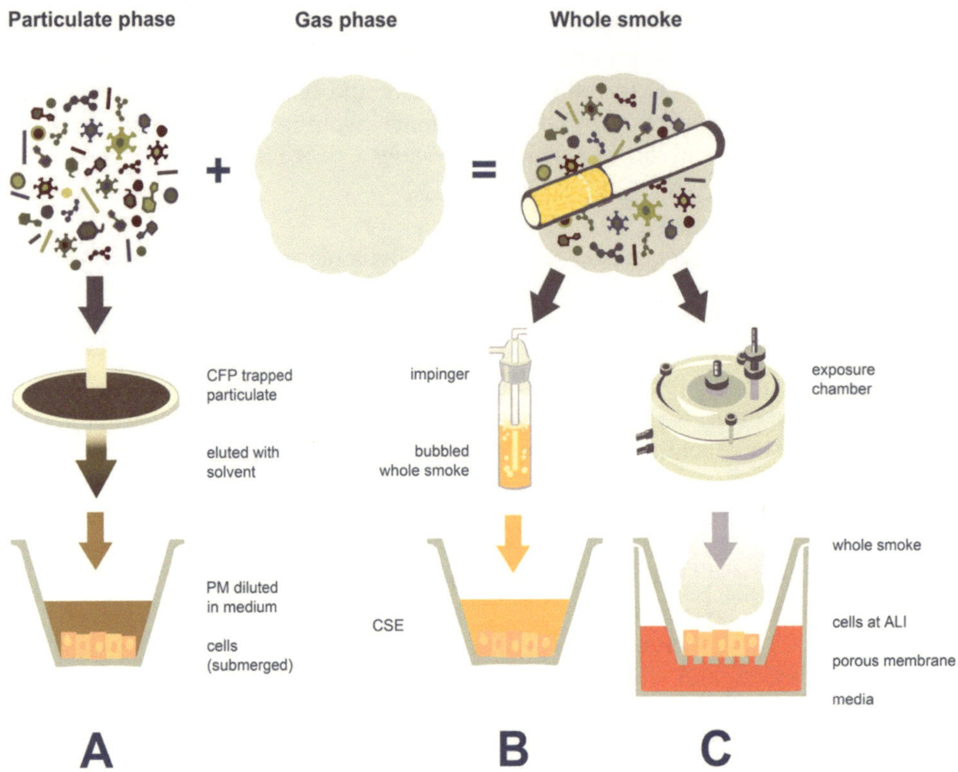

Fig. 4. Three general methods of generating smoke for *in vitro* testing: (A) particulate matter (PM), (B) Aqueous cigarette smoke extracts (CSE) and (C) whole smoke.

Cigarette smoke aqueous extracts (CSE) are collected using impingers, a piece of glassware designed to hold a liquid medium and which can be attached to a smoking machine. As the machine puffs on the cigarette, whole smoke is drawn through the impinger, bubbles through and dissolves into the cell culture medium or buffer within it (Figure 4B). The CSE can be diluted and added to cells in submerged culture conditions (St-Laurent et al., 2009). The benefit of this method is that it captures both particulate and gas phases of smoke, although there is uncertainty as to exactly which chemicals are trapped effectively and at what concentrations. Currently we are performing analyses on the collected CSE to quantify and qualify its composition. As before, cell cultures exposed to CSE are submerged and again this type of exposure method lacks in physiological relevance to the human lung. However, this method is useful when exposing endothelial cell types or anchorage-independent cell types where a submerged exposure is preferred.

Lastly, cells can be exposed to whole smoke within a specially designed exposure chamber which holds cells at the ALI (Maunders et al., 2007; Phillips et al., 2005; Thorne et al., 2009). This exposure method was developed in response to the challenges of making *in vitro* exposures akin to the *in vivo* situation. ALI exposures are more physiologically relevant, where the cells or tissues are exposed apically to smoke and supported on an insert (porous membrane) basally with cell culture medium (Figure 4C), resembling more closely the *in vivo* configuration. This method has many advantages over the previous two methods described, and is especially relevant to *in vitro* models of COPD using mono or bilayer models, 3D lung tissue constructs or whole lung slices, all of which can be supported at the ALI. Furthermore, assessments can be made on the contribution of the gas phase alone within this exposure set-up, simply by placing a CFP in-line of smoke generation to occlude the particulate phase from the exposure chamber. There are many types of exposure chambers designed to be used in conjunction with smoking machines for this purpose; they are available commercially, ranging in design and complexity, and will be described later.

4.3 Smoking machines

Laboratories within academia, specialist tobacco research groups, pharmaceutical and tobacco industries generally use smoke engines to reliably generate cigarette smoke for *in vitro* studies. Ranging in design, engineering, capability and price, all are intended to generate, dilute and deliver whole cigarette smoke to one or multiple exposure chambers housing cells at the ALI. Examples include the Borgwaldt RM20S smoking machine (Figure 5), (Adamson et al, in submission, Kaur et al., 2010; Maunders et al., 2008, Phillips et al., 2005; Thorne et al., 2009), the Borgwaldt RM 1/G and LM1 single port diluter (Clunes, 2008), the Burghart Mimic Smoker-01® (Scian et al., 2009) and the Vitrocell® VC 10® Smoking Robot (www.vitrocell.com). These machines vary in design and capability but in principle their purpose is shared. The specification on how the cigarette is smoked by the machine, or smoking regime, has been standardised. For example, the ISO regime states cigarette puff volume is 35ml, taken over 2 seconds every minute and that the vents on the filter paper are unblocked. In contrast, the Canadian Intense/Health Canada regime takes a 55ml puff over 2 seconds, every 30 seconds, and the vents are blocked (usually with a ring of tape). Furthermore, various smoking machines are freely programmable and are even capable of human smoking puffing profiles. As a result of many years of development, some of these devices are very sophisticated and capable of smoking cigarettes with a high level of repeatability and reproducibility.

4.4 Exposure chambers

As with smoking machines, there are many different types of exposure chamber to be used with *in vitro* cultures. There is a great diversity available and range significantly in design, sophistication, physiological resemblance, ease of use, flexibility in exposure design, fragility, sterility, price and compatibility with an individual smoking machine. An exposure chamber in its basic form is a container housing cells grown on a cell culture dish or commercially available insert, with an inlet for smoke to pass through and interact with the cultures. Simple examples include a small hermetic chamber big enough for a 12-wellplate containing two holes for ventilation and a small fan for smoke distribution (St-Laurent et al., 2009), or a rocking platform system which exposes half a submerged culture at a time to whole smoke as the liquid is rocked side to side (Bombick et al., 1997). Very sophisticated and engineered examples include Cultex® Laboratories exposure modules (Aufderheide & Mohr, 2000) and Vitrocell® linear modules (Walsh et al., 2008); both of which are commonly used with the Vitrocell® VC 10® Smoking Robot, and have special design features such as individual warmed media supply to each cell culture insert within the chamber, and specialised chamber docking to the dilution systems of the smoking robot.

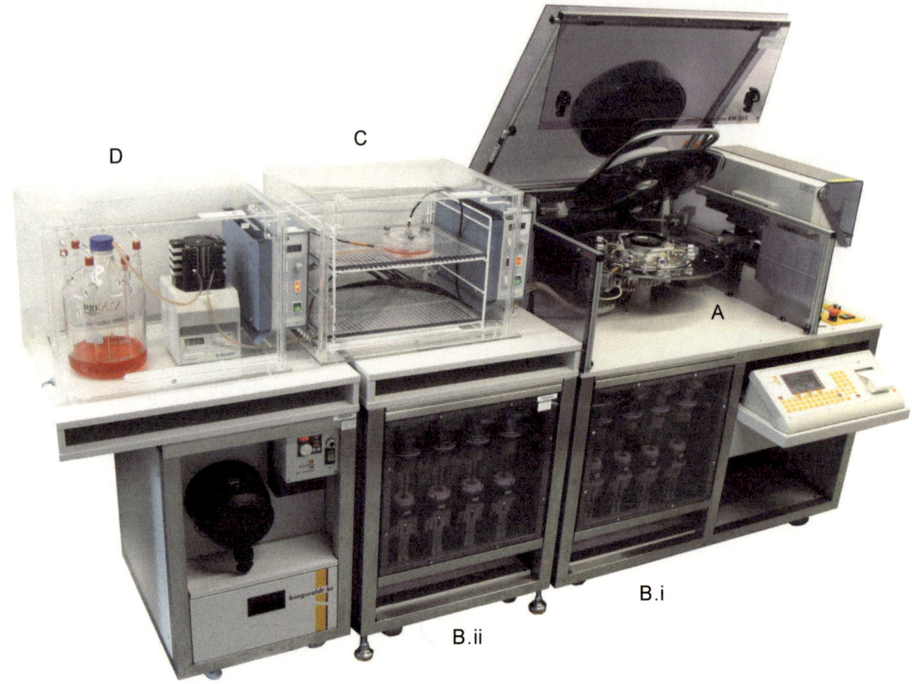

Fig. 5. The Borgwaldt RM20S eight syringe smoking machine. (A) cigarette smoke generator; (B.i) integral 4-syringe unit; (B.ii) additional 4-syringe unit to increase output; (C); incubator at 37°C to house exposure chambers containing cells/tissues at the ALI; (D) an incubator at 37°C holding the cell culture media which is supplied to the chambers using a pump (Adamson et al., in submission, http://www.bat-science.com/)

At BAT we have designed and developed an exposure chamber to enable ALI *in vitro* exposure to cigarette smoke and other aerosols (Phillips et al., 2005, Patent publication number WO 03/100417 A1). As shown in Figure 6 the exposure chamber is very simple in

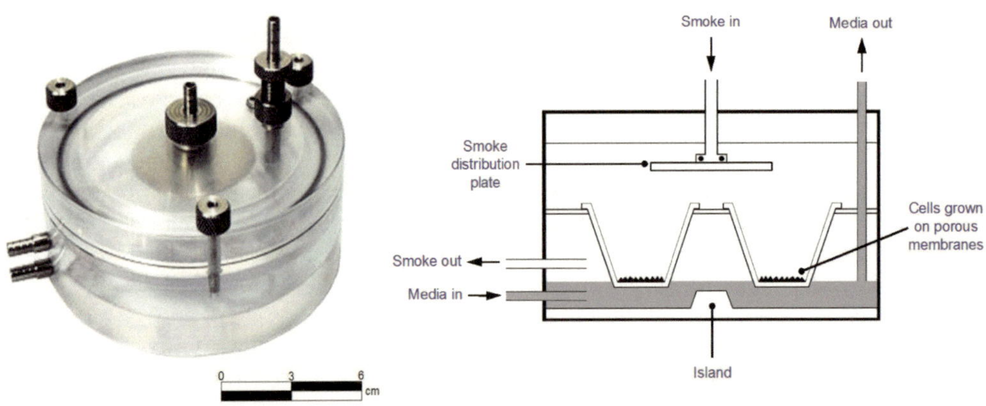

Fig. 6. BAT's exposure chamber, left, and a schematic cross-section, right (Adamson et al, in submission, http://www.bat-science.com)

design. It is therefore compact, robust, easy to clean and relatively economical. It can accommodate commercially available culture inserts, allowing flexibility in experimental design and replicate number: 3 large (24mm ø), 6 medium (12mm ø) or 8 small (6mm ø) fitting symmetrically in a single chamber simply by changing the insert support. Media is supplied into the chamber basally so it contacts with the porous membrane of the cell culture inserts, but does not flood the apical/air surface of the cultures. This chamber has been characterised and used extensively with Borgwaldt smoking machines (Adamson et al, in submission, Maunders et al., 2008, Phillips et al., 2005; Thorne et al., 2009) and most recently with the Vitrocell® VC10® smoking robot.

5. Conclusion and future research

As described in this chapter, there are many tools available to the biologist and toxicologist to evaluate and understand COPD disease processes and causative agents. There are advantages and disadvantages in the utility of these tools for risk and disease prediction. However it is important to note that each tool should be evaluated as a component part of an integrated or 'weight of evidence' approach and not solely in isolation. To add further reliability to the data and confirm the robustness of *in vitro* systems, there is a need to validate *in vitro* models of the whole respiratory system and appropriate exposure devices. This will only be achieved through closer working with the developers, users and producers of these systems along with better and more communication with regulators and opinion leaders in the field of *in vitro* testing and application.

At British American Tobacco, as part of our approach to tobacco harm reduction, we are developing a portfolio of appropriate pre-clinical assays for product assessment and investigating the components of cigarette smoke. We have described a number of these *in vitro* assays and presented an exposure system that is well characterised and demonstrates a physiologically relevant method of generating and exposing *in vitro* cultures to whole cigarette smoke at the ALI. This system allows all phases of cigarette smoke, particulate and gas, to be assessed separately or in combination with the possibility of assessing the effects of single aerosol or individual gas phase components. We propose to further use this system and our portfolio of *in vitro* models at BAT for the biological assessment and evaluation of future tobacco products designed to reduce the harmful effects of cigarette smoke. Furthermore, this exposure system could be a useful *in vitro* method in other industries for evaluating the effects of different aerosols and gaseous mixtures such as air pollutants, desiel particulates, inhaled pharmaceuticals, cosmetics and to examine occupational exposure scenarios.

6. References

Adamson, J.; Azzopardi, D.; Errington, G.; Dickens, C.; McAughey, J. & Gaça, M.D. (20XX). Characterisation and evaluation of a Borgwaldt RM20S 8-syringe smoking machine for in vitro cell culture investigations. In submission.

Araya, J.; Cambier, S.; Markovics, J. A.; Wolters, P.; Jablons, D.; Hill, A.; Finkbeiner, W.; Jones, K.; Broaddus, V. C.; Sheppard, D.; Barzcak, A.; Xiao, Y.; Erle, D. J. & Nishimura, S. L. (2007). Squamous metaplasia amplifies pathologic epithelial-mesenchymal interactions in COPD patients. *J.Clin.Invest*, Vol. 117, No. 11, pp. 3551-3562.

Aufderheide, M. & Mohr, U. (2000). CULTEX - an alternative technique for cultivation and exposure of cells of the respiratory tract to airborne pollutants at the air/liquid interface. *Exp. Toxicol. Pathol.*, Vol 52, pp265-270.

Baginski, T.K.; Dabbagh, K.; Satjawatcharaphong, C. & Swinney, D.C. (2006) Cigarette smoke synergistically enhances respiratory mucin induction by proinflammatory stimuli. *Am J.Respir.Cell Mol.Biol.*, Vol. 35, No. 2, pp. 165-174.

Barbosa, M.D.; Nguyen, Q.A.; Tchernev, V.T.; Ashley, J.A.; Detter, J.C.; Blaydes, S.M.; Brandt, S.J.; Chotai, D.; Hodgman, C.; Solari, R.C.; Lovett, M. & Kingsmore, S.F. (1996). Identification of the homologous Beige and Chediak-Higashi Syndrome genes. *Nature,* Vol. 382, pp. 262-265.

Barnes, P.J. (2007). Unexpected failure of anti-tumor necrosis factor therapy in chronic obstructive pulmonary disease. *Am. J. Respir. Crit Care Med.*, Vol. 175, pp. 866-867.

Bartalesi, B.; Cavarra, E.; Fineschi, S.; Lucattelli, M.; Lunghi, B.; Martorana, P.A. & Lungarella, G. (2005). Different lung responses to cigarette smoke in two strains of mice sensitive to oxidants. *Eur. Respir. J.*, Vol. 25, pp. 15-22.

Beck, G.J.; Doyle, C.A.; Schachter, E.N. (1981). Smoking and lung function. *Am. Rev. Respir.Dis,*. Vol. 123, pp. 149-155.

Blank, F.; Rothen-Rutishauser, B. & Gehr, P. (2007). Dendritic cells and macrophages form a transepithelial network against foreign particulate antigens. *Am J.Respir.Cell Mol.Biol.*, Vol. 36, No. 6, pp. 669-677.

Blank, F.; Wehrli, M., Lehmann, A.; Baum, O.; Gehr, P.; von Garnier, C.& Rothen-Rutishauser B.M. (2011). Macrophages and dendritic cells express tight junction proteins and exchange particles in an in vitro model of the human airway wall. *Immunobiology*, Vol. 216, pp. 86-95.

Bombick E, Ayres PH, Doolittle DJ (1997) Cytotoxicity assessment of whole smoke and vapour phase of mainstream and sidestream cigarette smoke from three Kentucky reference cigarettes. Tox Met 7: 177-190

Boucher, R.C.; Johnson, J.; Inoue, S.; Hulbert, W. & Hogg, J.C. (1980). The effect of cigarette smoke on the permeability of guinea pig airways. *Lab Invest.*, Vol. 43, No. 1, pp. 94-100.

Carney, D.N.; Gazdar, A.F.; Bepler, G.; Guccion, J.G.; Marangos, P.J.; Moody, T.W.; Zweig, M.H. & Minna, J.D. (1985). Establishment and identification of small cell lung cancer cell lines having classic and variant features. *Cancer Res.*, Vol. 45, No. 6, pp 2913-23.

Castell, J.V.; Donato, M.T. & Gomez-Lechon, M.J. (2005). Metabolism and bioactivation of toxicants in the lung. The in vitro cellular approach. *Exp.Toxicol.Pathol.*, Vol. 57 Suppl 1, pp. 189-204.

Chowdhury, F.; Howat, W.J.; Phillips, G.J. & Lackie, PM. (2010). Interactions between endothelial cells and epithelial cells in a combined cell model of airway mucosa: effects on tight junction permeability. *Exp Lung Res.*, Vol. 36, No. 1, pp. 1-11.

Churg, A.; Tai, H.; Coulthard, T.; Wang, R. & Wright, J.L. (2006). Cigarette smoke drives small airway remodeling by induction of growth factors in the airway wall. *Am. J. Respir. Crit Care Med.*, Vol. 174, pp. 1327-1334.

Churg, A.; Wang, R.; Wang, X.; Onnervik, P.O.; Thim, K. & Wright, J. L. (2007). Effect of an MMP-9/MMP-12 inhibitor on smoke-induced emphysema and airway remodelling in guinea pigs. *Thorax,* Vol. 62, pp.706-713.

Clunes, L.; Bridges, B.; Alexis, N. & Tarran, R. (2008). In vivo versus in vitro airway surface liquid nicotine levels following cigarette smoke exposure. *J Anal Toxicol.,* Vol. 32, No. 3, pp. 201–207.

Cosio, M.G.; Hale, K.A. & Niewoehner, D.E.(1980). Morphologic and morphometric effects of prolonged cigarette smoking on the small airways. *Am Rev.Respir.Dis.,* Vol. 122, No. 2, pp. 265-21.

Cosio, M.G.; Majo, J. & Cosio, M.G. (2002). Inflammation of the airways and lung parenchyma in COPD: role of T cells. *Chest,* Vol. 121, pp. 160S-165S.

Cozens, A.L.; Yezzi, M.J.; Kunzelmann, K.; Ohrui, T.; Chin, L.; Eng, K.; Finkbeiner, W.E.; Widdicombe, J.H. & Gruenert, D.C. (1994). CFTR expression and chloride secretion in polarized immortal human bronchial epithelial cells. *Am J.Respir.Cell Mol.Biol.,* Vol. 10, No. 1, pp. 38-47.

D'Armiento, J.; Dalal, S.S.; Okada, Y.; Berg, R.A. & Chada, K. (1992). Collagenase expression in the lungs of transgenic mice causes pulmonary emphysema. *Cell.,* Vol. 71, pp. 955-961.

Davidson, D.J.; Gray, M.A.; Kilanowski, F.M.; Tarran, R.; Randell, S.H.; Sheppard, D.N.; Argent, B.E. & Dorin, J.R. (2004). Murine epithelial cells: isolation and culture. *J.Cyst.Fibros.,* Vol. 3, Suppl. 2, pp. 59-62.

de Santi, M.M.; Martorana, P.A.; Cavarra, E. & Lungarella, G. (1995). Pallid mice with genetic emphysema. Neutrophil elastase burden and elastin loss occur without alteration in the bronchoalveolar lavage cell population. *Lab Invest.* Vol. 73, No. 1, pp. 40-47.

Driscoll, T.; Nelson, D.I.; Steenland, K.; Leigh, J.; Concha-Barrientos, M.; Fingerhut, M. & Pruss-Ustun, A. (2005). The global burden of non-malignant respiratory disease due to occupational airborne exposures. *Am. J. Ind. Med.* Vol. 48, pp. 432-445.

Elbert, K.J.; Schafer, U.F.; Schafers, H.J.; Kim, K.J.; Lee, V.H. & Lehr, C.M. (1999). Monolayers of human alveolar epithelial cells in primary culture for pulmonary absorption and transport studies. *Pharm.Res.,* Vol. 16, No. 5, pp. 601-608.

Elliott, M.K.; Sisson, J.H.; West, W.W. & Wyatt, T.A. (2006). Differential *in vivo* effects of whole cigarette smoke exposure versus cigarette smoke extract on mouse ciliated tracheal epithelium. *Exp.Lung Res..,* Vol. 32, No. 3-4, pp. 99-118.

Epithelix: Our Products. Updated 2011. Date of access: 18th March 2011. Available from: http://www.epithelix.com/content/view/4/4/lang,en/.

Fisher, R.L.; Smith, M.S.; Hasal, S.J.; Hasal, K.S.; Gandolfi, A.J. & Brendel, K. (1994). The use of human lung slices in toxicology. *Hum.Exp.Toxicol.,* Vol. 13, No. 7, pp. 466-471.

Fletcher, C. & Peto, R. The natural history of chronic airflow obstruction. (1977). *Br. Med. J.,* Vol. 1. pp. 1645-1648.

Foronjy, R.F.; Mirochnitchenko, O.; Propokenko, O.; Lemaitre, V.; Jia, Y.; Inouye, M.; Okada, Y. & D'Armiento, J.M. (2006). Superoxide dismutase expression attenuates cigarette smoke- or elastase-generated emphysema in mice. *Am. J. Respir. Crit Care Med.*, Vol. 173, pp. 623-631.

Forbes, B. & Ehrhardt, C. (2005). Human respiratory epithelial cell culture for drug delivery applications. *Eur.J.Pharm.Biopharm.*, Vol. 60, No. 2, pp. 193-205.

Freeman, B.A. & O'Neil, J.J. (1984). Tissue slices in the study of lung metabolism and toxicology. *Environ.Health Perspect.*, Vol. 56, pp. 51-60.

Fuchs, S.; Hollins, A.J.; Laue, M.; Schaefer, U.F.; Roemer, K.; Gumbleton, M. & Lehr, C.M. (2003). Differentiation of human alveolar epithelial cells in primary culture: morphological characterization and synthesis of caveolin-1 and surfactant protein-C. *Cell Tissue Res.*, Vol. 311, No. 1, pp. 31-45.

Global Initiative for Chronic Obstructive Lung Disease. Guidelines: Global strategy for the diagnosis, management and prevention of chronic obstructive pulmonary disease,. Updated 2010. Date of access: 21st March 2010, Available from: http://www.goldcopd.org

Gray, A.C.; McLeod, J.D. & Clothier, R.H. (2007). A review of in vitro modelling approaches to the identification and modulation of squamous metaplasia in the human tracheobronchial epithelium. *Altern.Lab Anim.*, Vol. 35, No. 5, pp. 493-504.

Gray, T.E.; Guzman, K.; Davis, C.W.; Abdullah, L.H. & Nettesheim, P. (1996). Mucociliary differentiation of serially passaged normal human tracheobronchial epithelial cells. *Am J.Respir.Cell Mol.Biol.*, Vol. 14, No. 1, pp. 104-112.

Green, M.C.; Sweet, H.O. & Bunker, L.E. (1976). Tight-skin, a new mutation of the mouse causing excessive growth of connective tissue and skeleton. *Am. J. Pathol.*, Vol. 82, pp. 493-512.

Gross, P.; Babyak, M.A.; Tolker, E. & Kaschak, M. (1964). Enzymatically produced pulmonary emphysema; a preliminary report. *J. Occup. Med.*, Vol. 6, pp. 481-484.

Hackett, N.R.; Heguy, A.; Harvey, B.G.; O'Connor, T.P.; Luettich, K.; Flieder, D.B.; Kaplan, R. & Crystal, R.G. (2003). Variability of antioxidant-related gene expression in the airway epithelium of cigarette smokers. *Am J.Respir.Cell Mol.Biol.*, Vol. 29, No. 3 Pt 1, pp. 331-343.

Harrigan, J.A.; Vezina, C.M.; McGarrigle, B.P.; Ersing, N.; Box, H.C.; Maccubbin, A.E. & Olson, J.R. (2004). DNA adduct formation in precision-cut rat liver and lung slices exposed to benzo[a]pyrene. *Toxicol.Sci.*, Vol. 77, No. 2, pp. 307-314.

Haswell, L.E.; Hewitt, K.; Thorne, D.; Richter, A. & Gaça, M.D. (2010). Cigarette smoke total particulate matter increases mucous secreting cell numbers in vitro: A potential model of goblet cell hyperplasia. *Tox In Vitro.*, Vol. 24, No. 3, pp. 981-987.

Hautamaki, R.D.; Kobayashi, D.K.; Senior, R., & Shapiro, S.D. (1997). Requirement for macrophage elastase for cigarette smoke-induced emphysema in mice. *Science.* Vol. 277, pp. 2002-2004.

Hermanns, M.I.; Unger, R.E.; Kehe, K.; Peters, K. & Kirkpatrick, C.J. (2004). Lung epithelial cell lines in coculture with human pulmonary microvascular endothelial cells: development of an alveolo-capillary barrier in vitro. *Lab Invest.* Vol. 84, No. 6, pp. 736-52.

Hermanns, M.I.; Fuchs, S.; Bock, M.; Wenzel, K.; Mayer, E.; Kehe, K.; Bittinger, F. & Kirkpatrick, C. J. (2009). Primary human coculture model of alveolo-capillary unit to study mechanisms of injury to peripheral lung. *Cell Tissue Res.*, Vol. 336, No. 1, pp. 91-105.

Hoffmann, D.; Djordjevic, M.V. & Hoffmann, I. (1997). The changing cigarette. *Prev. Med.*, Vol. 26, pp. 427-434

Hogg, J.C.; Chu, F.; Utokaparch, S.; Woods, R.; Elliott, W.M.; Buzatu, L.; Cherniack, R.M.; Rogers, R.M.; Sciurba, F.C.; Coxson, H.O. & Pare, P.D. (2004). The Nature of Small-Airway Obstruction in Chronic Obstructive Pulmonary Disease. *N. Engl. J. Med.*, Vol. 350, pp. 2645-2653.

Innes, A.L.; Woodruff, P. G.; Ferrando, R. E.; Donnelly, S.; Dolganov, G.M.; Lazarus, S.C. & Fahy, J.V. (2006). Epithelial mucin stores are increased in the large airways of smokers with airflow obstruction, *Chest*, Vol. 130, No. 4, pp. 1102-1108.

Jeffery, P.K. (2000). Comparison of the Structural and Inflammatory Features of COPD and Asthma. Giles F. Filley Lecture. *Chest*, Vol. 117, pp. 251S-260S.

Johnson, M.D.; Schilz, J.; Djordjevic, M.V.; Rice, J.R. & Shields, P.G. (2009) Evaluation of In Vitro Assays For Assessing the Toxicity of Cigarette Smoke and Smokeless Tobacco. *Cancer Epidemiol Biomarkers Prev*. Vol. 18, No. 12, pp. 3263-304.

Kaur, N.; Lacasse, M.; Roy, JP. ; Cabral, JL.; Adamson, J.; Errington, G.; Waldron K.C.; Gaça, M. & Morin. A. (2010). Evaluation of precision and accuracy of the Borgwaldt RM20S (®) smoking machine designed for in vitro exposure. *Inhal Tox.*, Vol. 22, No. 14, pp. 1174-1183.

Kielty, C.M.; Raghunath, M.; Siracusa, L.D.; Sherratt, M.J.; Peters, R.; Shuttleworth, C.A. & Jimenez, S.A. (1998). The tight skin mouse: demonstration of mutant fibrillin-1 production and assembly into abnormal microfibrils. *J. Cell Biol.*, Vol. 140, pp.1159-1166.

Kim, V.; Rogers, T.J. & Criner, G. J. (2008). New concepts in the pathobiology of chronic obstructive pulmonary disease. *Proc Am Thorac Soc.*, Vol. 5, No. 4, pp. 478-485.

Kode, A.; Yang, S.R. & Rahman, I. (2006). Differential effects of cigarette smoke on oxidative stress and proinflammatory cytokine release in primary human airway epithelial cells and in a variety of transformed alveolar epithelial cells. *Respir.Res.*, Vol. 7, pp. 132.

Komori, M.; Inoue, H.; Matsumoto, K.; Koto, H.; Fukuyama, S.; Aizawa, H. & Hara, N. (2001). PAF mediates cigarette smoke-induced goblet cell metaplasia in guinea pig airways. *Am. J. Physiol Lung Cell Mol. Physiol.*, Vol. 280, pp. L436-L441.

Korpi-Steiner, N.L.; Valkenaar, S.M.; Bates, M.E.; Evans, M.D.; Gern, J.E. & Bertics, P.J. (2010). Human monocytic cells direct the robust release of CXCL10 by bronchial epithelial cells during rhinovirus infection. *Clin.Exp.Allergy.*, Vol. 40, No. 8, pp. 1203-1213.

Lappalainen, U.; Whitsett, J.A.; Wert, S.E.; Tichelaar, J.W. and Bry, K. (2005). Interleukin-1beta causes pulmonary inflammation, emphysema, and airway remodeling in the adult murine lung. *Am. J. Respir. Cell Mol. Biol.*, Vol. 32, pp. 311-318.

Laugesen, M. & Fowles, J. (2005). Scope for regulation of cigarette smoke toxicity according to brand differences in toxicant emissions. *J. N. Z. Med J.*, Vol. 118, No. 1213

Lee, T.C.; Wu, R.; Brody, A.R.; Barrett, J.C. & Nettesheim, P. (1984). Growth and differentiation of hamster tracheal epithelial cells in culture. *Exp.Lung Res.*, Vol. 6, No. 1, pp. 27-45.

Lee, C.G.; Homer, R.J.; Cohn, L.; Link, H.; Jung, S.; Craft, J.E.; Graham, B.S.; Johnson, T.R. & Elias, J.A. (2002). Transgenic overexpression of interleukin (IL)-10 in the lung causes mucus metaplasia, tissue inflammation, and airway remodeling via IL-13-dependent and -independent pathways. *J. Biol. Chem.*, Vol. 520, No. 277, pp. 35466-35474.

Lehmann, A.D.; Daum, N.; Bur, M.; Lehr, C.M., Gehr, P. & Rothen-Rutishauser, B.M. (2011). An *in vitro* triple cell co-culture model with primary cells mimicking the human alveolar epithelial barrier. *Eur.J.Pharm.Biopharm.* Vol. 77, No. 3, pp. 398-406.

Lin, J.C.; Talbot, S.; Lahjouji, K.; Roy, JP.; Senecal, J.; Couture, R. & Morin, A. (2010) Mechanism of cigarette smoke-induced kinin B(1) receptor expression in rat airways. *Peptides*, Vol. 31, No. 10, pp. 1940-1945.

Liu, C.; McAdam, K. & Perfetti, T.A. (2010). Some Recent Topics in Cigarette Smoke Science, In: Special Issue for Free Radical Chemistry in Cigarette Smoke and Smoking Related Diseases, Guest Editors: Chuan Liu and Kevin G. McAdam, Bentham Sciences, Publishing. In Press

Liu, X.; Luo, M.; Zhang, L.; Ding, W.; Yan, Z. & Engelhardt, J.F. (2007). Bioelectric properties of chloride channels in human, pig, ferret, and mouse airway epithelia. *Am J.Respir.Cell Mol.Biol.*, Vol. 36, No. 3, pp. 313-323.

Liu, Y.; Gao, W. & Zhang, D. (2010). Effects of cigarette smoke extract on A549 cells and human lung fibroblasts treated with transforming growth factor-beta1 in a coculture system. *Clin.Exp.Med.*, Vol. 10, No. 3, pp. 159-16.

Ma, R.; Wang, Y.; Cheng, G.; Zhang, H.Z.; Wan, H.Y. & Huang, S.G. (2005). MUC5AC expression up-regulation goblet cell hyperplasia in the airway of patients with chronic obstructive pulmonary disease. *Chin Med.Sci.J.*, Vol. 20, No. 3, pp. 181-184.

MacNee, W. (2005). Pathogenesis of chronic obstructive pulmonary disease. *Proc Am Thorac Soc.*, Vol. 2, No. 4, pp. 258-266.

Mattek: The EpiAirway™ Tissue Model. Updated 2011. Date of Access: 21st March 2011, Available from: http://www.mattek.com/pages/products/epiairway .

Maunders, H.; Patwardhan, S.; Phillips, J.; Clack, A. & Richter, A. (2007). Human bronchial epithelial cell transcriptome: Gene expression changes following acute exposure to whole cigarette smoke in vitro. *Am J Physi - Lung Cell Mol Phys.* Vol. 292, No. 5, pp. L1248-L1256

McCartney, A.C.; Fox, B.; Partridge, T.A.; Macrae, K.D.; Tetley, T.D.; Phillips, G.J. and Guz, A. (1988). Emphysema in the blotchy mouse: a morphometric study. *J. Pathol.*, Vol. 156, pp. 77-81.

Mossman, B.T.; Lounsbury, K.M. & Reddy, S.P. (2006). Oxidants and signaling by mitogen-activated protein kinases in lung epithelium. *Am J.Respir.Cell Mol.Biol.*, Vol. 34, No. 6, pp. 666-669.

Newland, N. & Ricther, A. (2008). Agents associated with lung inflammation induce similar responses in NCI-H292 lung epithelial cells. *Tox In Vitro.* Vol. 22, No.7, pp 1782-8

Newland, N. Baxter, A. Hewitt, K. & Minuet, E. (2011). CYP1A1/1B1 and CYP2A6/2A13 activity is conserved in cultures of differentiated primary human tracheobronchial epithelial cells. *Tox In Vitro.* In Press

Nikula, K.J. & Green, F.H. (2000). Animal models of chronic bronchitis and their relevance to studies of particle-induced disease. *Inhal. Toxicol.* Vol. 12, Suppl. 4, pp. 123-153.

Noguchi, C.; Umino, T.; Miyazaki, Y.; Jinta, T.; Usui, Y. & Yoshizawa, Y. (2007). TGF-beta and glutathione promote tissue repair in cigarette smoke induced injury. *J.Med.Dent.Sci.*, Vol. 54, No. 1, pp. 109-116.

Ostrowski, L.E.; Randell, S.H.; Clark, A.B.; Gray, T.E. & Nettesheim, P. (1995). Ciliogenesis of rat tracheal epithelial cells in vitro. *Methods Cell Biol.*, Vol. 47, pp. 57-63.

Oswald, N.C. & Medvei, V.C. (1995). Chronic bronchitis; the effect of cigarette-smoking. *Lancet.* Vol. 269, pp. 843-844.

Papritz, M.; Pohl, C.; Wübbeke, C.; Moisch, M.; Hofmann, H.; Hermanns, M.I.; Thiermann, H.; Kirkpatrick, C.J. & Kehe, K. (2010). Side-specific effects by cadmium exposure: apical and basolateral treatment in a coculture model of the blood-air barrier. *Toxicol Appl Pharmacol.* Vol. 245, No. 3, pp. 361-9.

Pare, P.D.; Wiggs, B.R.; James, A.; Hogg, J.C. & Bosken, C. (1991). The comparative mechanics and morphology of airways in asthma and in chronic obstructive pulmonary disease. *Am. Rev. Respir. Dis.*, Vol. 143, pp. 1189-1193.

Parrish, A.R.; Gandolfi, A.J. & Brendel, K. (1995). Precision-cut tissue slices: applications in pharmacology and toxicology. *Life Sci.*, Vol. 57, No. 21, pp. 1887-1901.

Pauwels, R.A.; Buist, A.S.; Ma, P.; Jenkins, C. R. & Hurd, S.S. (2001). Global strategy for the diagnosis, management, and prevention of chronic obstructive pulmonary disease: National Heart, Lung, and Blood Institute and World Health Organization Global Initiative for Chronic Obstructive Lung Disease (GOLD): executive summary. *Respir.Care.*, Vol. 46, No. 8, pp. 798-825.

Phillips, J.; Kluss, B.; Richter, A. & Massey, E.D. (2005). Exposure of bronchial epithelial cells to whole cigarette smoke: assessment of cellular responses. *ATLA.*, Vol. 33, No. 3, pp 239-248.

Pohl, C.; Hermanns, M.I.; Uboldi, C.; Bock, M.; Fuchs, S.; Dei-Anang, J.; Mayer, E.; Kehe, K.; Kummer, W. & Kirkpatrick, C.J. (2009). Barrier functions and paracellular integrity in human cell culture models of the proximal respiratory unit. *Eur.J.Pharm.Biopharm.*, Vol. 72, No. 2, pp. 339-349.

Rodgman, A. & Perfetti, T.A. (2008). *The Chemical Components of Tobacco and Tobacco Smoke.* CRC Press, ISBN 9781420078831, Florida, USA.

Rogers, D.F. & Jeffery, P.K. (1986). Inhibition of cigarette smoke-induced airway secretory cell hyperplasia by indomethacin, dexamethasone, prednisolone, or hydrocortisone in the rat. *Exp. Lung Res.*, Vol. 10, pp. 285-298.

Rogers, D.F. (2007). Physiology of airway mucus secretion and pathophysiology of hypersecretion. *Respir.Care.*, Vol. 52, No. 9, pp. 1134-1149.

Roh, G.S.; Yi, C.O.; Cho, Y.J.; Jeon, B.T.; Nizamudtinova, I.T.; Kim, H.J.; Kim, J.H.; Oh, Y.M.; Huh, J.W.; Lee, J.H.; Hwang, Y.S.; Lee, S.D. & Lee, J.D. (2010). Anti-inflammatory effects of celecoxib in rat lungs with smoke-induced emphysema. *Am. J. Physiol Lung Cell Mol. Physiol,.* Vol. 299, pp. L184-L191.

Rothen-Rutishauser, B.M.; Kiama, S.G., & Gehr, P. (2005) A three-dimensional cellular model of the human respiratory tract to study the interaction with particles. *Am J.Respir.Cell Mol.Biol.*, Vol. 32, No. 4, pp. 281-289.

Saetta, M.; Turato, G.; Baraldo, S.; Zanin, A.; Braccioni, F.; Mapp, C.E.; Maestrelli, P.; Cavallesco, G.; Papi, A. & Fabbri, L.M. (2000). Goblet cell hyperplasia and epithelial inflammation in peripheral airways of smokers with both symptoms of chronic bronchitis and chronic airflow limitation. *Am J.Respir.Crit Care Med.*, Vol. 161, No. 3, pp. 1016-1021.

Schwab, U.E.; Fulcher, M.L.; Randell, S.H.; Flaminio, M.J. & Russell, D.G. (2010). Equine bronchial epithelial cells differentiate into ciliated and mucus producing cells in vitro. *In Vitro Cell Dev.Biol.Anim.*, Vol. 46, No. 2, pp. 102-106.

Scian, M.J.; Oldham, M.J.; Kane, D.B.; Edmiston, J.S. & McKinney, W.J. (2009). Characterization of a whole smoke in vitro exposure system (Burghart Mimic Smoker-01). *Inhal Toxicol.*, Vol. 21, No. 3, pp. 234-43.

Sethi, J.M. & Rochester, C.L. (2000). Smoking and chronic obstructive pulmonary disease. *Clin. Chest Med.*, Vol. 21, pp. 67-86, viii.

Shao, M.X.; Nakanaga, T. & Nadel, J.A. (2004). Cigarette smoke induces MUC5AC mucin overproduction via tumor necrosis factor-alpha-converting enzyme in human airway epithelial (NCI-H292) cells. *Am J.Physiol Lung Cell Mol.Physiol.*, Vol. 287, No. 2, pp. L420-L427.

Shapiro, S.D. (2000). Animal Models for COPD. *Chest*, Vol. 117, pp. 223S-227S.

Simet, S.M.; Sisson, J.H.; Pavlik, J.A.; Devasure, J.M.; Boyer, C.; Liu, X.; Kawasaki, S.; Sharp, J.G.; Rennard, S.I. & Wyatt, T.A. (2010). Long-term cigarette smoke exposure in a mouse model of ciliated epithelial cell function. *Am J.Respir.Cell Mol.Biol.*, Vol. 43, No. 6, pp. 635-640.

Sisson, J.H.; Stoner, J.A.; Ammons, B.A. & Wyatt, T.A. (2003). All-digital image capture and whole-field analysis of ciliary beat frequency. *J.Microsc.*, Vol. 211, No. Pt 2, pp. 103-111.

Sisson, J.H.; Tuma, D.J. & Rennard, S.I. (1991). Acetaldehyde-mediated cilia dysfunction in bovine bronchial epithelial cells. *Am J.Physiol.*, Vol. 260, No. 2, Pt 1, pp. L29-L36.

Smith, K.R.; Uyeminami, D.L.; Kodavanti, U.P.; Crapo, J.D.; Chang, L.Y. & Pinkerton, K.E. (2002). Inhibition of tobacco smoke-induced lung inflammation by a catalytic antioxidant. *Free Radic. Biol. Med.*, Vol. 33, pp. 1106-1114.

Sporty, J.L.; Horalkova, L. & Ehrhardt, C. (2008). *In vitro* cell culture models for the assessment of pulmonary drug disposition. *Expert.Opin.Drug Metab Toxicol.*, Vol. 4, No. 4, pp. 333-345.

St-Laurent, J.; Proulx, L.I.; Boulet, L.P. & Bissonnette, E. (2009). Comparison of two in vitro models of cigarette smoke exposure. *Inhal Tox.,* Vol. 21, No. 13, pp. 1148-1153.

Sussan, T.E., Rangasamy, T., Blake, D.J., Malhotra, D., El-Hadda, H., Bedja, D.,Yates, M.S., Kombairaju, P., Yamamoto, M., Liby, K.T.,Sporn, M.B., Gabrielson, K.L., Champion, H.S., Tuder, R.M., Kensler, T.W. & Bisal, S. (2009). Targeting Nrf2 with the triterpenoid CDDO-imidazolide attenuates cigarette smoke-induced emphysema and cardiac dysfunction in mice. *Proc Natl Acad Sci USA.;* Vol 106, No. 1, pp250-255.

Takubo, Y.; Guerassimov, A.; Ghezzo, H.; Triantafillopoulos, A.; Bates, J.H.; Hoidal, J.R. & Cosio, M.G. (2002) Alpha1-antitrypsin determines the pattern of emphysema and function in tobacco smoke-exposed mice: parallels with human disease. *Am. J. Respir. Crit Care Med.,* Vol. 166, pp.1596-1603.

Thorne, D.; Wilson, J.; Kumaravel, T.S.; Massey, E.D. & McEwan, M. (2009). Measurement of oxidative DNA damage induced by mainstream cigarette smoke in cultured NCI-H292 cells. *Mut Res.,* Vol. 673, No. 1, pp.3-8.

Torvinen, M.; Campwala, H. & Kilty, I. (2007). The role of IFN-gamma in regulation of IFN-gamma-inducible protein 10 (IP-10) expression in lung epithelial cell and peripheral blood mononuclear cell co-cultures. *Respir Res.* Vol. 8, pp. 80.

Verra, F.; Escudier, E.; Lebargy, F.; Bernaudin, J.F.; De, C.H. & Bignon, J. (1995). Ciliary abnormalities in bronchial epithelium of smokers, ex-smokers, and nonsmokers. *Am J.Respir.Crit Care Med.,* Vol. 151, No. 3 Pt 1, pp. 630-634.

Wang, Z.; Zheng, T.; Zhu, Z.; Homer, R.J.; Riese, R.J.; Chapman, H.A. Jr.; Shapiro, S.D. & Elias, J.A. (2000). Interferon gamma induction of pulmonary emphysema in the adult murine lung. *J. Exp. Med.,* Vol. 192, pp. 1587-1600.

Whole smoke. Updated 2011. Date of access 18th March 2011. Available from:http://www.batscience.com/groupms/sites/BAT_7AWFH3.nsf/vwPages WebLive/DO7AXGRG?opendocument&SKN=1

Witherden, I.R.; Vanden Bon, E. J.; Goldstraw, P.; Ratcliffe, C.; Pastorino, U. & Tetley, T.D. (2004). Primary human alveolar type II epithelial cell chemokine release: effects of cigarette smoke and neutrophil elastase. *Am J.Respir.Cell Mol.Biol.,* Vol. 30, No. 4, pp. 500-509.

Wohlsen, A.; Martin, C.; Vollmer, E.; Branscheid, D.; Magnussen, H.; Becker, W.M.; Lepp, U. & Uhlig, S. (2003). The early allergic response in small airways of human precision-cut lung slices. *Eur.Respir.J.,* Vol. 21, No. 6, pp. 1024-1032.

Wright, J.L.; Ngai, T. & Churg, A. (1992). Effect of long-term exposure to cigarette smoke on the small airways of the guinea pig. *Exp. Lung Res.,* Vol. 18, pp.105-114.

Wright, J.L; Farmer, S.G. & Churg, A. (2002). Synthetic serine elastase inhibitor reduces cigarette smoke-induced emphysema in guinea pigs. *Am J Respir Crit Care Med.* Vol. 166, No. 7, pp. 954-60.

Wright, J.L.; Postma, D.S.; Kerstjens, H.A.; Timens, W.; Whittaker, P. & Churg, A. (2007). Airway remodeling in the smoke exposed guinea pig model. *Inhal. Toxicol.,* Vol. 19, pp. 915-923.

Wright, J.L. & Churg, A. (2008). Short-term exposure to cigarette smoke induces endothelial dysfunction in small intrapulmonary arteries: analysis using guinea pig precision cut lung slices. *J.Appl.Physiol.*, Vol. 104, No. 5, pp. 1462-1469.

Wright, J.L. & Churg, A. (2010). Animal models of cigarette smoke-induced chronic obstructive pulmonary disease. *Expert. Rev. Respir. Med.*, Vol. 4, pp. 723-734.

Yoshida, T. & Tuder, R.M. (2007). Pathobiology of cigarette smoke-induced chronic obstructive pulmonary disease. *Physiol Rev.*, Vol. 87, pp. 1047-1082.

Zheng, T.; Zhu, Z.; Wang, Z.; Homer, R.J.; Ma, B.; Riese, R.J. Jr.; Chapman, H.A. Jr.; Shapiro, S.D. & Elias, J.A. (2000). Inducible targeting of IL-13 to the adult lung causes matrix metalloproteinase- and cathepsin-dependent emphysema. *J. Clin. Invest.*, Vol. 106, pp. 1081

4

Cigarette Smoking and Lower Respiratory Tract Infection

Fernando Saldías and Orlando Díaz
Departamento de Enfermedades Respiratorias,
Facultad de Medicina, Pontificia Universidad Católica de Chile
Chile

1. Introduction

Acute bronchitis, one of the most common diagnoses in ambulatory care medicine, accounted for approximately 2.5 million visits to U.S. physicians in 1998 (Slusarcick & McCaig, 2000). This condition consistently ranks as one of the top ten diagnoses for which patients seek medical care, with cough being the most frequently mentioned symptom necessitating office evaluation (Knutson & Braun, 2002; Saldías et al., 2007). The diagnosis is based on clinical findings, without standardized diagnostic signs and sensitive or specific confirmation laboratory tests (Oeffinger et al., 1997).

Acute bronchitis is usually caused by a viral infection, especially by influenza, parainfluenza and respiratory syncytial virus, it is also caused by adenovirus, coronavirus and rhinovirus (Marrie, 1998). When microbiological studies are performed, less than 10-20% of patients will have evidence of acute bacterial infection (Macfarlane et al., 2001). Thus, *Bordetella pertussis, Mycoplasma pneumoniae* and *Chlamydia pneumoniae* have been clearly established as causes of acute bronchitis. But there is no clear evidence that *Streptococcus pneumoniae, Haemophilus influenzae* or *Moraxella catarrhalis* cause acute bronchitis in adults without underlying lung disease; studies have failed to distinguish between colonization and acute infection (Ramirez-Ronda et al., 1981; Treanor & Hayden, 2000). However, these bacteria are important causes of superinfections after acute viral respiratory illnesses (Hament et al., 1999; Peltola & McCullers, 2004).

The devastating health impact of cigarette smoking is well known (Kuper et al., 2002; Stewart et al., 2008). Despite ongoing efforts to reduce smoking prevalence, over 1.1 billion people continue to smoke, representing one-sixth of the world's population (Jha et al., 2002). Cigarette smoking is a major risk factor for premature mortality due to cancer, cardiovascular and cerebrovascular disease, and chronic obstructive pulmonary disease (Dye & Adler, 1994). About half of all smokers will develop a serious smoking-related illness, such as chronic obstructive pulmonary disease (COPD), which is characterized by irreversible airway obstruction, or cardiovascular disease. Furthermore, about 1–5% of smokers will develop a smoking-related malignancy, mostly lung adenocarcinoma or other epithelial cell tumours. But cigarette smoking also appears to be a major risk factor for respiratory tract infections (Marcy & Merrill, 1987). Both active and passive cigarette smoke exposure increase the risk of infections. Passive exposure to tobacco smoke in children contributes significantly to morbidity and mortality (Cheraghi & Salvi, 2009). Children in particular, seem to be the most susceptible population for the harmful effects of environmental tobacco smoke (ETS). Exposure to ETS amongst children at homes have been reported to vary from 27.6% in Africa, 34.3% in South East Asia, 50.6% in Western Pacific, and up to 77.8% in Europe (Warren et al., 2008). The morbidity and mortality of infectious diseases associated to smoking are not widely appreciated by physicians. The mechanism of increased susceptibility to infections in smokers is multifactorial and includes alteration of the structural (Dye & Adler, 1994; Marcy & Merrill, 1987) and immunologic host defenses (Sopori et al., 1994; Sopori et al., 1998). We reviewed the epidemiology of smoking-related lung infections and the mechanisms by which smoking increases the risk of infection.

2. Mechanisms by which cigarette smoking may predispose to respiratory infections

The specific mechanisms by which cigarette smoking increases the risk of respiratory infections are incompletely understood (Saldías et al., 2007; Domagala-Kulawik, 2008). They are multifactorial and probably interactive in their effects. Mechanisms by which smoking increases the risk of infections include structural changes in the respiratory tract (Dye & Adler, 1994) and a decrease in immune response (Sopori et al., 1998).

2.1 Structural changes caused by smoking

The ciliated respiratory epithelium, the main target of most respiratory viruses, is the first line of defense against harmful environmental agents and protects by sweeping particles away in the overlying mucus gel layer, phagocytosing and killing some pathogens, maintaining a barrier through tight junctions and priming, activating and recruiting other immune cells. Cigarette smoke and many of its components produce structural changes in the respiratory tract. These changes include peribronchiolar inflammation and fibrosis, increased mucosal permeability, impairment of the mucociliary clearance, changes in pathogen adherence, and disruption of the respiratory epithelium (Dye & Adler, 1994). These changes are thought to predispose to the development of upper and lower respiratory tract infections, which may amplify the cigarette smoke–induced lung inflammation. A number of components of cigarette smoke, including acrolein, acetaldehyde, formaldehyde, free radicals produced from chemical reactions within the cigarette smoke, and nitric oxide, may contribute to the observed structural alterations in the airway epithelial cells (Marcy & Merrill, 1987).

Smoke directly compromises the integrity of this physical barrier, increases the permeability of the respiratory epithelium and impairs mucociliary clearance (Dye & Adler, 1994; Jones et al., 1980; Burns et al., 1989). Although cigarette smoke has been shown to activate epithelial cells to produce pro-inflammatory mediators (Mio et al., 1997), it attenuates the *in vitro* production of pro-inflammatory mediators by epithelial cells following stimulation with pathogen-associated molecular patterns (PAMPs), such as lipopolysaccharide or double-stranded RNA (Laan et al., 2004; Bauer et al., 2008). Smoke also induces direct oxidative damage to membrane lipids and causes extensive single-strand DNA breaks, triggering repair and apoptotic cascades (Kim et al., 2004). Thus, cigarette smoke acutely suppresses the respiratory epithelium and chronically can cause damage, inflammation and may ultimately transform it.

2.2 Effect of cigarette smoke on the lung and systemic immunity

Cigarette smoke has been shown to affect a wide range of host defense mechanisms (Sopori et al., 1994). However, findings between studies can be controversial and sometimes contradictory, probably because of differences in smoking history, genetic susceptibility and socioeconomic status (such as exercise, nutrition, occupation and ambient air quality, which can modify disease). Similar issues apply to animal models and *in vitro* systems, in which parameters of smoke exposure, such as duration, frequency and mode vary markedly between studies (Domagala-Kulawik, 2008; Stämpfli & Anderson, 2009). Accordingly, as the patterns of smoke exposure are so varied individually and geographically, no single experimental smoke exposure system can replicate the diversity of human smoking patterns, and each experimental system probably reflects only facets of the overall picture.

2.2.1 Cell-mediated immune responses

White blood cell count and distribution in peripheral blood. Smokers usually exhibit an elevated peripheral white blood cell count, around 30% higher than that of nonsmokers (Friedman et al., 1973; Yeung & Buncio, 1984; Tollerud et al., 1989; Mili et al., 1991). It has been shown a significant relationship between the white blood cell count in smokers and the plasma concentration of nicotine (Taylor et al., 1986). It has been suggested that nicotine induced catecholamine release might be the mechanism for this effect (Friedman et al., 1973). Other studies support the hypothesis that cigarette smoking causes bone marrow stimulation (Van Eeden & Hogg, 2000). It has been suggested that proinflammatory factors released from alveolar macrophages, such as tumor necrosis factor α, interleukin (IL) 1, IL-8, and granulocyte-macrophage colony-stimulating factor, are probably responsible for the stimulation of bone marrow by cigarette smoking. It has been reported the same relationship between cigarette smoking and increased leukocyte count in adolescents, indicating that there appears to be a rapid effect of cigarette smoking on white blood cell count that is unlikely to be due to smoking induced chronic disease conditions as seen in adult smokers (Tell et al., 1985).

Reports of the effects of smoking on the different subsets of lymphocyte T cells are conflicting. Light to moderate smokers were reported to have a significant increase in CD3+ and CD4+ counts and a trend toward increased CD8+ lymphocyte count (Miller et al., 1982; Hughes et al., 1985; Tollerud et al., 1989; Mili et al., 1991). By contrast, studies of heavy smokers (over 50 pack-years) reported a decrease in CD4+ and a significant increase in CD8+ cell counts. Thus, the decrease observed in the ratio of CD4+ to CD8+ lymphocytes in heavy smokers was due predominantly to an increase of CD8+ cells (Ginns et al., 1982). These effects appeared to be reversible as soon as 6 weeks after smoking cessation (Miller et al., 1982). Other studies have reported no difference in the CD4+ and CD8+ lymphocyte counts among moderate smokers (Costabel et al., 1986). Since CD4+ cells facilitate B-cell proliferation and differentiation and immunoglobulin synthesis, the decrease in this subset observed in heavy smokers might contribute to the increased susceptibility to infections in this population.

Airways and lung parenchyma. Bronchoalveolar lavage studies have demonstrated a marked decrease in the absolute number of CD4+ cells, and an increase in CD8+ cells with a lower CD4+/CD8+ cell ratio in moderate smokers vs nonsmokers (Leatherman et al., 1984; Costabel et al., 1986; Wewers et al., 1998). No significant changes in these variables in the peripheral blood were found in this population of moderate smokers, in contrast with the findings in heavy smokers discussed previously. Thus, changes in lymphocyte population in the bronchoalveolar lavage in smokers may disclose pathologic changes earlier than in blood. Moreover, these findings suggest that smokers have a deficit in cell-mediated immunity in the lung alveolus, a site critical in the first-line defense against infection.

The retention of CD8+ T cells in the lungs of chronic smokers warrants particular attention as it is a hallmark of COPD and it is known that these cells can activate alveolar macrophages to produce matrix metalloproteinase 12, a potent elastin-degrading enzyme that has been linked to emphysema (Hautamaki et al., 1997; Grumelli et al., 2004). Furthermore, CD8+ T cells are required for inflammation and tissue destruction in smoke-induced emphysema in mice (Maeno et al., 2007). Cigarette smoke has also been found to promote the retention of virus-specific CD8+ memory effector T cells, but to weaken their defensive ability (Gualano et al., 2008).

Smoking is also associated with significant increases in the percentage of macrophages in bronchoalveolar lavage fluid (Wewers et al., 1998). Owing to their strategic positioning within the alveolar space, alveolar macrophages have a key role in sensing and eliminating microbial agents early in the course of an infection. Cigarette smoking increases the number of alveolar macrophages (Sopori et al., 1998) and activates them to produce pro-inflammatory mediators, reactive oxygen species and proteolytic enzymes (de Boer et al., 2000; Russell et al., 2002), thereby providing a cellular mechanism that links smoking with inflammation and tissue damage. Similar to its effects on the respiratory epithelium, cigarette smoke compromises the ability of alveolar macrophages to phagocytose bacteria (King et al., 1988; Berenson et al., 2006) and apoptotic cells (Hodge et al., 2007) and to sense PAMPs (Drannik et al., 2004; Chen et al., 2007; Gaschler et al., 2008). Importantly, cigarette smoke may not simply suppress the function of alveolar macrophages as previously suggested, but instead might skew their inflammatory mediator profile. The nature of the skewing may be a determinant of disease susceptibility. Accordingly, one study reported a distinctive state of activation of alveolar macrophages in smokers that distinguished them from those in non-smokers (Woodruff et al., 2005). This highlights a key emerging concept – smoke may induce partial M1 deactivation or partial M2 activation of macrophages. The balance and intensity of this skewing has direct implications for the immune system and its response to disease because effective host defense requires a macrophage activation programme that is appropriate for the particular type of pathogen and because M1-type macrophages can cause marked lung damage (emphysema), whereas M2-type macrophages are linked to tumour progression. The molecular mechanisms of altered alveolar macrophage responsiveness and skewing are not presently understood but they are at least partially reversible by exposure to the reduced form of glutathione, which implicates oxidative damage of effector pathways. The infection risk is compounded by host deficiencies or polymorphisms in innate and adaptive immune response genes, in particular those encoding pattern recognition receptors, such as mannose-binding lectin, and their signal transduction intermediates (Becker & O'Neill, 2007).

In the lungs, dendritic cells (DCs), which are the most potent antigen-presenting cells and are indispensable for the initiation of T cell-mediated immune responses (Mellman & Steinman, 2001), are probably highly susceptible to smoke-induced effects because of their anatomical position (in the lumen and directly beneath the epithelium of the lung) (McComb et al., 2008). Although it is known that the DC-directed chemokine CX3CL1 is upregulated in emphysema (McComb et al., 2008), there are only a few studies assessing the effects of smoking on lung DCs in humans and animal models (Tsoumakidou et al., 2008). Clinical studies suggest that the number of mature DCs is reduced in the large airways of patients with COPD who smoke (Jahnsen et al., 2006). Following smoking cessation, the numbers of mature DCs increase and are similar to non-smoking healthy controls. By contrast, the number of immature DCs is increased in the small airways of patients with COPD compared with individuals who have never smoked and individuals who smoke but do not have COPD (McComb et al., 2008). These data indicate that smoking behavior may affect DC numbers and maturity state.

Leukocytes function. Polymorphonuclear leukocytes from the peripheral blood of smokers exhibit depressed migration and chemotaxis compared with PMNs from nonsmokers (Noble & Penny, 1975; Corberand et al., 1979). The motility and chemotaxis of PMNs are depressed in the oral cavity of smokers compared with nonsmokers (Eichel & Shahrik, 1969; Noble & Penny, 1975). The whole cigarette smoke, its gas phase and the water-soluble fraction are potent inhibitors of PMN chemotaxis (Bridges et al., 1977). Of the water-soluble fraction of cigarette smoking, the unsaturated aldehydes (acrolein and crotonaldehyde) were the major contributors to the inhibitor properties. The non-volatile components of cigarette smoking also inhibit chemotaxis by a mechanism that differs from that of the unsaturated aldehydes present in the vapour phase of smoke (Bridges et al., 1977; Bridges & Hsieh, 1986). The non-volatile component did not inhibit migration. Nicotine had no effect on PMN migration and chemotaxis (Sasagawa et al., 1985). Macrophages from the lungs of smokers have a greater inhibitory effect on lymphocyte proliferation than macrophages from the lungs of nonsmokers. Thus, the immunosuppressive effects of the macrophages on cell-mediated immune response are increased in smokers (Holt, 1987). The release of cytokines (TNFα, IL-1, IL-2 and IL-6) from macrophages may also be altered in smokers (McCrea et al., 1994; Twigg et al., 1994; Ouyang et al., 2000; Hagiwara et al., 2001). Hydroquinone, the phenolic compound in cigarette tar, had the most potent inhibitory effect of these cytokines, whereas nicotine had little effect. The cytokines IL-1 and IL-6 are important in the host defense against infection (Smith, 1988; Luster et al., 1999). Animal studies have shown that depletion of these cytokines increases susceptibility to bacterial pneumonia. Since PMNs play a significant role in host defense against acute bacterial infections, an impairment of PMN functions by smoke may contribute to the increased susceptibility of smokers to systemic infections, including bacterial pneumonia.

Lymphocyte functions. Natural killer (NK) cell activity in peripheral blood has been reported to be reduced in smokers compared with nonsmokers (Ferson et al., 1979; Hughes et al., 1985; Tollerud et al., 1989; Nair et al., 1990). These alterations appear to be reversible, since NK activity in ex-smokers was similar to that of a never-smoking group compared with smokers (Silverman et al., 1975; Hersey et al., 1983). The recovery period was relatively short, as little as 6 weeks (Miller et al., 1982; Hughes et al., 1985). Since NK cells are important in the early surveillance response against viral infections and resistance against microbial infections (Herberman & Holden, 1978; Herberman, 1980), impairment of NK cell activity by cigarette smoking is a potential mechanism for the increased incidence of infections among smokers.

Mounting evidence suggests that natural killer cells have an important role in innate host defense against microbial agents and in protective antitumour immune surveillance. This is achieved by direct cytotoxicity through perforin and granzymes, CD95 ligand-induced apoptosis and pro-inflammatory cytokine and chemokine release (Tollerud et al., 1989;

Hamerman et al, 2005). Several studies have shown that NK cell numbers and activity are decreased in smokers compared with non-smokers (Swann et al., 2007). Exposure to cigarette smoke attenuates the cytotoxic activity and cytokine production of NK cells in humans and mice (Lu et al., 2006; Mian et al., 2008), thereby linking NK cell defects to increased infection risk and cancer.

Animal studies have shown that nicotine inhibits the antibody-forming cell response through impairment of antigen-mediated signalling in T cells and suppression of intracellular calcium response (Geng et al., 1995; Geng et al., 1996; Sopori et al., 1998). It has been suggested that nicotine through activation of protein tyrosine kinases and depletion of inositol-1,4,5-trisphosphate-sensitive calcium stores in T cells could be a major immunosuppressive component in cigarette smoking (Kalra et al., 2000).

2.2.2 Humoral immune system

Peripheral blood. The effects of cigarette smoking on humoral immunity have been studied extensively (Sopori et al., 1994; Sopori et al., 1998). Several studies have found that smokers had serum immunoglobulin levels (IgA, IgG, and IgM) 10% to 20% lower than those of nonsmokers (Dales et al., 1974; Ferson et al., 1979; Gerrard et al., 1980; Andersen et al., 1982). It has been shown that IgA, IgG, and IgM levels are higher among former smokers than current smokers and increased with duration of smoking cessation (Mili et al., 1991). This suggests that the effect is reversible, with a return toward the immunoglobulin levels of nonsmokers. It has been reported that three months after subjects stopped smoking, IgG and IgM but not IgA levels have increased compared with levels during smoking (Hersey et al., 1983).

Lung parenchyma. The IgG content of bronchial fluids was found to be twice higher in smokers than nonsmokers (Onari et al., 1978; Hersey et al., 1983). A selective increase in immunoglobulin levels could be explained either by stimulation of local immunoglobulin production or by exudation of plasma immunoglobulin into alveolar spaces in response to inhaled cigarette smoke (Warr et al., 1977). The availability of opsonic antimicrobial antibodies is essential for optimal function of phagocytes to take up and contain bacteria (Reynolds, 1988). The antibody response to a variety of antigens, such as influenza virus infection and vaccination is depressed in cigarette smokers (Finklea et al., 1971).

Autoimmunity has been proposed as a cause of smoke-induced lung disease. B cells are abundant in smoke-induced lung disease, and their roles, although obscure, are probably greatly underestimated. Cigarette smoke serves as an adjuvant, possibly because it is a potent inducer of granulocyte/macrophage colony-stimulating factor production in the lungs, which enhances the ability of DCs to present antigen and probably to induce TH_2 type-biased immune responses (Trimble et al, 2009).

3. Smoking and respiratory infections

Given the complex nature of the immune system, in which unaffected defense mechanisms may compensate for local deficiencies, it is difficult to predict how the impact of cigarette smoke on specific host defense pathways affects the overall responses to microbial agents (Domagala-Kulawik, 2008). Specifically, it is unclear whether the increased risk of infection observed in smokers is due to increased susceptibility to microbial agents, an inability to effectively clear infectious agents or exaggerated pro-inflammatory responses to microbial agents (owing to changes in immune homeostasis), thereby evoking symptoms of infection. Similar considerations apply to acute exacerbations of COPD that are due to bacterial and viral infections (Sethi & Murphy, 2001; Wedzicha, 2004; Papi et al., 2006) and to microbial colonization of the airways, which occurs in approximately one third of patients with COPD (Patel et al., 2002).

3.1 Viral infections

Environmental tobacco smoke exposure increases significantly the risk of lower respiratory tract infections in children, especially maternal smoking (Table 1). Using mouse models, it has been investigated the effects of cigarette smoke on inflammatory processes, viral clearance and secondary immune protection following influenza virus infection (Robbins et al., 2006; Gualano et al., 2008; Kang et al., 2008). Cigarette smoke exposure was found to be associated with exacerbated pro-inflammatory responses to influenza virus, although neither the rate of viral clearance nor the development of influenza virus-specific memory responses were compromised. Hence, cigarette smoke mainly affects primary antiviral inflammatory processes, whereas secondary immune protection remains intact (Robbins et al., 2006). The heightened inflammatory response was associated with increased production of pro-inflammatory mediators and mortality. Furthermore, one study (Kang et al., 2008) showed that increased inflammation led to accelerated emphysema formation and airway fibrosis, providing evidence that altered responsiveness to viral agents may contribute to the pathogenesis of emphysema.

Common cold. Several epidemiological studies support the association between smoking and the prevalence of colds and lower respiratory tract symptoms. In a prospective cohort study that examined a large group of US Army recruits found an increased risk of upper respiratory tract infection in smokers (relative risk: 1.5; 95% confidence interval [CI], 1.1-1.8) (Blake et al., 1988). It has been reported that smoking status is predictive of the development of clinical colds when healthy volunteers are exposed intranasally to a low dose of respiratory viruses (Cohen et al., 1993). Viral suspensions were installed into the nares and infections were diagnosed on the basis of viral isolation, virus-specific antibody, and clinical findings. Smokers had a significantly higher incidence of acute infection (clinical cold) than nonsmokers (OR: 2.23; 95% CI, 1.03-4.82). Among virologically confirmed infected individuals, smoking was associated with a higher likelihood of symptoms leading to a clinical diagnosis (OR: 1.83; 95% CI, 1.00-3.36). The relationship between smoking and increased symptoms from viral respiratory infections could be explained by impairment of immune processes that limit viral replication or enhancement of inflammatory processes involved in the production of symptoms.

Influenza. Several studies have confirmed the relationship between cigarette smoking and the risk of influenza infections (Finklea et al., 1969). Influenza infections are more severe, with more cough, acute and chronic phlegm production, breathlessness, and wheezing in smokers. Female smokers in the Israeli Army had increased risk of influenza (OR: 1.44; 95% CI, 1.03-2.01) and complications associated to influenza infection compared with nonsmokers (Kark & Lebiush, 1981). In another study, the incidence of influenza in healthy young male recruits was higher among smokers (OR: 2.42; 95% CI, 1.53-3.83) (Kark et al., 1982). Influenza was more severe among smokers, with a dose-related increase in rate: 30% in nonsmokers, 43% in light smokers, and 54% in heavy smokers ($p<0.001$). Overall, 31.2% (95% CI, 16.5-43.1) of influenza cases were attributed to cigarette smoking.

Enhanced bacterial adherence has been documented for respiratory cells infected, with influenza A virus being responsible for viral-bacterial combination pneumonia (Hament et al., 1999). Studies have suggested that inflammatory activation of platelet-activating factor is an important factor in the attachment and invasion of cells by pneumococcal strains. Cigarette smoking alters platelet-activating factor metabolism and may contribute to the increased incidence of bacterial superinfection in people who develop influenza (Miyaura et al., 1992; Ichimaru & Tai, 1992).

Study	Design/Population	Sample size	Outcome
1) Jedrychowski & Flak.	Cohort study in children from Poland.	1,129	Maternal smoking during pregnancy and postnatal exposure to ETS increase risk of acute respiratory infections.
2) Li et al.	Meta-analysis study including 13 studies.		ETS exposure increases risk of serious LRTI at early life.
3) Gürkan et al.	Case control study in children from Turkey.	58	ETS exposure increases risk of respiratory syncytial virus bronchiolitis.
4) Boyce et al.	Retrospective cohort study in children from USA.	248,652	Increase risk for RSV brochiolitis hospitalization at first year of life.
5) Pardo Crespo et al.	Case-reference study in children from Spain.	885	Maternal smoking increase the risk of hospitalization for LRTI.
6) Albernaz et al.	Nested case-control study in infants from Brazil.	5,304	Maternal smoking increase the risk of hospitalization for bronchiolitis.
7) Nielsen et al.	Retrospective case-control study in infants from Denmark.	1,252	Maternal smoking during pregnancy increase the risk of hospitalization for RSV infection.
8) Zlotkwaska & Zedja.	Cross sectional study in children from Poland.	1,561	ETS exposure increases risk of bronchitis, wheeze and attacks of dyspnoea.
9) Pattenden et al.	Cross sectional study in children from Austria.	53,879	Parental smoking increase wheeze, asthma, bronchitis and nocturnal cough.
10) Baker et al.	Cohort study in children from Czech Republic.	452	ETS exposure increases incidence of LRTI.
11) Keskinoglu et al.	Case control study in children from Turkey.	300	ETS exposure increases incidence of LRTI.
12) Chatzimicael et al.	Cross sectional study from Greece.	586	ETS exposure increases risk of upper and lower respiratory tract infections.
13) Fríguls et al.	Cohort study in children from England and Spain.	1,611	Prenatal and post natal tobacco exposure increase risk of upper and lower respiratory tract infections.

References: 1) *Environ Health Prospect* 1997;105:302-6; 2) *Pediatr Pulmonol* 1999;27:5-13.; 3) *Eur J Epidemiol* 2000;16:465-8; 4) *J Pediatr* 2000;137:865-70; 5) *An Esp Pediatr* 2000;53:339-45; 6) *Rev Saude Publica* 2003;37:485-93; 7) *Acta Paediatr* 2003;92:1314-21; 8) *Eur J Epidemiol* 2005;20:719-27; 9) *Tob Control* 2006;15:294-301; 10) *Environ Health Perspect* 2006;114:1126-32; 11) *Eur J Pediatr* 2007;166:455-9; 12) *Indian J Pediatr* 2008;75:335-40; 13) *Arch Bronconeumol* 2009;45:585-90.

Table 1. The environmental tobacco smoke (ETS) exposure increases the risk of lower respiratory tract infections (LRTI) in children.

Although influenza was more severe in smokers, antibody levels to A(H1N1) antigen were not significantly higher than those of nonsmokers. Moreover, influenza antibodies wane more rapidly in smokers than in nonsmokers (Finklea et al., 1971). This finding suggests that smokers are not only at a high risk of influenza, but have an increased susceptibility to new attacks afterward (Kark et al., 1982). Influenza rates are similar in vaccinated smokers and nonsmokers. However, influenza vaccination can be considered to be more efficacious in smokers than nonsmokers because the infection rates are higher in unvaccinated smokers (Cruijff et al., 1999).

Respiratory syncytial virus bronchiolitis. Respiratory syncytial virus (RSV) infection is very common in early life; over 95% of children have been infected by two years of age. RSV infections are responsible for over 100,000 hospital admissions in the United States annually, mostly affecting infants (Moler & Ohmit, 1999). Of RSV-related admissions, 7% to 21% will require ventilatory support because of respiratory insufficiency (Everard & Milner, 1992). Therefore, RSV infection imposes a significant burden on children early in life. Maternal smoking exposure has been shown to reduce lung function in children, and several studies suggest that this effect on lung function is attributable primarily to exposure during pregnancy (intrauterine cigarette smoke exposure) (Hofhuis et al., 2003). Maternal smoking during pregnancy may impair in utero airway development or alter lung elastic properties. It has been shown that maternal cigarette smoking, especially postnatal, increase the severity of RSV bronchiolitis infection in infants (Gürkan et al., 2000; Lanari et al., 2002; Bradley et al., 2005). As a preventive measure, it has been reported a protective effect of long-term breastfeeding on the risk of lower respiratory tract infection during the first year of life, especially in children exposed to environmental tobacco smoke (Nafstad et al., 1996).

Passive smoking and respiratory tract infections in childhood. A study in 1974 reported that infants of mothers who smoked had significantly more admissions for bronchitis or pneumonia than infants of non-smoking mothers (Harlap & Davies, 1974). The excess bronchitis and pneumonia increased with increased number of cigarettes smoked by the mother. This excess was mainly seen in infants aged 6 to 9 months. Another study (Colley et al., 1974), also found that the incidence of pneumonia and bronchitis in the first year of life was associated with parents' smoking habits; the incidence was lowest where both parents were non-smokers, highest where both smoked, and lay between these two levels where only one parent smoked. During the following three decades, a large number of investigations have reported associations between parental smoking and occurrence of lower respiratory tract illness in young children (Table 1). A systematic review (Strachan & Cook, 1997) of around 50 studies in children up to 3 years, including 38 studies used for quantitative analysis, has confirmed these findings. There was consistency in the findings between the community and hospital studies. Pooled ratios were found to be 1.57 for smoking by either parent and 1.72 for maternal smoking. The reviewers also found that there was a significantly increased risk from smoking by other household members in families where the mother did not smoke (odds ratio 1.29). In most of the studies also a dose-response relationship was evident, and the associations with paternal smoking were still present after adjustment for confounding factors. From earlier studies, it appeared that the risk was higher during the first 6 months of life, and gradually decreased to slightly above normal by age 3 years. However, later studies (Taylor & Wadsworth, 1987) have found similar relationships between maternal smoking and lower respiratory illness in children up to 5 years of age. Exposure to passive smoking also seems to increase the risk for acute respiratory tract infections in older children (Jedrychowski & Flak, 1997). A dose-response between the degree of exposure to environmental tobacco smoke and acute respiratory infection was found in a cohort of 9-year-old children. Passive smoking combined with allergy nearly tripled the risk of acute respiratory tract infections (odds ratio 3.39).

3.2 Bacterial infections

Similarly, cigarette smoke exposure was also found to be associated with increased inflammation following challenge with bacterial agents such as *Pseudomonas aeruginosa* and non-typeable *H. influenzae* (Drannik et al., 2004; Gaschler et al., 2009), two pathogens that are associated with COPD exacerbations. Cigarette smoke was associated with increased bacterial burden in mice infected with *P. aeruginosa*, whereas bacterial burden was decreased in smoke-exposed animals following infection with non-typeable *H. influenzae*. Changes in the bactericidal activity of alveolar macrophages may contribute to increased bacterial burden (Drannik et al., 2004), but it is unclear how infection with non-typeable *H. influenzae* induces decreased bacterial levels; the mechanisms of this are currently being investigated. Preliminary data suggest that increased levels of immunoglobulins in the bronchoalveolar lavage of smoke-exposed animals might have contributed to this phenomenon. This finding provides evidence that compensatory mechanisms may outweigh certain deficiencies and help to explain why not all smokers suffer from severe chest infections. As discussed above, smoke affects all people who are exposed to it, but the degree and severity is modified by many susceptibility determinants.

Pneumococcal pneumonia. Cigarette smoking is a substantial risk factor for pneumococcal pneumonia, especially in patients with chronic obstructive pulmonary disease. However, even without chronic obstructive pulmonary disease, smoking is a major risk factor. In a population based surveillance study (Pastor et al., 1995), smoking was strongly associated with invasive pneumococcal disease in healthy young and middle aged adults, for whom pneumococcal vaccination is not currently recommended. Among such individuals with invasive pneumococcal disease, 47% were current smokers. The odds ratio (OR) for invasive pneumococcal disease was 2.6 (95% CI, 1.9-3.5) for smokers in the 24-to 64-year age group and 2.2 (95% CI, 1.4-3.4) for smokers 65 years or older. The attributable risk from smoking was 31% and 13% in these 2 groups, respectively.

A population based case-control study (Nuorti et al., 2000) showed that smoking was the strongest independent risk factor for invasive pneumococcal disease among immunocompetent adults. The OR was 4.1 (95% CI, 2.4-7.3) for active smoking and 2.5 (95% CI, 1.2-5.1) for passive smoke exposure in nonsmokers compared with nonexposed nonsmokers. The attributable risk in this population was 51% for cigarette smoking and 17% for passive smoking. The risk of pneumococcal disease declined to nonsmoker levels 10 years after cessation. In another case-control study, current smoking was associated with a nearly 2-fold risk of community-acquired pneumonia (OR: 1.88; 95% CI, 1.11-3.19), where 32% of the risk was attributable to cigarette smoking (Almirall et al, 1999). There was a trend toward a dose-response relationship: A 50% reduction in the OR was reported 5 years after cessation of smoking.

In vitro adherence of *Streptococcus pneumoniae* to buccal epithelial cells has been shown to be increased in cigarette smokers (Raman et al., 1983). This increased adherence may persist for up to three years after smoking cessation. Since increased adherence of bacteria to surface cells is an established pathogenic step for bacterial colonization and infection in the lung, this may contribute to the increased risk of respiratory infection that exists in cigarette smokers.

Legionnaires disease. Legionnaires disease is a life-threatening lower respiratory tract infection responsible for 1% to 3% of community-acquired pneumonia. Diverse environmental factors have been identified, and cigarette smoking appears to be an independent risk factor (Doebbeling & Wenzel, 1987; Straus et al., 1996). The risk of legionnaires disease was significantly increased for smoking (OR: 3.48; 95% CI, 2.09-5.79), specially for persons without an underlying disease (OR: 7.49; 95% CI, 3.2-17.1) (Straus et al., 1996).

Otitis media and exposure to secondhand tobacco smoke. Long term tobacco smoke exposure is a risk factor for otitis media and bronchitis in children (Richardson, 1988). In a case-control study, children with recurrent otitis media more commonly had exposure to secondhand smoke (OR: 1.88; 95% CI, 1.02-3.49; p=0.04). A prospective follow-up of the case group showed no significant difference in the clinical course of the children who were exposed to secondhand smoke (Kitchens, 1995). In other study, passive smoking was a significant risk factor for otitis media with effusion and recurrent otitis media (Ilicali et al, 1999). But only maternal smoking was a significant factor ($p<0.001$). Moreover, in utero exposure to cigarette smoke was associated with an increased risk of otitis media. In a study (Stathis et al, 1999), acute ear infections were associated with the mother's consumption of 1 to 9 cigarettes (OR: 1.6; 95% CI, 1.1-2.5), 10 to 19 cigarettes (OR: 2.6, 95% CI, 1.6-4.2), and 20 or more cigarettes (OR: 3.3; 95% CI, 1.9-5.9) per day during pregnancy. For subacute ear infections, an association was present with the mother's consumption of 10 to 19 cigarettes (OR: 2.6; 95% CI, 1.4-5.0) and 20 or more cigarettes (OR: 2.8; 95% CI, 1.3-6.0). In utero exposure to 20 or more cigarettes per day was also associated with an increased risk of ear surgery by 5 years after delivery (OR: 2.9; 95% CI, 1.3-6.6).

Tuberculosis. Developing tuberculosis disease involves two distinct transitions, with their corresponding risk factors: the transition from being exposed to being infected and the transition from being infected to developing disease. Several studies have shown that smoking is a risk factor for tuberculin skin test reactivity, skin test conversion, and the development of active tuberculosis (Table 2). It has been reported an increased relative risk of development of tuberculosis for heavy smokers compared with nonsmokers (RR: 2.17; 95%CI, 1.29-3.63) (Yu et al., 1988). After adjusting for age and heavy drinking, smokers of 20 years' or greater duration had 2.6 times (95% CI, 1.1-5.9) the risk of nonsmokers for tuberculosis (Buskin et al., 1994). It has been found a strong association between active smoking and the risk of pulmonary tuberculosis (Alcaide et al., 1996). Both studies showed a dose-response relationship with the number of cigarettes consumed daily. In other study, current smokers had a nearly 2-fold increased risk compared with never-smokers (OR: 1.87; 95% CI, 0.73-4.80) (McCurdy et al., 1997).

A large case-control study in India examined smoking and tuberculosis in men between 35 and 69 years of age (Gajalakshmi et al., 2003). The tuberculosis prevalence risk ratio was 2.9 (95% CI, 2.6-3.3) for ever-smokers compared with never-smokers, and the prevalence was higher with a higher level of cigarette consumption. The authors found that the smoking attributable fraction of deaths from tuberculosis was 61%, greater than the fraction of smoking-attributable deaths from vascular disease or cancer. In a study among children living with a patient with active pulmonary tuberculosis, passive smoking confirmed by measurement of urinary cotinine levels was a strong risk factor for the development of active tuberculosis (OR: 5.39; 95% CI, 2.44-11.91) (Altet et al., 1996).

Study	Design/Population	Outcome
1) Yu GP et al.	Cross sectional study of risk factors associated to pulmonary TB diagnosis in adults, China.	RR of pulmonary TB for heavy smokers: 2.2 (95%CI 1.3-3.6).
2) Buskin SE et al.	Case-control study of risk factors for diagnosis of active TB among adults, USA.	OR for smokers ≥30 years: 2.6 (95%CI 1.1-5.9).
3) Alcaide J et al.	Case-control study investigating the impact of active and passive smoking on risk of developing active TB among infected young adults, Barcelona, Spain.	OR for young adults exposed to smoke: Active smoking: 3.6 (95%CI 1.4-9.2). Active and passive smoking: 5.1 (95%CI 1.9-13.2). Dose response: 1-20 cig/day: 3.0 (p<0.05). > 20 cig/day: 13.0 (p<0.001).
4) Altet MN et al.	Case-control study investigating the impact of passive smoking on risk of developing active TB among infected children, Barcelona, Spain.	OR for those exposed to passive smoke: 5.4 (95%CI 2.4-11.9). Dose response: 1-20 cig/day : 1.6 (95%CI 0.7-2.6). 21-40 cig/day: 4.0 (95%CI 1.5-9.8). > 40 cig/day: 7.8 (95%CI 3.4-17.6).
5) Tocque K et al.	Case-control study that investigates the impact of smoking on risk of pulmonary TB, Liverpool, England.	OR for smokers ≥ 30 years: 2.3 (95%CI 1.2-4.2).
6) Kolappan C & Gopi P.	Case-control study investigating the impact of smoking on diagnosis with pulmonary TB among men, India.	OR for smokers: 2.2 (95%CI 1.3-3.9) Dose response based on quantity and years smoked compared to non-smokers (p<0.0001).
7) Tekkel M et al.	Case-control study that investigates the risk factors for new diagnosis of pulmonary TB among individuals over age 15, Estonia.	OR of pulmonary TB diagnosis for smokers: Current smoker: 4.6 (95%CI 2.4-8.7) Former smoker: 2.3 (95%CI 1.0-5.1)
8) Leung CC et al.	Cross-sectional study to assess the impact of smoking on epidemiology and characteristics of TB, Hong Kong.	OR of developing TB among ever-smoker: 2.4 (95%CI 1.7-3.4).
9) Miguez-Burbano et al.	Case-control study that investigates the impact of long-term smoking on development of TB in HIV-1 infected patients, Miami, USA.	RR for long-term smokers (≥20 y): 3.0 (p=0.04).
10) Ariyothai N et al.	Case-control study investigating the impact of smoking (active and passive) on risk of pulmonary TB in HIV-negative individuals over age 15, Thailand.	OR for those exposed to tobacco smoke: Current active smokers: 2.7 (95%CI 1.0-7.0) Ever-active, >10 years 3.0 (95%CI 1.1-8.2) Ever-active, >10 cig/day: 4.0 (95%CI 1.3-12.6)
11) Crampin A et al.	Case-control study to examine risk factors for diagnosis with tuberculosis in individuals at least 15 years old, Malawi.	OR for smokers compared to never smokers: Ex-smokers: 1.6 (95%CI 0.7-3.2) < 5 cig/day: 0.9 (95%CI 0.5-1.7) ≥ 5 cig/day: 1.3 (95%CI 0.7-2.4)
12) Leung CC et al.	Prospective study of adults ≥65 years old to investigate the relationship between smoking and TB, Hong Kong.	Hazard ratios compared to never-smokers: Active tuberculosis: Current smoker: 2.6 (95%CI 1.9-3.7) Ex-smoker: 1.4 (95%CI 1.0-2.0)
13) Lienhardt C et al.	Case-control study to investigate host and environmental factors potentially associated with risk of developing smear-positive pulmonary tuberculosis in individuals >15 years, West Africa.	OR for smokers compared to never-smokers: Past smokers: 2.4 (95%CI 1.5-3.8) Current smokers: 3.1 (95%CI 2.4-4.2)
14) Tipayamongkholgul M et al.	Case-control study to examine risk factors associated with TB in BCG immunized children, Bangkok, Thailand.	Passive exposure to tobacco smoke was significantly associated with TB: OR: 9.31 (95%CI 3.14-27.58)

References: 1) *Tubercle* 1988;69:105-12 ; 2) *Am J Pub Health* 1994;84:1750-6; 3) *Tuber Lung Dis* 1996; 77:112-6; 4) *Tuber Lung Dis* 1996;77:537-44; 5) *Eur Respir J* 2001;18:959-64; 6) *Thorax* 2002;57:964-6; 7) *Int J Tuberc Lung Dis* 2002;6:887-94; 8) *Int J Tuberc Lung Dis* 2003;7:980-6; 9) *Addict Biol* 2003;8:39-43; 10) *Southeast Asian J Trop Med Public Health* 2004;35:219-27; 11) *Int J Tuberc Lung Dis* 2004;8:194-203; 12) *Am J Respir Crit Care Med* 2004;170:1027-33; 13) *Int J Epidemiol* 2005;34:914-23; 14) *Southeast Asian J Trop Med Public Health* 2005;36:145-50.

Table 2. Tobacco smoking and active tuberculosis (TB).

The biological basis by which tobacco smoking increases tuberculosis risk may be through a decrease in immune response, mechanical disruption of cilia function, defects in macrophage immune responses, and/or CD4+ lymphopenia, increasing the susceptibility to pulmonary tuberculosis (Rich & Ellner, 1994; Onwubalili et al., 1987).

4. Conclusion

Smoking appears to be an important risk factor for the acquisition of a lower respiratory tract infection (bronchitis, influenza, pneumonia, tuberculosis). This link is likely mediated by smoking's adverse effects on respiratory defenses (structural and immune system changes induced by smoking). Considering the high rates of morbidity and mortality from pneumonia, tuberculosis and influenza, as well as the economic consequences of work days lost from lesser respiratory infections, the merits of smoking cessation are clear. The fact that smokers have been shown to be less likely than nonsmokers to undergo vaccination and yet are probably at higher risk for influenza and pneumococcal infections highlights the importance of targeting this group for vaccination. The available epidemiological evidence, from studies worldwide, indicates a dose-response relationship between smoking and tuberculosis and that the association is likely to be a causal one. This provides a compelling reason for smoking cessation measures to be undertaken to combat the scourge of tuberculosis, particularly in developing countries. Physicians should educate their smoking patients about their increased risk of respiratory infections, the importance of appropriate vaccinations, and the benefits of smoking cessation.

5. References

Alcaide J, Altet MN, Plans P, Parrón I, Folguera L, Saltó E, et al. Cigarette smoking as a risk factor for tuberculosis in young adults: a case-control study. *Tuber Lung Dis* 1996;77:112-6.

Almirall J, González CA, Balanzó X, Bolíbar I. Proportion of community-acquired pneumonia cases attributable to tobacco smoking. *Chest* 1999;116:375-9.

Altet MN, Alcaide J, Plans P, Taberner JL, Saltó E, Folguera LI, et al. Passive smoking and risk of pulmonary tuberculosis in children immediately following infection. A case-control study. *Tuber Lung Dis* 1996;77:537-44.

Andersen P, Pedersen OF, Bach B, Bonde GJ. Serum antibodies and immunoglobulins in smokers and nonsmokers. *Clin Exp Immunol* 1982;47:467-73.

Bauer CM, Dewitte-Orr SJ, Hornby KR, Zavitz CC, Lichty BD, Stämpfli MR, et al. Cigarette smoke suppresses type I interferon-mediated antiviral immunity in lung fibroblast and epithelial cells. *J Interferon Cytokine Res* 2008;28:167-9.

Becker CE, O'Neill LA. Inflammasomes in inflammatory disorders: the role of TLRs and their interactions with NLRs. *Semin Immunopathol* 2007;29:239-48.

Berenson CS, Garlipp MA, Grove LJ, Maloney J, Sethi S. Impaired phagocytosis of nontypeable *Haemophilus influenzae* by human alveolar macrophages in chronic obstructive pulmonary disease. *J Infect Dis* 2006;194:1375-84.

Black JH 3rd. Evidence base and strategies for successful smoking cessation. *J Vasc Surg* 2010;51:1529-37.

Blake GH, Abell TD, Stanley WG. Cigarette smoking and upper respiratory infection among recruits in basic combat training. *Ann Intern Med* 1988;109:198-202.

Bradley JP, Bacharier LB, Bonfiglio J, Schechtman KB, Strunk R, Storch G, et al. Severity of respiratory syncytial virus bronchiolitis is affected by cigarette smoke exposure and atopy. *Pediatrics* 2005;115:e7-14.

Bridges RB, Kraal JH, Huang LJ, Chancellor BM. Effects of tobacco smoke on chemotaxis and glucose metabolism of polymorphonuclear leukocytes. *Infect Immun* 1977;15:115-23.

Bridges RB, Hsieh L. Effects of cigarette smoke fractions on the chemotaxis of polymorphonuclear leukocytes. *J Leukoc Biol* 1986;40:73-85.

Burns AR, Hosford SP, Dunn LA, Walker DC, Hogg JC. Respiratory epithelial permeability after cigarette smoke exposure in guinea pigs. *J Appl Physiol* 1989;66: 2109-16.

Buskin SE, Gale JL, Weiss NS, Nolan CM. Tuberculosis risk factors in adults in King County, Washington, 1988 through 1990. *Am J Public Health* 1994; 84:1750-6.

Chen H, Cowan MJ, Hasday JD, Vogel SN, Medvedev AE. Tobacco smoking inhibits expression of proinflammatory cytokines and activation of IL-1R-associated kinase, p38, and NF-κB in alveolar macrophages stimulated with TLR2 and TLR4 agonists. *J Immunol* 2007;179:6097-106.

Cheraghi M, Salvi S. Environmental tobacco smoke (ETS) and respiratory health in children. *Eur J Pediatr* 2009;168:897-905.

Cohen S, Tyrrell DA, Russell MA, Jarvis MJ, Smith AP. Smoking, alcohol consumption, and susceptibility to the common cold. *Am J Public Health* 1993;83: 1277-83.

Colley JR, Holland WW, Corkhill RT. Influence of passive smoking and parental phlegm on pneumonia and bronchitis in early childhood. *Lancet* 1974;2:1031-4.

Corberand J, Nguyen F, Do AH, Dutau G, Laharrague P, Fontanilles AM, et al. Effect of tobacco smoking on the functions of polymorphonuclear leukocytes. *Infect Immun* 1979;23:577-81.

Costabel U, Bross KJ, Reuter C, Rühle KH, Matthys H. Alterations in immunoregulatory T-cell subsets in cigarette smokers. A phenotypic analysis of bronchoalveolar and blood lymphocytes. *Chest* 1986;90:39-44.

Cruijff M, Thijs C, Govaert T, Aretz K, Dinant GJ, Knottnerus A. The effect of smoking on influenza, influenza vaccination efficacy and on the antibody response to influenza vaccination. *Vaccine* 1999;17:426-32.

Dales LG, Friedman GD, Siegelaub AB, Seltzer CC. Cigarette smoking and serum chemistry tests. *J Chronic Dis* 1974;27:293-307.

de Boer WI, Sont JK, van Schadewijk A, Stolk J, van Krieken JH, Hiemstra PS. Monocyte chemoattractant protein 1, interleukin 8, and chronic airways inflammation in COPD. *J Pathol* 2000;190:619-26.

Doebbeling BN, Wenzel RP. The epidemiology of *Legionella pneumophila* infections. *Semin Respir Infect* 1987;2:206-21.

Domagala-Kulawik J. Effects of cigarette smoke on the lung and systemic immunity. *J Physiol Pharmacol* 2008;59(Suppl 6):19-34.

Drannik AG, Pouladi MA, Robbins CS, Goncharova SI, Kianpour S, Stämpfli MR. Impact of cigarette smoke on clearance and inflammation after *Pseudomonas aeruginosa* infection. *Am J Respir Crit Care Med* 2004;170:1164-71.

Dye JA, Adler KB. Effects of cigarette smoke on epithelial cells of the respiratory tract. *Thorax* 1994;49:825-34.

Eichel B, Shahrik HA. Tobacco smoke toxicity: loss of human oral leukocyte function and fluid-cell metabolism. *Science* 1969;166:1424-8.

Everard ML, Milner AD. The respiratory syncytial virus and its role in acute bronchiolitis. *Eur J Pediatr* 1992;151:638-51.

Ferson M, Edwards A, Lind A, Milton GW, Hersey P. Low natural killer–cell activity and immunoglobulin levels associated with smoking in human subjects. *Int J Cancer* 1979;23:603-9.

Finklea JF, Sandifer SH, Smith DD. Cigarette smoking and epidemic influenza. *Am J Epidemiol* 1969;90:390-9.

Finklea JF, Hasselblad V, Riggan WB, Nelson WC, Hammer DI, Newill VA. Cigarette smoking and hemagglutination inhibition response to influenza after natural disease and immunization. *Am Rev Respir Dis* 1971;104:368-76.

Friedman GD, Siegelaub AB, Seltzer CC, Feldman R, Collen MF. Smoking habits and the leukocyte count. *Arch Environ Health* 1973;26:137-43.

Gajalakshmi V, Peto R, Kanaka TS, Jha P. Smoking and mortality from tuberculosis and other diseases in India: retrospective study of 43000 adult male deaths and 35000 controls. *Lancet* 2003;362:507-15.

Gaschler GJ, Zavitz CC, Bauer CM, Skrtic M, Lindahl M, Robbins CS, et al. Cigarette smoke exposure attenuates cytokine production by mouse alveolar macrophages. *Am J Respir Cell Mol Biol* 2008;38:218-26.

Gaschler GJ, Skrtic M, Zavitz CC, Lindahl M, Onnervik PO, Murphy TF, et al. Bacteria challenge in smoke-exposed mice exacerbates inflammation and skews the inflammatory profile. *Am J Respir Crit Care Med* 2009;179:666-75.

Geng Y, Savage SM, Johnson LJ, Seagrave J, Sopori ML. Effects of nicotine on the immune response. I. Chronic exposure to nicotine impairs antigen receptor-mediated signal transduction in lymphocytes. *Toxicol Appl Pharmacol* 1995;135: 268-78.

Geng Y, Savage SM, Razani-Boroujerdi S, Sopori ML. Effects of nicotine on the immune response. II. Chronic nicotine treatment induces T cell anergy. *J Immunol* 1996;156:2384-90.

Gerrard JW, Heiner DC, Ko CG, Mink J, Meyers A, Dosman JA. Immunoglobulin levels in smokers and non-smokers. *Ann Allergy* 1980;44:261-2.

Ginns LC, Goldenheim PD, Miller LG, Burton RC, Gillick L, Colvin RB, et al. T-lymphocyte subsets in smoking and lung cancer: Analysis of monoclonal antibodies and flow cytometry. *Am Rev Respir Dis* 1982;126:265-9.

Grumelli S, Corry DB, Song LZ, Song L, Green L, Huh J, et al. An immune basis for lung parenchymal destruction in chronic obstructive pulmonary disease and emphysema. *PLoS Med* 2004;1(1):e8.

Gualano R, Hansen MJ, Vlahos R, Jones JE, Park-Jones RA, Deliyannis G, et al. Cigarette smoke worsens lung inflammation and impairs resolution of influenza infection in mice. *Respir Res* 2008;9:53.

Gürkan F, Kiral A, Dağli E, Karakoç F. The effect of passive smoking on the development of respiratory syncytial virus bronchiolitis. *Eur J Epidemiol* 2000;16:465-8.

Hagiwara E, Takahashi KI, Okubo T, Ohno S, Ueda A, Aoki A, et al. Cigarette smoking depletes cells spontaneously secreting Th(1) cytokines in the human airway. *Cytokine* 2001;14: 121-6.

Hament J, Kimpen JL, Fleer A, Wolfs TF. Respiratory viral infection predisposing for bacterial disease: a concise review. *FEMS Immunol Med Microbiol* 1999;26: 189-95.

Hamerman JA, Ogasawara K, Lanier LL. NK cells in innate immunity. *Curr Opin Immunol* 2005;17:29-35.

Harlap S, Davies AM. Infant admissions to hospital and maternal smoking. *Lancet* 1974;1:529-32.

Hautamaki RD, Kobayashi DK, Senior RM, Shapiro SD. Requirement for macrophage elastase for cigarette smoke-induced emphysema in mice. *Science* 1997;277:2002-4.

Herberman RB, Holden HT. Natural cell-mediated immunity. *Adv Cancer Res* 1978;27:305-77.

Herberman RB. *Natural Cell–Mediated Immunity Against Tumors*. New York, NY: Academic Press; 1980.

Hersey P, Prendergast D, Edwards A. Effects of cigarette smoking on the immune system. Follow-up studies in normal subjects after cessation of smoking. *Med J Aust* 1983;2:425-9.

Hodge S, Hodge G, Ahern J, Jersmann H, Holmes M, Reynolds PN. Smoking alters alveolar macrophage recognition and phagocytic ability: implications in chronic obstructive pulmonary disease. *Am J Respir Cell Mol Biol* 2007;37:748-55.

Hofhuis W, De Jongste JC, Merkus PJ. Adverse health effects of prenatal and postnatal tobacco smoke exposure on children. *Arch Dis Child* 2003;88:1086-90.

Holt PG. Immune and inflammatory function in cigarette smokers. *Thorax* 1987;42: 241-9.

Hughes DA, Haslam PL, Townsend PJ, Turner-Warwick M. Numerical and functional alterations in circulatory lymphocytes in cigarette smokers. *Clin Exp Immunol* 1985;61:459-66.

Ichimaru T, Tai HH. Alteration of platelet activating factor (PAF) metabolism in rat pulmonary alveolar macrophages and plasma by cigarette smoking. *Prostaglandins Leukot Essent Fatty Acids* 1992;47:123-8.

Ilicali OC, Keleş N, Değer K, Savaş I. Relationship of passive cigarette smoking to otitis media. *Arch Otolaryngol Head Neck Surg* 1999;125:758-62.

Jahnsen FL, Strickland DH, Thomas JA, Tobagus IT, Napoli S, Zosky GR, et al. Accelerated antigen sampling and transport by airway mucosal dendritic cells following inhalation of a bacterial stimulus. *J Immunol* 2006;177:5861-7.

Jedrychowski W, Flak E. Maternal smoking during pregnancy and postnatal exposure to environmental tobacco smoke as predisposition factors to acute respiratory infections. *Environ Health Perspect* 1997;105:302-6.

Jha P, Ranson MK, Nguyen SN, Yach D. Estimates of global and regional smoking prevalence in 1995, by age and sex. *Am J Public Health* 2002;92:1002-6.

Jones JG, Minty BD, Lawler P, Hulands G, Crawley JC, Veall N. Increased alveolar epithelial permeability in cigarette smokers. *Lancet* 1980;1:66-8.

Kalra R, Singh SP, Savage SM, Finch GL, Sopori ML. Effects of cigarette smoke on immune response: chronic exposure to cigarette smoke impairs antigen-mediated signaling in T cells and depletes IP3-sensitive Ca(2+) stores. *J Pharmacol Exp Ther* 2000;293:166-71.

Kang MJ, Lee CG, Lee JY, De la Cruz CS, Chen ZJ, Enelow R, Elias JA. Cigarette smoke selectively enhances viral PAMP- and virus-induced pulmonary innate immune and remodeling responses in mice. *J Clin Invest* 2008;118:2771-84.

Kark JD, Lebiush M. Smoking and epidemic influenza-like illness in female military recruits: a brief survey. *Am J Public Health* 1981;71: 530-2.

Kark JD, Lebiush M, Rannon L. Cigarette smoking as a risk factor for epidemic A(H1N1) influenza in young men. *N Engl J Med* 1982;307:1042-6.

Kim H, Liu X, Kobayashi T, Conner H, Kohyama T, Wen FQ, et al. Reversible cigarette smoke extract-induced DNA damage in human lung fibroblasts. *Am J Respir Cell Mol Biol* 2004;31:483-90.

King TE Jr, Savici D, Campbell PA. Phagocytosis and killing of *Listeria monocytogenes* by alveolar macrophages: smokers versus nonsmokers. *J Infect Dis* 1988;158:1309-16.

Kitchens GG. Relationship of environmental tobacco smoke to otitis media in young children. *Laryngoscope* 1995;105:1-13.

Knutson D, Braun C. Diagnosis and management of acute bronchitis. *Am Fam Physician* 2002;65:2039-44.

Kuper H, Adami HO, Boffetta P. Tobacco use, cancer causation and public health impact. *J InternMed* 2002;251:455-66.

Laan M, Bozinovski S, Anderson GP. Cigarette smoke inhibits lipopolysaccharide-induced production of inflammatory cytokines by suppressing the activation of activator protein-1 in bronchial epithelial cells. *J Immunol* 2004;173:4164-70.

Lanari M, Giovannini M, Giuffré L, Marini A, Rondini G, Rossi GA, et al. Prevalence of respiratory syncytial virus infection in Italian infants hospitalized for acute lower respiratory tract infections, and association between respiratory syncytial virus infection risk factors and disease severity. *Pediatr Pulmonol* 2002;33:458-65.

Leatherman JW, Michael AF, Schwartz BA, Hoidal JR. Lung T cells in hypersensitivity pneumonitis. *Ann Intern Med* 1984;100:390-2.

Lu L, Lind EF, Gondek DC, Bennett KA, Gleeson MW, Pino-Lagos K, et al. Mast cells are essential intermediaries in regulatory T-cell tolerance. *Nature* 2006;442: 997-1002.

Luster MI, Simeonova PP, Gallucci R, Matheson J. Tumor necrosis factor alpha and toxicology. *Crit Rev Toxicol* 1999;29:491-511.

Lynch JP 3rd, Zhanel GG. *Streptococcus pneumoniae*: epidemiology and risk factors, evolution of antimicrobial resistance, and impact of vaccines. *Curr Opin Pulm Med* 2010;16:217-25.

Macfarlane J, Holmes W, Gard P, Macfarlane R, Rose D, Weston V, et al. Prospective study of the incidence, aetiology and outcome of adult lower respiratory tract illness in the community. *Thorax*. 2001;56:109-14.

Maeno T, Houghton AM, Quintero PA, Grumelli S, Owen CA, Shapiro SD. CD8+ T cells are required for inflammation and destruction in cigarette smoke-induced emphysema in mice. *J Immunol* 2007;178:8090-6.

Marcy TW, Merrill WW. Cigarette smoking and respiratory tract infection. *Clin Chest Med* 1987;8:381-91.

Marrie TJ. Acute bronchitis and community acquired pneumonia. In: Fishman AP, Elias JA, eds. *Fishman's Pulmonary diseases and disorders*. 3rd ed. New York: McGraw-Hill, 1998:1985-95.

McComb JG, Ranganathan M, Liu XH, Pilewski JM, Ray P, Watkins SC, et al. CX3CL1 up-regulation is associated with recruitment of CX3CR1+ mononuclear phagocytes and T lymphocytes in the lungs during cigarette smoke-induced emphysema. *Am J Pathol* 2008;173:949-61.

McCrea KA, Ensor JE, Nall K, Bleecker ER, Hasday JD. Altered cytokine regulation in the lungs of cigarette smokers. *Am J Respir Crit Care Med* 1994;150: 696-703.

McCurdy SA, Arretz DS, Bates RO. Tuberculin reactivity among California Hispanic migrant farm workers. *Am J Ind Med* 1997;32:600-5.

Mellman I, Steinman RM. Dendritic cells: specialized and regulated antigen processing machines. *Cell* 2001;106:255-8.

Mian MF, Lauzon NM, Stämpfli MR, Mossman KL, Ashkar AA. Impairment of human NK cell cytotoxic activity and cytokine release by cigarette smoke. *J Leukoc Biol* 2008;83:774-84.

Mili F, Flanders WD, Boring JR, Annest JL, Destefano F. The associations of race, cigarette smoking, and smoking cessation to measures of the immune system in middle-aged men. *Clin Immunol Immunopathol* 1991;59:187-200.

Miller LG, Goldstein G, Murphy M, Ginns LC. Reversible alterations in immunoregulatory T cells in smoking. Analysis by monoclonal antibodies and flow cytometry. *Chest* 1982;82:526-9.

Mio T, Romberger DJ, Thompson AB, Robbins RA, Heires A, Rennard SI. Cigarette smoke induces interleukin-8 release from human bronchial epithelial cells. *Am J Respir Crit Care Med* 1997;155:1770-6.

Miyaura S, Eguchi H, Johnston JM. Effect of a cigarette smoke extract on the metabolism of the proinflammatory autacoid, platelet-activating factor. *Circ Res* 1992;70:341-7.

Moler FW, Ohmit SE. Severity of illness models for respiratory syncytial virus-associated hospitalization. *Am J Respir Crit Care Med* 1999;159:1234-40.

Nafstad P, Jaakkola JJ, Hagen JA, Botten G, Kongerud J. Breastfeeding, maternal smoking and lower respiratory tract infections. *Eur Respir J* 1996;9:2623-9.

Nair MP, Kronfol ZA, Schwartz SA. Effects of alcohol and nicotine on cytotoxic functions of human lymphocytes. *Clin Immunol Immunopathol* 1990;54:395-409.

Noble RC, Penny BB. Comparison of leukocyte count and function in smoking and nonsmoking young men. *Infect Immun* 1975;12:550-5.

Nuorti JP, Butler JC, Farley MM, Harrison LH, McGeer A, Kolczak MS, et al; Active Bacterial Core Surveillance Team. Cigarette smoking and invasive pneumococcal disease. *N Engl J Med* 2000; 342:681-9.

Oeffinger KC, Snell LM, Foster BM, Panico KG, Archer RK. Diagnosis of acute bronchitis in adults: a national survey of family physicians. *J Fam Pract* 1997;45: 402-9.

Onari K, Seyama A, Inamizu T, Kodomari N, Takaishi M, Yorioka N, et al. Immunological study on cigarette smokers. Part I. Serum protein pattern in smokers. *Hiroshima J Med Sci* 1978;27:113-8.

Onwubalili JK, Edwards AJ, Palmer L. T4 lymphopenia in human tuberculosis. *Tubercle* 1987;68:195-200.

Ouyang Y, Virasch N, Hao P, Aubrey MT, Mukerjee N, Bierer BE, et al. Suppression of human IL-1 beta, IL-2, IFN-gamma, and TNF-alpha production by cigarette smoke extracts. *J Allergy Clin Immunol* 2000;106:280-7.

Papi A, Bellettato CM, Braccioni F, Romagnoli M, Casolari P, Caramori G, et al. Infections and airway inflammation in chronic obstructive pulmonary disease severe exacerbations. *Am J Respir Crit Care Med* 2006:173:1114-21.

Pastor P, Medley F, Murphy TV. Invasive pneumococcal disease in Dallas County, Texas: results from population-based surveillance in 1995. *Clin Infect Dis* 1998;26: 590-5.

Patel IS, Seemungal TA, Wilks M, Lloyd-Owen SJ, Donaldson GC, Wedzicha JA. Relationship between bacterial colonisation and the frequency, character, and severity of COPD exacerbations. *Thorax* 2002;57:759-64.

Peltola VT, McCullers JA. Respiratory viruses predisposing to bacterial infections: role of neuraminidase. *Pediatr Infect Dis J* 2004;23(1 Suppl):S87-97.

Raman AS, Swinburne AJ, Fedullo AJ. Pneumococcal adherence to the buccal epithelial cells of cigarette smokers. *Chest* 1983;83:23-7.

Ramirez-Ronda CH, Fuxench-López Z, Nevárez M. Increased pharyngeal bacterial colonization during viral illness. *Arch Intern Med* 1981;141:1599-603.

Reynolds HY. Immunoglobulin G and its function in the human respiratory tract. *Mayo Clin Proc* 1988;63:161-74.

Rich EA, Ellner JJ. Pathogenesis of tuberculosis. In: Friedman LN, ed. *Tuberculosis: Current Concepts and Treatment*. Boca Raton, Fla: CRC Press; 1994: 27-31.

Richardson MA. Upper airway complications of cigarette smoking. *J Allergy Clin Immunol* 1988;81:1032-5.

Robbins CS, Bauer CM, Vujicic N, Gaschler GJ, Lichty BD, Brown EG, Stämpfli MR. Cigarette smoke impacts immune inflammatory responses to influenza in mice. *Am J Respir Crit Care Med* 2006;174:1342-51.

Russell RE, Thorley A, Culpitt SV, Dodd S, Donnelly LE, Demattos C, et al. Alveolar macrophage-mediated elastolysis: roles of matrix metalloproteinases, cysteine, and serine proteases. *Am J Physiol Lung Cell Mol Physiol* 2002;283:L867-L73.

Saldías F, Méndez JI, Ramírez D, Díaz O. Tobacco smoke and risk of respiratory infection. *Rev Chil Enf Respir* 2007;23:179-87.

Saldías F, Méndez JI, Ramírez D, Díaz O. Predictive value of history and physical examination for the diagnosis of community-acquired pneumonia in adults: a literature review. *Rev Med Chil* 2007;135:517-28.

Sasagawa S, Suzuki K, Sakatani T, Fujikura T. Effects of nicotine on the functions of human polymorphonuclear leukocytes in vitro. *J Leukoc Biol* 1985;37:493-502.

Schultz-Cherry S, Jones JC. Influenza vaccines: the good, the bad, and the eggs. *Adv Virus Res* 2010;77:63-84.

Sethi S, Murphy TF. Bacterial infection in chronic obstructive pulmonary disease in 2000: a state-of-the-art review. *Clin Microbiol Rev* 2001;14:336-63.

Silverman NA, Potvin C, Alexander JC Jr, Chretien PB. In vitro lymphocyte reactivity and T-cell levels in chronic cigarette smokers. *Clin Exp Immunol* 1975; 22:285-92.

Slusarcick AL, McCaig LF. National hospital ambulatory medical care survey: 1998 outpatient department summary. Hyattsville, Md.: U.S. Dept. of Health and Human Services, Centers for Disease Control and Prevention, National Center for Health Statistics, 2000; DDHS publication no. (PHS) 2000-1250/0-0520.

Smith KA. Interleukin-2: inception, impact, and implications. *Science* 1988;240: 1169-76.

Sopori ML, Goud NS, Kaplan AM. Effect of tobacco smoke on the immune system. In: Dean JH, Luster AE, Kimer M, eds. *Immunotoxicology and Immunopharmacology.* New York, NY: Raven Press; 1994:413-32.

Sopori ML, Kozak W, Savage SM, Geng Y, Soszynski D, Kluger MJ, et al. Effect of nicotine on the immune system: possible regulation of immune responses by central and peripheral mechanisms. *Psychoneuroendocrinology* 1998;23:189-204.

Stämpfli MR, Anderson GP. How cigarette smoke skews immune responses to promote infection, lung disease and cancer. *Nat Rev Immunol* 2009;9:377-84.

Stathis SL, O'Callaghan DM, Williams GM, Najman JM, Andersen MJ, Bor W. Maternal cigarette smoking during pregnancy is an independent predictor for symptoms of middle ear disease at five years' postdelivery. *Pediatrics* 1999; 104:e16.

Stewart SL, Cardinez CJ, Richardson LC, Norman L, Kaufmann R, Pechacek TF, et al. Surveillance for cancers associated with tobacco use -- United States, 1999-2004. *MMWR Surveill Summ* 2008;57:1-33.

Strachan DP, Cook DG. Health effects of passive smoking. 1. Parental smoking and lower respiratory illness in infancy and early childhood. *Thorax* 1997;52:905-14.

Straus WL, Plouffe JF, File TM Jr, Lipman HB, Hackman BH, Salstrom SJ, et al; Ohio Legionnaires Disease Group. Risk factors for domestic acquisition of legionnaires disease. *Arch Intern Med* 1996; 156:1685-92.

Swann JB, Coquet JM, Smyth MJ, Godfrey DI. CD1-restricted T cells and tumor immunity. *Curr Top Microbiol Immunol* 2007;314:293-323.

Taylor B, Wadsworth J. Maternal smoking during pregnancy and lower respiratory tract illness in early life. Arch Dis Child 1987;62:786-91.

Taylor RG, Woodman G, Clarke SW. Plasma nicotine concentration and the white blood cell count in smokers. *Thorax* 1986;41:407-8.

Tell GS, Grimm RH Jr, Vellar OD, Theodorsen L. The relationship of white cell count, platelet count, and hematocrit to cigarette smoking in adolescents: the Oslo Youth Study. *Circulation* 1985;72:971-4.

Tollerud DJ, Clark JW, Brown LM, Neuland CY, Mann DL, Pankiw-Trost LK, et al. Association of cigarette smoking with decreased numbers of circulating natural killer cells. *Am Rev Respir Dis* 1989;139:194-8.

Tollerud DJ, Clark JW, Brown LM, Neuland CY, Mann DL, Pankiw-Trost LK, et al. The effects of cigarette smoking on T cell subsets. A population-based survey of healthy caucasians. *Am Rev Respir Dis* 1989;139:1446-51.

Treanor JJ, Hayden FG. *Viral infections.* In: Murray JF, ed. Textbook of respiratory medicine. 3d ed. Philadelphia: Saunders, 2000:929-84.

Trimble NJ, Botelho FM, Bauer CM, Fattouh R, Stämpfli MR. Adjuvant and anti-inflammatory properties of cigarette smoke in murine allergic airway inflammation. *Am J Respir Cell Mol Biol* 2009;40:38-46.

Tsoumakidou M, Demedts IK, Brusselle GG, Jeffery PK. Dendritic cells in chronic obstructive pulmonary disease: new players in an old game. *Am J Respir Crit Care Med* 2008;177:1180-6.

Twigg HL 3rd, Soliman DM, Spain BA. Impaired alveolar macrophage accessory cell function and reduced incidence of lymphocytic alveolitis in HIV-infected patients who smoke. *AIDS* 1994;8:611-8.

US Department of Health and Human Services. *The Health Consequences of Involuntary Exposure to Tobacco Smoke: A Report of the Surgeon General.* (US Department of Health and Human Services, Centers for Disease Control and Prevention, National Center for Chronic Disease Prevention and Health Promotion, Office on Smoking and Health, 2004).

Van Eeden SF, Hogg JC. The response of human bone marrow to chronic cigarette smoking. *Eur Respir J* 2000;15:915-21.

Warr GA, Martin RR, Sharp PM, Rossen RD. Normal human bronchial immunoglobulins and proteins: effects of cigarette smoking. *Am Rev Respir Dis* 1977;116:25-30.

Warren CW, Jones NR, Peruga A, Chauvin J, Baptiste JP, Costa de Silva V, et al. Global youth tobacco surveillance, 2000–2007. *MMWR Surveill Summ* 2008;57:1-28.

Wedzicha JA. Role of viruses in exacerbations of chronic obstructive pulmonary disease. *Proc Am Thorac Soc* 2004;1:115-20.

Wewers MD, Diaz PT, Wewers ME, Lowe MP, Nagaraja HN, Clanton TL. Cigarette smoking in HIV infection induces a suppressive inflammatory environment in the lung. *Am J Respir Crit Care Med* 1998;158:1543-9.

Woodruff PG, Koth LL, Yang YH, Rodriguez MW, Favoreto S, Dolganov GM, et al. A distinctive alveolar macrophage activation state induced by cigarette smoking. *Am J Respir Crit Care Med* 2005;172:1383-92.

Yeung MC, Buncio AD. Leukocyte count, smoking, and lung function. *Am J Med* 1984;76:31-37.

Yu GP, Hsieh CC, Peng J. Risk factors associated with the prevalence of pulmonary tuberculosis among sanitary workers in Shanghai. *Tubercle* 1988;69:105-12.

5

Bronchitis and Environment

Ayse Emel Önal and Ahmet Abbasoglu
Istanbul University, Istanbul Medical Faculty
Turkey

1. Introduction

Acute bronchitis is an inflammation of the big bronchi mucosa that develops and heals rapidly in fifteen days at the latest. Coughing that lasts more than five days is the cardinal symptom. Production of sputum and fever exists in cases with an infectious cause. Chronic bronchitis is defined having sputum production for three months or more, two years in a row. The prevailing complaint is dyspnea. Bronchitis occurs with the inhaling of the infectious agents or physicochemical agents via the airway. Environmental factors are effective in the development of bronchitis.

2. Etiology in bronchitis

2.1 Infectious causes

2.1.1 Bacteria

H Influenzae, S pneumonia, M catarrhalis account for 70% of all exacerbations and 85-95% of bacterial exacerbations. After those responsible Staphylococcus aureus, Pseudomonas aeruginosa, opportunist gram-negatives and mycoplasmma pneumonia are the most frequent bacterial agents in order of frequency. (Ball, 1995; Boldy et al., 1990; Johnson et al., 1997; MacKay et al., 1996). Mycoplasma pneumoniae, Chlamydophila pneumoniae rarely contribute to the causes of acute bronchitis (Wenzel & Fowler, 2006).

2.1.2 Viruses

Influenza/parainfluenza viruses, Respiratory syncytial virus, rhinoviruses and coronaviruses account for 30% of all acute infective exacerbations (Ball, 1995; Boldy et al., 1990; Jonsson et al., 1997; MacKay et al., 1996).

2.2 Chemical causes

Relationship between the consumption of domestic coal per acre in 1952 and the average annual death rates from bronchitis of males aged 45-64 years from 1950 to 1952, in 83 counted boroughs of England and Wales are one of the first studies that put emphasis on air pollution in developing bronchitis. In this study as the consumption of domestic coal per acre had increased, deaths from bronchitis also increased. (Daly C,1954). Industrial pollution is a major precipitant in air pollution. Before the death incidents due to smogs that took place in 1950s and 1960s in London and Los Angeles, Reid and Fairbairn had previously defined the relationship between fog and work absenteeism due to bronchitis among London postmen during the 1940s. During the 1950s in Great Britain, it's been showed that there is a correlation between the measurements of sulphur dioxide and deaths due to bronchitis in all the years for men that are over 45 and in some of the years also in women. (Pemberton & Goldberg, 1954). The basis of warming and pollutants from industry are particulate matter and sulphurdioxide. In Donora (Pennsylvania), London and New York, in 1940s, 50s and 60s episodes of severe air pollution resulted from sulfur dioxideand particulate matter (1996). Clean Air Act was created in 1971 in the United States six criteria air pollutant, ozone, particulate matter, sulfur dioxide, nitrogen dioxide, lead, and 189 units were identified toxic or hazardous air pollutant (Clean Air Act., 1971)..

The main components of particulate matter are sulfates, carbonmaterials, nitrates, trace elements and water. (Dockery & Pope, 1994) Of those pollutants Sulphur dioxide (SO2) and respirable particulate material up to 10 microns (PM10) in diameter are most frequently held responsible for the contamination and health effects. Therefore, in routine measurements they are considered first. According to NAAQS (National Ambient Air Quality Standards) standards and limit values for pollutants that affect health primarily are: Annual Arithmetic Mean for Sulfur Dioxide (SO2) 0:03 ppm(80µg/m3), 24 hour limit is 0:14 ppm (365µg/m3), Suspended Particulate Matter (PM10) limit value for the annual arithmetic average is 50 µg/m3, boundary value for 24 Hours is 150µg/m3 (Evyapan, 2010).

Children are more affected by air pollution than adults. Because 80% of alveoli forms postnatally and full development of the lungs continues until the age of six to eight. (Dietert RR at al, 2000; Plopper &Fonucchi, 2000).

Research linking air pollution with morbidity and mortality indicates the strongest effects on the very young and the elderly (Picciotto IH et al., 2007). In their study of 2010 Benrayeb and colleagues investigate the relationship between air pollution in France and individuals over 65 with bronchitis-like symptoms . In this study they found a 10% and a 23% increase in usual cough for a 10 $\mu g/m^3$ increment in PM_{10} and a 1 $\mu g/m^3$ increment in SO_2 respectively, and a 23% increase in usual phlegm for a 1 $\mu g/m^3$ increase in SO_2.. A more pronounced effect of SO_2 and PM10 was observed in women on cough and phlegm. (Bentayeb et al., 2010).

Especially exhaust fumes by vehicles are being held responsible of ambient air pollution more than industrialization, and warming up (Bates, 1995; Ana et al., 2000, ISDE, 2003). The WHO study in the three countries, investigated the effects on health of air pollution from traffic, PM10 was found to be the most harmful pollutant. The chronic bronchitis incidence of whom are over 25 years attributed to total air pollution cases or days are 6 200 for Austria, 36700 for France, 4 200 for Switzerland. These patients under the age of 15 for bronchitis or days, are 47700, 450000, and 45400 respectively. Within These the cases or days attributed to the road traffic for over the age of 25 chronic bronchitis patients are 2700 for Austria, 20400 for France, 22000 for Switzerland, for bronchitis patients under age 15 are 20600, 250000, and 24100 respectively (ISDE,2003). Besides ambient air pollution quality of indoor air pollution (Kurmi et al., 2010, Galeone et al., 2008, Padhi&Padhy, 2008) and the cigarette smoke (Pirastu et al., 2009; Vial, 1986) are important environmental factors responsible for the formation of bronchitis. Biomass fuels that are used at homes (Ekici et al., 2005; Özbay et al., 2001; Kiraz et al., 2003; Akhtar et al., 2007), solid fuels (Kurmi et al., 2010, Galeone et al., 2008, Padhi&Padhy, 2008) that form these are counted for the chemical elements of the environment. In the meta-analysis that Kurmi had done, there were positive associations between the use of solid fuels and COPD and chronic bronchitis. Pooled estimates for different types of fuel show that exposure to wood smoke while performing

domestic work presents a greather risk of COPD (Chronic obstructive pulmonary disease) and chronic bronchitis than other fuels. In many areas of Africa, Central America, South-East Asia, and South Asia, more than 90% of rural homes use solid fuel as the primary cooking and/or heating fuel. Of these fuels the use of biomass and wood, coal causes chronic bronchitis more than charcoal (Kurmi et al., 2010). In the study of Padhi and Padhy, children whom biomass is used in their homes and suffering from respiratory tract infection are compared to children whom in the homes liquified petroleum gas (LPG) is used and have respiratory tract infections. Impaired lung function were more for users of biomass. (Padhi&Padhy,2008). The outcome of this study shows that the use of biomass as a cooking fuel produces high concentrations of CO, CO_2, NO, NO_2, SO_2 and SPM in the indoor environment in comparison to LPG. A questionnaire survey of children aged between 9 and 12 years in Turkey, which included spirometry, found that coal users had more day/night cough, and that those using wood-burning stoves had the lowest values of FVC, FEV, PEFR, and FEF25 (forced expiratory flow rate at 25 % of lung volume) (Güneser at al, 1994). In Turkey since the 1970s warming, industrialization and road traffic have caused outdoor air pollution. In 1970's in Ankara, in 1980's in İstanbul, especially with the 1973 oil crisis, when the use of lignite coal has increased air pollution has increased too. (Evyapan, 2010).
Sulphurdioxide which forms as a result of the combustion of coal, petrol and fuel oil is the most common aetiology of bronchitis (Hapcıoglu et al., 2006; Schwela, 2010). Sulphur dioxide increases the mucosal permeability of the trachea and bronchi, inhibits the ciliary movements and mucous transport (Güler&Cobanoglu, 1997). Water soluble gases, sulfur dioxide and ammonia are absorbed via bronchi, ozone and nitrogen gases which are relatively non-absorbable are effective on the alveolar region that is not covered with the mucosa (Güler&Cobanoglu, 1997). Large particles, 50 micrometers in diameter in the breathing air are usually struck with the nose and pharynx. Small particles of 10 micrometres can reach alveoli. The relation between PM10 or PM2.5 exposure and acute health effects is linear at concentrations below 100 micrograms/m3 (Schhwela, 2000). There are studies that didn't determine a (Patenden et al., 2006) correlation between nitrogen dioxide and bronchitis as well as that do (Schwela, 2010). A statistically significant relationship is confirmed between polycyclic aromatic hydrocarbons (PAHs) that are greater than 2.5 microgram in diameter and the bronchitis observed in children between 3-4.5 years (Picciotto et al., 2007).
Acute and chronic bronchitis is observed often in the workers working in the fields exposed to dust and hazardous gases. Analysis of epidemiological data from the 1930s and 1940s confirmed the impression of a strong link between occupation and chronic bronchitis. In the 1950s and early 1960s, irreversible airflow limitation and emphysema, which are funtional and pathological abnormalities associated with chronic bronchitis, were shown to be increased among mineworkers. The preventability of occupation related disease influence researchers about chronic bronchitis and environmental exposure (Trupin at al, 2003). In the study of Trupin et al. post occupational exposure significantly increased the likelhood of chronic obstructive pulmonary disease, independent of the effects of smoking. One of five cases of COPD may be attributable to occupational exposures. In this study 42% of 189 subjects self reported vapours, gases, dusts or fumes. 29% of them exposed combustion by products, 23% ınorganic dusts or fumes, 15% organic dusts. Job exposure matrix, exposure probability is 69% low, 24% intermediate, 6% high (Trupin et al., 2003). Some of the branch of industry-economic activity along with cigarette smoking that are held responsible for chronic bronchitis are fields that cause exposure to asbestos, cement, grain working, textile

industry (cotton, hemp, flax dust) and welding (irritant gases, metal fumes, dusts) (Benowitz & Hua, 2004). The most commonly held minerals responsible for chronic bronchitis are coal, oil mist, silica, synthetic vitreous fibers, portland cement and metals are osmium, vanadium, welding fumes (Balmes, 2004).

2.3 Physical causes

It is known that bronchitis has always been initiated with cold weather and high humidity (Fletcher at al, 1959). The units such as school and barracks where communal life are cause the agents to spread easily and let epidemias break out (Schima&Adachi, 2000; Chen at al, 1998; Aydogdu&Assan, 2005; Kak, 2007). The presence of an crowded environment, with close interaction between individuals, increases the risk of persons being exposed to various respiratory secretions and potentially infectious respiratory viruses (Kak, 2007). Bronchitis is related to seasons and change of air. In a study conducted in Ankara the lowness of the daily temperature and of the amount of precipitation increases the risk of wheezing (Yalçın, 2010). High humidity and air pressure, and low temperature (Hapcıoglu et al., 2006) increases the incidence of bronchitis (Chen et al., 2008). In the study of Hapcıoglu et al. when the meteorological and pollution parameters were evaluated by multiple variable stepwise regression analysis, it can be seen that the only variable that explaints the COPD admissions is temperature (Other variables were pressure, humiditiy, S02, CO, NO, NO2 and PM10). Authors noted that seasonal variations exist for COPD admissions. They reported that they found admissions more in autumn, spring and winter when summer seasonal values are taken as reference (Hapcıoglu et al., 2006). In the study of Chen et al. chronic bronchitis was mainly concentrated in August and September. They explained this situation with the sudden change from cold to hot during the use of air-condition. Weather change was an important factor, especially when temperature change rapidly, and the daily average temperature fell more than 3°C bronchitis occur (Chen et al., 2008). The important factor was the amplitude of the temperature change was small, but the temperature changed frequently. When the activity of cold and warm air is sudden or frequent, there is a greater incidence of disease. This occured when hot and cold weather appeared alternately, but the fluctuation was under 3° C (Chen et al., 2008). It's been thought that the changes happening in the bronchi enable the viruses and bacteria to effect mucosa of the bronchi with relative ease.

3. Epidemiology

When looked at the relationship of bronchitis with age, small airway inflammation are observed more often in kids 6 months to 4 years old, acute bronchitis are more often in children and adolescents, whereas chronic bronchitis prevalance increases with age in adults and elderly (Chen et al., 2008). In the study of Picciotto, the overall rates for lower respiratory illness, bronchitis, and croup in children under 2 years of age were 83, 55 and 27 per 1000 child-months, respectively (or expressed equivalently, 8.3%, 5.5%, and 2.7% per month (Picciotto, 2007). Bronchitis rates in this age group were also higher in children of mothers with lower education, and children from homes with adults who smoke, or homes in which coal was used for heating or cooking. Current or recent breast-feeding was protective, as was older maternal age. In a study conducted in China, 5.9% of patients who has chronic bronchitis and asthma are between the age of 51-55, 16.2 % are seen in age 71 to 75 (Chen et al., 2008). In a study done in Boston the prevalance of chronic bronchitis is 4.5%

(Bhattacharyya, 2009). In Istanbul among the children whose mean age is 13 the bronchitis (acute and chronic) frequency is found to be 6.5% in the health problems they are aware of (Onal et al., 2009). In Nigeria school-age children reported over 10% for prevalence of bronchitis (Ana GR at al, 2009). Bronchitis is more common in young children, especially under the first age (Chen at al, 2008); The frequency increases with age after middle age, children and the elderly more easily had bronchitis (Prieto, 2007). In the study established with postal workers, in London, in 1959, Fletcher and his colleagues were found cough and sputum more in men than in women. Symptoms increases with age in men. Ventilatory capacity was significantly impaired in the men. The authors suggest these results is related to more cigarette smoking (Fletcher, 1959).

4. Diagnosis

The clinical symptoms of bronchitis are coughing, expectoration and fever with an infectious aetiology. In acute bronchitis coughing will go on for more than five days and recovers in two weeks. Bronchitis which take longer than 3 months for two consecutive years are called chronic bronchitis (Fletcher et al., 1959, Kilburn, 1998). Coughing and expectoration are seldom seen in chronic bronchitis. Dyspnea is the most important symptom and wheezing the most important sign. Ever since Badham (1808) first introduced the word bronchitis to medical literature it has been customary to include dyspnoea together with cough and expectoration as an essential symptom of bronchitis. Oswald (1958) describes two types of disability of bronchitis; breathlessness and exacerbations of infection; the presence of either of which justifies the diagnosis. Pemberton (1956) and Ogilvie and Newell (1957) accepted cough and sputum as evidence of bronchitis in earliest phase. To admit the diagnosis of bronchitis all those who have persistent cough and sputum is essential from the point of view of preventive medicine (Fletcher et al., 1959) . Today, some clinicians considered that making a diagnosis of bronchitis based on defined criteria for chronic sputum production is easy, but has limited clinical value (Clausen, 1990). For the differential diagnosis the chest radiograph is necessary. The studies continue about the place of high-resolution computed tomography in the diagnosis (Gupta et al., 2009). The respiratory functions are disturbed in patients. The measurements made by spirometer (difficult to conduct in children younger than 6 years old). Forced vital capacity (FVC), forced expiratory volume (FEV) and peak expiratory flow rate (PEFR) shows reversible decrease (Padhi&Padhy, 2008; Schwela, 2010). Evidence of airflow obstruction forced expiratory volume in one second (FEV1) less than 80% of the predicted value, and FEV1/FVC less than 70%, with an increase of less than 10% in FEV1 after inhalation of a β-agonist aerosol indicate COPD (Zalacain et al.,1999).

5. Treatment

The treatment of acute bronchitis is symptomatic. Nonsteroid antiinflammatory drugs and nasal decongestants are recommended. In the clinical studies conducted during the treatment of acute bronchitis the antibiotics are ineffective. In the case of bronchitis which produce sputum antibiotic treatment is appropriate to be administered according to the culture-antibiogram result. H. Influenzae infections give better reponse to amoxicillin and ciprofloxacine, while erythromycin, azithromycin and amoxicillin are more effective in S. Pneumoniae infections (Ball,1995). Humidifying treatment hastens the recovery of the illness. Short and long acting bronchodilators (beta-2 agonists) are effective in chronic bronchitis. The epidemiologic studies conducted found out that there is a correlation with the air pollution (especially suspended particulate matter PM10-PM2.5) and the use of bronchodilator drugs (Schwela, 2000).

Results of placebo-controlled trials of efficacy of antibiotic therapy in acute exacerbations of chronic bronchitis show that in defined exacerbations, the patients benefit significantly from antibiotic therapy. Patients who had exacerbations characterized by increses in dyspnea, sputum production, and sputum purulence. In 1987 Anthonisen and coworkers either demonstrate that in the group of patients who take amoxycillin, co-trimoxazole or doxycycline the clinical succes is %68, otherwise in the placebo group clinical succes was %55. In Allegras' study, the clinical succes of patients who take co-amoxyclavin was %86, otherwise in placebo group was %50 (Ball, 1995).

6. Prevention

Quitting smoking, staying out of foggy, dusty, smudge environment is important for prevention and treatment. Quitting smoking is possible with pharmacological treatment such as bupropion HCL and varenicline. Nicotine replacement therapy is possible with nicotine tape, nicotine gum and nicotine sublingual tablet. Measures against occupational exposure should be taken if necessary. Haveing a flu vaccination once a year and having the vaccinations in the routine vaccination program of children and elderly (such as pneumococcus and H. influenzae vaccination) is important in prevention of bronchitis.

7. References

Ball P, Epidemiology and Treatment of chronic bronchitis and its exacerbations, Chest,108:2:Suppl:S43-52, 1995.

Boldy DA, Skimore SJ, Ayres JG, Acute bronchitis in the community : Clinical features, infective factors, changes in pulmonary function and bronchial reactivity to histamine, Respir Med 84:377, 1990.

Jonsson JS, Sigurdsson JA, Kristinsson KG et al., Acute bronchitis in adults. How close do we come to its aetiology in general practice? Scand J Health Care, 15:156, 1997.

MacKay DN, Treatment of acute bronchitis in adults without underlying lung disease, J Gen İntern Med, 11:557, 1996.

Wenzel RP, Fowler AA, III. Clinical practice, Acute bronchitis, N Eng J Med, 355:2125, 2006.

Daly C, Air pollution and bronchitis, British Medical Journal, sept 18, 687-688, 1954.

Pemberton J, Goldberg C, Air pollution and bronchitis, British Medical Journal,4:568-570, 1954.

No author listed, Health effects of outdoor air pollution. Committee of the Environmental and Occupational Health Assembly of the American Thoracic Society, Am J Crit Med, 153(1):3-50, 1996.

Clean Air Act. 33 United States Code Sec.1241 Et Esq., 1971 Astım Allerji İmmunoloji 2005;3(2):77-85.
http://www.aai.org.tr/managete/UploadedFiles/%202005-02/77_85.pdf
23.11.2010

Dockery DW, Pope III CA. Acute respiratory effects of particulate air pollution. Annual Review of Public Health 1994 ; 15 : 107 – 132 .
http://www.annualreviews.org/doi/pdf/10.1146/annurev.pu.15.050194.000543

Tekbaş ÖF. Air pollution and its' health effect, in Environmental Health, GATA Basımevi, p:153-165, Ankara, 2010.

Dietert RR, Etzel RA, Chen D et al. Workshop to identify critical windows of exposure for children's health: Immune and respiratory systems work group summary, Environ Health Perspective, 108:Supp 3:483-490, 2000.

Plopper CG, Fonucchi MV, Do urban environmental pollutants exacerbate childhood lung diseases? Environ Health Perspect, 108:252-253, 2000.

Picciotto IH, Baker RJ, Yap PS, Dostal M, Joad JP, Lipsett M, Greenfield T, Herr CEW, Benes I, Shumway RH, Pinkerton KE, Sram R, Early chilhood lower respiratory ilness and air pollution, Environ Health Perspect, 115(10):1510-1518, 2007.

Bentayeb M, Hemler C, Raherison C, et al. Bronchitis-like symptoms and proximity air pollution in French elderly, Respiratory Medicine, 104:880-888, 2010.

Bates DV, The effects of air pollution on children, Environ Health Perspect. 103 Supp 6:49-53, 1995.

Ana GR, Shendell DG, Odesi TA, Sridhar MK, Identification and initial characterization of prominent air pollution sources and respiratory health at secondary schools in Ibadan, Nigeria, J Asthma, 46(7):670-676, 2009.

ISDE, International Society of Doctors fort he Environment, Ed: Silberschmidt G, Translation : Şahin Ü, Transportation, Environment, Health, ÇİHD, İTO, p:18, 2003.

Kurmi OP, Semple S, Simkhada P, Smithy WCS, Ayres JG, COPD and chronic bronchitis risk of indoor air pollution from solid fuel:a systematic review and meta-analysis, Thorax, 65:221-228,2010.

Galeone C, Pelucchi C, La Vecchia C, Negri E, Bosetti C, Hu J, Indoor air pollution from solid fuel use, chronic lung diseases and lung cancer in Harbin, Northeast China, Eur J Cancer Prev. 17(5):473-478, 2008.

Padhi BK, Padhy PK, Domestic fuels, indoor air pollution, and children's health, Ann N Y Acad Sci, 1140:209-217, 2008.

Pirastu R, Bellu C, Greco P, Pelosi U, Pistelli R, Accetta G, Biggeri A, Indoor exposure to environmental tobacco smoke and dampness: respiratory symptoms in Sardinian children-DRIAS study, Environ Res 109(1):59-65, 2009.

Vial WC. Cigarette smoking and lung disease, Am J Med Sci, 291(2):130-142,1986.

Bates DV, The effects of air pollution on children, Environ Health Perspect. 103 Suppl 6:49-53, 1995.

Ekici A, Ekici M, Kurtipek E at al, Obstructive airway diseases in women exposed to biomass smoke, Environ Res. Sep;99(1):93-8, 2005.

Ozbay B, Uzun K, Arslan H at al, Funcyional and radiological impairment in women highly exposed to indoor biomass fuels, Respirology, 6(3):255-258, 2001.

Kiraz N, Kart L, Demir R at al, Chronic pulmonary disease in rural women exposed to biomass fumes, Clin Invest Med, 26:243-248, 2003.

Akhtar T, Ulah Z, Khan MH at al, Chronic bronchitis in women using solid biomass fuel in rural Peshawar, Pakistan, Chest, 132(5):1472-1475, 2007.

Güneser SA, Atıcı A, Alpaslan N, Cinaz P, Effects of indoor environmental factors on respiratory systems of children, J. Trop. Pediatr. 40:14-16, 1994.

Evyapan F. Air pollution in Turkey, and health effect on respiratory system, www.toraks.org.tr/pdf/hava_kir_semp/hava_kirliligi.pdf

Hapcıoglu B, İşsever H, Koçyiğit E, Dişçi R, Vatansever S, Özdilli K, The effect of air pollution and meteorological parameters on chronic obstructive pulmonary disease at an Istanbul hospital. Indoor and Built Environment, 15:2:147-153, 2006.

Güler Ç, Çobanoğlu Z, Chemicals and the Environment, T. C., Ministry of Health, Public Health Project Coordinator, Environmental Health Basic Source Serie, Ankara, 1997.

Patenden S, Hoek G, Braun-Fahrlander C, Forastiere F, Kosheleva A, Neuberger M, Fletcher T, NO2 and children's respiratory symptoms in the PATY study, Occup Environ Med, 63(12):828-835, 2006.

Trupin L, Earnest G, San Pedro M et al., The occupational burden of chronic obstructive pulmonary disease, Eur Respir J, 22:462-469, 2003.

Benowitz NL, Hua F, Smoking & Occupational Health, in Occupational & Environmental Medicine, Ed:Ladou J, fourth edition, Mc Graw Hill Medical, New York, 2004, p;715.

Balmes JR, Occupational Lung Diseases,in Occupational & Environmental Medicine, Ed:Ladou J, fourth edition, Mc Graw Hill Medical, New York, p;330, 2004.

Fletcher CM, Elmes PC, Fairbairn AS, Wood CH, The significance of respiratory symptoms and the diagnosis of chronic bronchitis in a working popularion, British Medical Journal, 29:257-266, 1959.

Shima M, Adachi M, Effect of outdoor and indoor nitrogen dioxide on respiratory symptoms in schoolchildren, Int J Epidemiol. 29(5):862-70, 2000.

Chen PC, Lai YM, Wang JD et al. Adverse effect of air pollution on respiratory health of primary school children in Taiwan, Environ Health Perspect. 106(6):331-5, 1998.

Aydoğdu H, Assan A: Monitoring of Fungi and Bacteria in the Indoor Air of Primary Schools in Edirne City, Turkey: Indoor and Built Environment: 14:5:411-425, 2005.

Kak V, Infections in confined spaces: Cruise ships, military barracks, and college dormitories, Infectious Disease Clinics of North America, 21:3:773-784, 2007.

Yalçın P, Applications of environmental medicine in social pediatrics, 3th Congress of Environmental Medicine, Proceedings Book, p: 157, 23-25 June 2010.

Chen X, Cao Q, Liu C, Xu C, Research on meteorological conditions and their relayed diseases in Hefei, China, Annals of the New York Academy of Sciences, 1140:86-90, 2008.

Bhattacharyya N, Does annual temperature influence the prevalence of otolaryngologic respiratory diseases? Laryngoscope, 119(10):1882-1886, 2009.

Onal AE, Erbil S, Gürtekin B, Ayvaz Ö, Özel S, Cevizci S, Güngör G, Perception of Self Health Among primary school students and their knowledge of health matters, Nobel Medicus, 5:2:24-28, 2009.

Prieto C MJ, Mancilla F P, Astudillo O P at al, Excess respiratory diseases in children and elderly people in a community of Santiago with high particulate air pollution. Rev Med Chil. 2007 Feb;135(2):221-228. www.ncbi.nlm.nih.gov/pubmed/17406741

Kilburn KH, Pulmonary Responses to Gases and Particles, in Public Health & Preventive Medicine, Ed: Wallace RB, Doebbeling BN, fourteenth edition, Appleton&Lange, Stamford, p:581-586, 1998.

Clausen JL, The diagnosis of emphysema, chronic bronchitis, and asthma, Clin Chest Med., 11(3):405-416, 1990.

Gupta PP, Yadav R, Verma M at al, High-resolution computed tomography features in patients with chronic obstructive pulmonary disease, Singapore Med, 50(2):193-200, 2009.

Zalacain R, Sobradillo V, Amiliba J at al, Predisposing factors to bacterial colonization in chronic obstructive pulmonary disease, Eur Respir J, 13:343-348, 1999.

Schwela D, Air pollution and health in urban areas, Rev Environ Health, 15(1-2):13-42, 2000.

6

Toxicity of Nanomaterials and Recent Developments in Lung Disease

R. Asmatulu
Department of Mechanical Engineering, Wichita State University
Fairmount, Wichita,
USA

1. Introduction

1.1 Background

Nanotechnology is the study of materials, compounds, devices, and/or systems at near atomic or molecular levels [1]. Usually, one of the dimensions of nanoproducts is between 1 nm and 100 nm length in scale. This emerging technology involves fabricating, imaging, measuring, modeling, and manipulating matter at this scale [2]. The goal of nanotechnology is to control individual atoms, molecules, or particles in order to significantly improve the physical, chemical, physicochemical, and biological properties of materials and devices for various humanitarian purposes. One of the most important aspects of nanotechnology is the greatly improved surface area-to-volume ratio at this level. It includes a broad range of highly multidisciplinary fields, such as engineering, materials science, colloidal science, physics, chemistry, pharmacy, medicine, and biology [3].

Nanomaterials can exhibit entirely different properties than their bulk-scaled conventional materials, enabling them to be appealing materials in many industrial applications [3]. For example, inert materials become catalytic materials (e.g., platinum and gold), opaque substances turn out to be transparent materials (e.g., carbon, copper), melting temperatures of solid materials are greatly reduced (e.g., gold, platinum, titanium), semiconductors become conductors (e.g., silicon, germanium), and non-combustible materials turn into combustible materials (e.g., aluminum) [1-3]. These fascinating behaviors of nanomaterials can be obtained only at nanoscale.

Nanomaterials, including nanoparticles, nanotubes, nanofibers, and nanocomposites, in the forms of metals and alloys, ceramics, polymers, and composites are all produced by nanotechnology processes and are considered to be the next generation of materials for manufacturing faster cars and planes, more powerful computers and satellites, more sensitive sensors, stronger materials for structural applications, and better micro- and nanochips and batteries [1]. This is because nanomaterials have outstanding mechanical, electrical, optical, magnetic, quantum mechanic, and thermal properties. Nanomaterials are already found in more than a thousand different products, including bacteria-free cloth, concrete, filtration units, sunscreen, car bumpers, tooth paste, polymeric coatings, solar and fuel cells, lithium-ion batteries, tennis rackets, wrinkle-resistant clothing, and optical, electronic, and sensing devices [2]. In the near future, the use of nanomaterials will drastically increase worldwide. It is expected that the global market growth of nanotechnology is on track to reach one trillion dollars, and 50 percent of all new products will be nanotechnology-oriented by the year 2015 [20,21].

1.2 Motivation

Throughout the manufacturing, transportation, storage, consumption, and waste disposal of nanomaterials, the air, water, soil, and food (e.g., vegetables, fruits, and animal products) can become contaminated, resulting in countless public concerns [8,22]. Nanoparticles can also remain airborne for hundreds of kilometers and penetrate humans, animals, and plant cells, causing many known and unknown side effects [4]. Nanomaterials mainly enter the human body by inhalation, ingestion, and/or contact through skin and persist in the system. Most human-made nanomaterials do not appear in the environment, so living organisms may not have an appropriate immune system to deal with these nanoscale products [5,8]. Recent studies show that when some nanomaterials of varying surface areas, sizes, shapes, charges and energy, and compounds interact with human and animal cells or organs, they can damage or kill those cells or organs, block blood flow, and cause serious diseases [6,7]. Illnesses associated with nanomaterials include bronchitis, asthma, lung and liver cancer, Parkinson's disease, Alzheimer's disease, Crohn's disease, heart disease, and colon cancer [4,5]. Understanding the mechanisms and causes of nanomaterials will allow us to find efficient cures for lung diseases and other related illnesses associated with nanomaterials and devices [8,9].

Since nanomaterials are a new set of materials produced by entirely new manufacturing techniques, there are currently no specific rules and regulations for many of them. Hence, these uncertainties bring nanoethics and bioethics in research, development, and education to seek and examine the potential risks and rewards of the applications of these materials, as well as societal, economic, moral, health, and other broader human implications of advances in this technology [23-27].

Objectives of this study are as follows: ***i***) to understand the surface properties of nanomaterials, ***ii***) to determine the effects of nanoscale surfaces on the lung and other related diseases associated with nanomaterials, ***iii***) to find possible protection methods for students, scientists, engineers, medical personnel, policymakers, and regulators working in the field, and *iv*) to inform these groups of people about progress and future developments in the field [4,]. Some of these objectives and future developments are summarized below.

2. Surface properties of nanomaterials

Surface chemistry, surface potential, surface area, and particle size are dominating factors in the toxicity of nanomaterials [4-8]. These materials can react with the body, stay inert, and/or interact with a system based on their surface properties, and they can settle in the body for a long period of time [9-11]. It has been stated that almost all properties of nanoparticles are entirely different than their bulk-size counterparts [2]. Since the properties of nanomaterials are completely different, their toxicity could be different as well. Recent toxicological studies have demonstrated that particles less than 100 nm induce toxicity in many cell-cultured human and animal models [4-11]. Figure 1 shows the comparison of rat macrophage cells (raw cells) with different particles. As can be seen, nanoparticles are several orders of magnitude smaller than human and animal cells. They can be even smaller than DNA, pathogens, proteins, and enzymes [1]. Previous studies confirm that the smaller the particle size, the higher the toxicity [8,14]. Note that human macrophages are approximately twice as large as rat macrophages, so nanoparticle penetration may be easier for human macrophages or other larger living entities.

The surface area of nanomaterials is exponentially high when the size is at nanoscale, so the surface chemistry (e.g., surface charge, zeta potential, and surface energy) of materials is drastically changed. The high surface area of nanomaterials means numerous unbonded atoms, resulting in huge surface interaction with surrounding tissues. Hence, surface chemistry can basically provide information about the mechanisms of biological toxicity of nanomaterials in cells [4,6]. For example, gold, silver, and platinum are chemically inactive and usually do not interact directly with the body at bulk scale. Allergic reactions and other toxic effects of these inert materials are at minimum level in bulk or at microscale. However, because of their size, the surface of nanoscale materials can be chemically activated to harm the surrounding cells or organs [4]. Some nanomaterials have higher surface-to-volume ratios, which can be also responsible for the shape-dependent surface reactivity and toxicity [12-17].

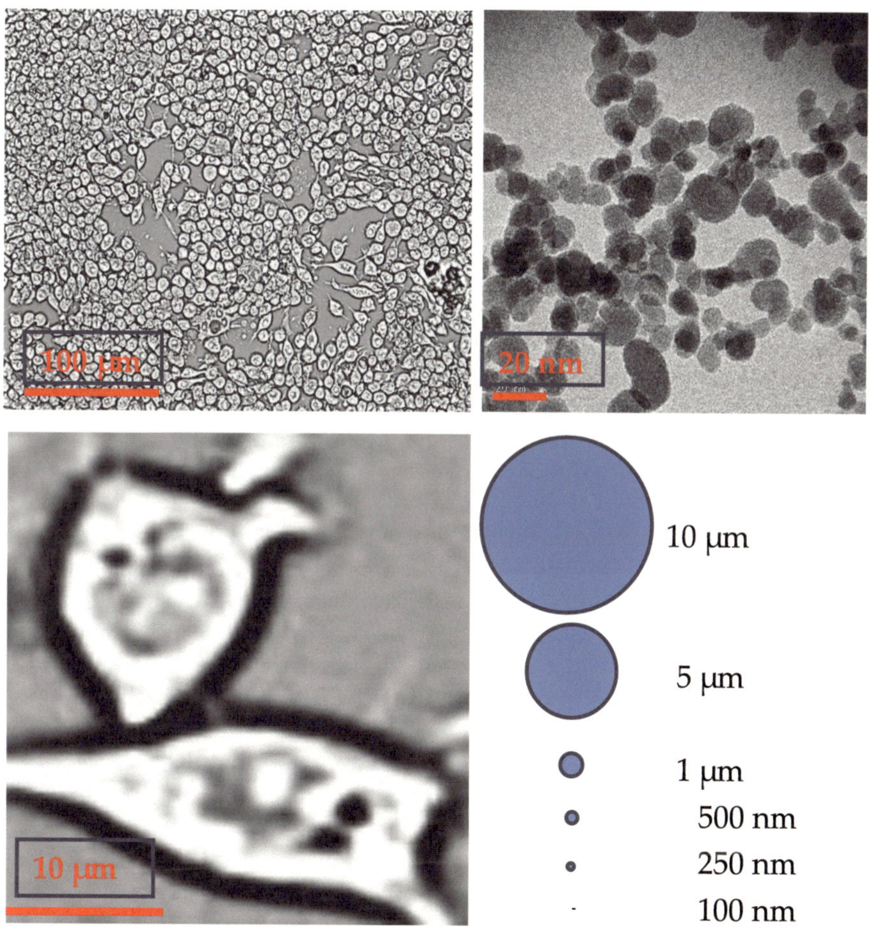

Fig. 1. Various images of cells and nanoparticles: A) rat raw cells (macrophages) at lower magnification, B) TEM image of magnetic nanoparticles with average diameter of 10 μm, C) comparison of raw macrophage cells, and D) drawings of particles at various size ranges.

Nanoparticles tend to aggregate due to intermolecular interactions, such as electrostatic, hydrophobic, and van der Waals, which makes the aggregation process easier [39]. Particle agglomeration, stability, and distribution can be related to surface charge and zeta potential values of nanoparticles in an aqueous media. The surface charge mainly regulates the stability of the nanoparticles [1]. At lower surface charges, nanoparticles usually agglomerate and make a larger cluster [2]. It has been reported that the toxicity of single particles is much higher than that of aggregated nanoparticles [4].

The toxicity of nanomaterials can be minimized using different chemical processes, such as surface treatment, modification, and functionalization [39-42]. In this way, surface energy and surface charge of nanoparticles can be changed via additions of chemicals (e.g., surfactants, electrolytes, and polymers). These chemicals include (but are not limited to) citric acid, tetramethyl ammonium hydroxide, gum Arabic, sodium dodecyl sulfate, and other carboxyl and amine functionalization groups. As a result, the surface functionalization process will help nanomaterials perform at less toxic levels in the body or in other applications [6,7].

3. Toxicity of nanomaterials and lung disease

Nanomaterials can enter the human body by various routes, such as breathing, eating, and touching the skin (Figure 2) [4-8,29,45]. Skin is the first defense barrier against the outside environment and is typically the first place on the body that is exposed to nanomaterial toxicity. Larger micron-scale particles normally cannot pass through skin and will not cause any health concerns. For the past few years, toxicological studies demonstrated that particles less than 100 nm in diameter induce toxicity in cell-cultured models as well as animal models [28-31]. It is also more difficult to remove nanoparticles from the body than the same kinds of larger particles. Table 1 shows the relationship between nanoparticle size and possible toxicity to living cells [8]. As is known, several kinds of sicknesses can be expected from nanomaterials that accumulate in the body, including inflammation of the airways, bronchitis, asthma, emphysema, lung cancer, neurodegenerative diseases, cardiovascular effects, liver cancer, Parkinson's disease, Alzheimer's disease, Crohn's disease, heart disease, and colon cancer [4,40].

Unless functionalized, most nanomaterials are not stable in in-vitro conditions, so their stability is dependent on several factors, such as pH, ionic strength, solubility, thermodynamic feasibility, concentration, kinetic facility of electron transfers, and redox conditions of biological media [5]. The toxicity of nanomaterials can occur through three different mechanisms in the body: ***i***) dissolution process of nanomaterials in biological media, ***ii***) catalyst properties of nanomaterials, and ***iii***) reduction and oxidation (Redox) evolution of the surfaces [4-6].

In one study, an organ exposed to nanoparticles was analyzed, and the results indicated that the smaller particles diffused into the respiratory system faster than microscale particles [5]. It was also found that nanoparticles penetrate into cells and, by transcytosis, across epithelial and endothelial cells and into lymph circulation to reach very sensitive parts of the body, such as the nervous system, bone marrow, brain, lymph nodes, spleen, and heart. This study concluded that surface coating and in-vivo surface modification could reduce the side effects of those nanoparticles [6,7]. Figure 3 shows the nanoparticles of a lead compound and scanning transmission electrograph of ceria nanoparticles exposed to clearing sludge [29,45].

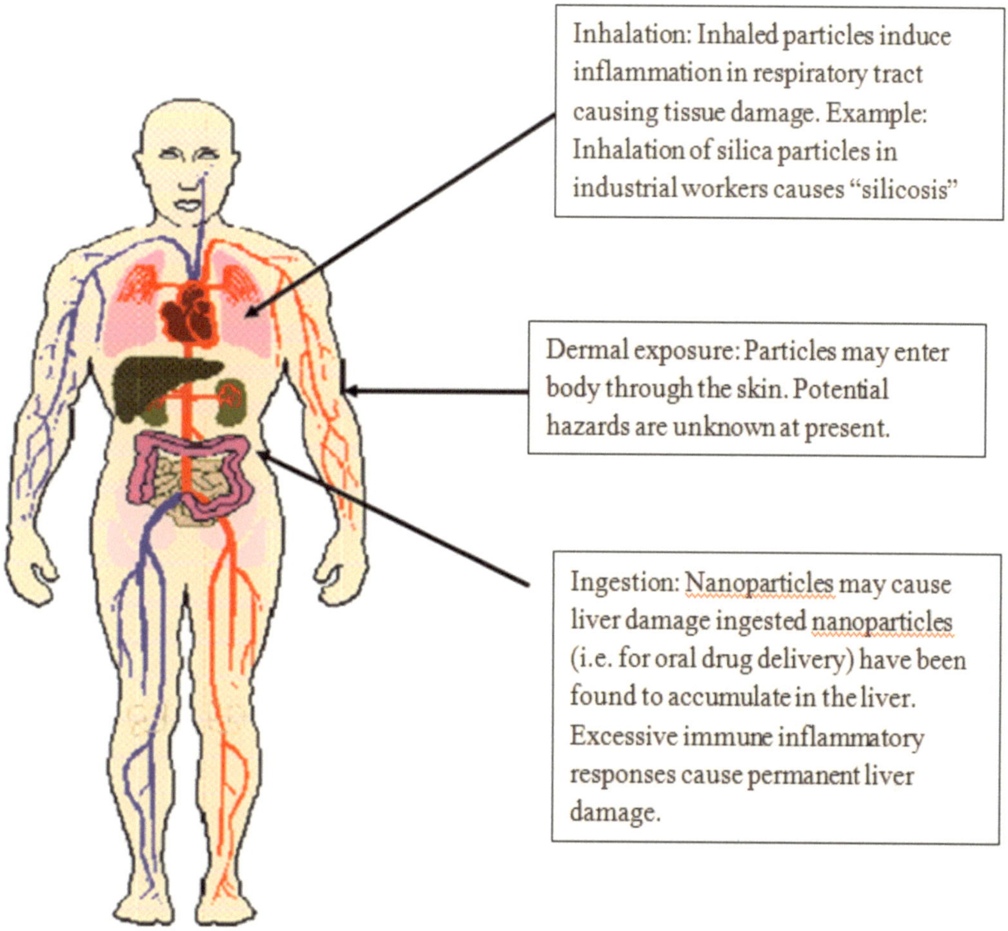

Fig. 2. Entrances of nanoscale materials into the body through inhalation, dermal exposure, and ingestion, resulting in many potential hazards [25].

Lung disease involves many illnesses, such as bronchitis, asthma, chronic obstructive pulmonary disease, influenza, pneumonia, tuberculosis, cancer, and many other breathing-related illnesses [5]. Recent studies have shown that some lung diseases, such as bronchitis and asthma, are directly linked to the uptake of nanomaterials. After the inhalation of nanomaterials, they can be deposited throughout the entire respiratory system, beginning in the nose to the inside of the lung, which has airways that transport air combined with nanomaterials in (mostly) and out (rarely) of the body. Because of the larger surface area of lungs, nanoparticles have a primary entry route. Although larger particles (more than 10 μm) tend to be deposited in the upper part of the respiratory system and removed easily by the body through coughing and sneezing, smaller nanoscale particles can reach the gas exchange surfaces and remain there for a longer period of time. This is where the real problem begins [8].

Broken surfaces and other damage in the lung and other parts of the respiratory system accelerate the penetration of nanomaterials into the surrounding tissue, resulting in faster-growing lung diseases [4]. Also, when nanoparticles enter the blood stream, they can be

Type of Material	Particle Size (nm)	Surface Area (m²/g)	Charge/Zeta Potential (mV)	Biological Toxicity
Alumina	116	13.37	45-50	Protein (BSA) adsorption with time
			(pH 5.5–6.5)	IEP shifts with pH and surface area
PEG Quantum Dots	10	–	–	Retention of Q dots in liver, spleen, and bone marrow
MWCNT	10–20	40–300	–	Cytotoxicity: alveolar macrophages at high dose
SWCNT	1.4	270	–	Cytotoxicity: alveolar macrophages at low dose;
				transient inflammatory and cell injury
Titania	300nm(rutile)	6	–	Short-term reversible inflammation
	Rods(20–233)	26.5	–	Short-term reversible inflammation
	(anatase rods)		–	Minor adverse lung tissue reaction
	Spherical(5–6)	169.4	–	Short-term reversible inflammation
	(anatase spherical powder)		–	Minor adverse lung tissue reaction
Quartz	1.5µn	4	–	High pulmonary toxicity
PTFE	20	–	–	Cell death–15 min. exposure
	130	–	–	No ill effects
Emulsifying Wax	74.7 ± 53.4 (neutral)	–	-14.1 ± 2.1	No BBB; permeation ability in low conc.
	127.1 ± 70.6 (anionic)	–	-59 ± 2.9	No BBB; permeation ability in low concentrations
	97.2 ± 68.9 (cataionic)	–	45.2 ± 3.5	Toxic at brain microvasculaturue endothelium
Ceria	3–5	–	–	Radio protection, nontoxic at low/medium dose
Yttria	50	–	–	Neuroprotection against oxidative stress

Table 1. Relationship between nanoparticle size and nanoparticle toxicity [8].

delivered to organs and tissues in the entire body, including the brain, heart, liver, kidneys, spleen, bone marrow, and nervous system [40]. Unlike larger particles, nanoparticles can reach the cell mitochondria and cell nuclei of these organs, which in turn cause DNA mutation and induce major structural damage and cell death [25,28,41]. In this case, particle size and shape are the major factors in determining particle toxicity.

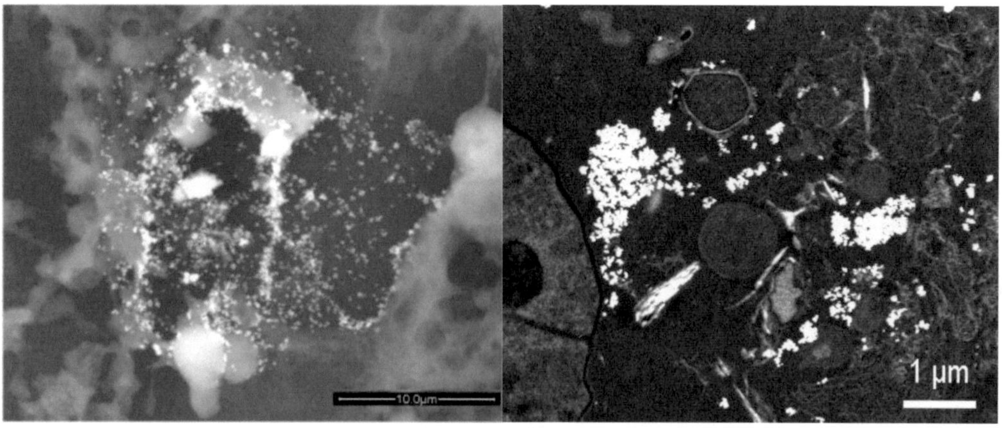

Fig. 3. Nanoparticles of lead compound located in lung where patient was affected by multiorgan granulomatosis (left), and scanning transmission electrograph of ceria nanoparticles exposed to clearing sludge (high-density cerium oxide nanoparticles are bright) (right) [29,45].

One latest study showed that, after 12 weeks of inhalation tests, small TiO_2 nanoparticles 20 nm in size were characterized by a longer retention time in the lungs of rats and increased translocation to interstitial sites than larger TiO_2 nanoparticles 250 nm in size [4,50-52]. Another study in healthy animals also showed that inhalation of metallic nanoparticles (less than 30 nm) into the circulatory system was much faster than that of non-metallic nanoparticles (between 4 nm and 200 nm) [53]. Although the mechanism of nanomaterial penetration is not fully understood, it is believed that nanoparticles can be absorbed by lung cells and induce local effects, leading to long-term consequences of airway inflammation, bronchitis, asthma, emphysema, lung cancer, neurodegenerative diseases, and cardiovascular effects [4-6].

Carbon-based nanomaterials (CBNs) in different forms of fullerenes, single- and multi-walled carbon nanotubes (SWCNTs and MWCNTs), and carbon nanoparticles and nanofibers are being used in a number of different applications [1-3]. The shape of CBNs is an important factor in determining its toxicity [42]. Some CBNs are structurally similar to asbestos, raising concerns that widespread use of carbon nanotubes may lead to mesothelioma, cancer of the lining of the lungs caused by an exposure to asbestos. In particular, the needle-like fiber shapes of CNTs are more toxic than other CBNs are to human skin fibroblasts [46-49]. MWCNTs and SWCNTs have strong chemical stability, and when inhaled, they cannot be easily dissolved in the body, which in turn could damage cells, DNA, and surrounding tissues [42-44]. Generally, SWCNTs are more toxic than MWCNTs because of their size [6]. Recent studies have also shown that sidewall-functionalized MWCNTs and SWCNTs were less toxic to human cells than those without functionalization. Also, it is interesting to note that CNTs synthesized by a catalytic chemical vapor deposition are not toxic to human umbilical vein endothelial cells [4,32-34]. Although nanomaterials have superior properties in various applications, they can be very dangerous if not properly handled. Toxicity of nanomaterials has not been completely identified yet, and most studies have mainly focused on acute and liver toxicity [4,49]. Long-term toxicity of nanomaterials and examination of chronic exposure must be studied in detail to understand the mechanisms involved. Even though several factors are involved in nanomaterial toxicity, more efforts and time are needed to conduct research on nanoscale products and lung and other diseases [6,50].

4. Protection methods

Hazard reduction of nanomaterials is necessary for students, engineers, and health professionals working on their production, processing, and analysis, as well as workers and consumers in contact with commercial products [5,35,36]. Table 2 provides a hierarchy of the exposure controls of nanomaterials at different categories, such as elimination, substitution, engineering, administration, and personal protective equipment [9,37].

Control Methods	Process, Equipment, and Tasks
Elimination	Change design to eliminate or minimize hazardous materials.
Substitution	Replace high-hazard material with a low one (e.g., environmental).
Engineering	Use isolation/enclosure, ventilation, filtration, and collection.
Administration	Adhere to procedures, policies, shift design, and new rules and regulations.
Personal Protective Equipment	Use respirators, clothing, gloves, goggles, and ear plugs.

Table 2. The hierarchy of exposure controls of nanomaterials and their controls [9,37].

The processing, equipment, and job tasks associated with the control methods are as follows: *i*) change the design to eliminate or minimize hazardous materials; *ii*) replace a high-hazard material with a low one; *iii*) use isolation, ventilation, filtration, and dust collection; *iv*) adhere to procedures, policies, shift design, and new rules and regulations; and *v*) use respirators, clothing, gloves, goggles, and ear plugs. Figure 4 shows some methods of protection that should be used during the production and use of nanomaterials [5,35], which are outlined as follows [4-6]:

- Students, workers, engineers, doctors, and scientist who are working with nanomaterials and devices are recommended to wear a disposable, typically plastic, body covering over their work clothes during high-exposure activities and to wear long gloves pulled over their sleeves to minimize wrist exposure and other contamination. Other recommendations are antistatic shoes to prevent ignition by static charges, and sticky mats at laboratory entrances to prevent the accidental transfer of nanomaterials in and out of the working area [5].

- The hazardous effects of nanomaterials need to be reduced during their production and processing. The waste of nanomaterials should be limited. Outputs are sometimes more hazardous than the products or wastes from such activities [5].
- Workers who inhale nanomaterials are advised to consume milk and unrefined sugar to reduce the toxicity level of nanomaterials [5].
- Nitrile gloves or wrist-length disposable nitrile gloves with extended sleeves must be worn during the handling of nanomaterials (Figure 4). These gloves need to be changed frequently[5].
- For eye protection, safety glasses with side shields must be on the face during the use of nanomaterials in the form of solids, liquids, and aerosols [5].
- Volumes of liquid-based nanomaterials must be limited to the milliliter range (< 200 ml) in a sealed container when not in use [5].
- Total particle masses must be limited to the milligram range (< 200 mg) and must be manipulated within a high efficient particulate air (HEPA)-filtered laboratory exhaust hood over water-soaked absorbent paper to capture any spilled materials [5].
- Containers of nanomaterials must be labeled with a sign indicating "NANOMATERIALS" [5].
- Nanomaterials are considered to be hazardous materials, so workers should follow all the safety rules necessary in the field and laboratory [5].
- The use of nanomaterials increasing worldwide brings with it several concerns for worker and user safety. Thus, new measurement devices should be developed and used in the specified areas where nanomaterials and devices are produced and utilized.

In addition to the previous information, the National Institute for Occupational Safety and Health (NIOSH) has provided sequential steps for students, workers, engineers, and others who are involved in nanotechnology-related teaching, research, and development [5,38]. These steps, shown in Figure 5, will potentially reduce the risk of exposing nanomaterials to personnel and consumers [5,38].

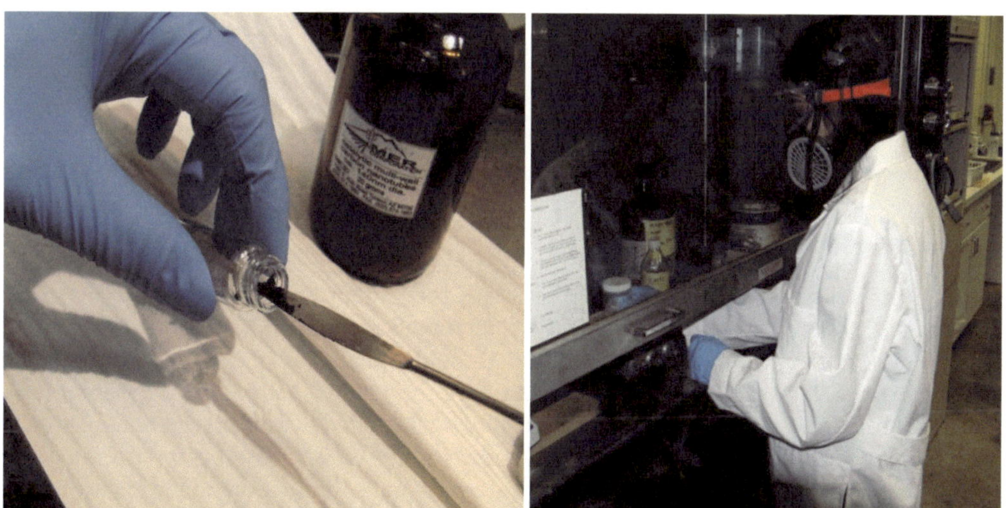

Fig. 4. Simple protection methods for using potentially hazardous engineered nanomaterials in laboratory conditions.

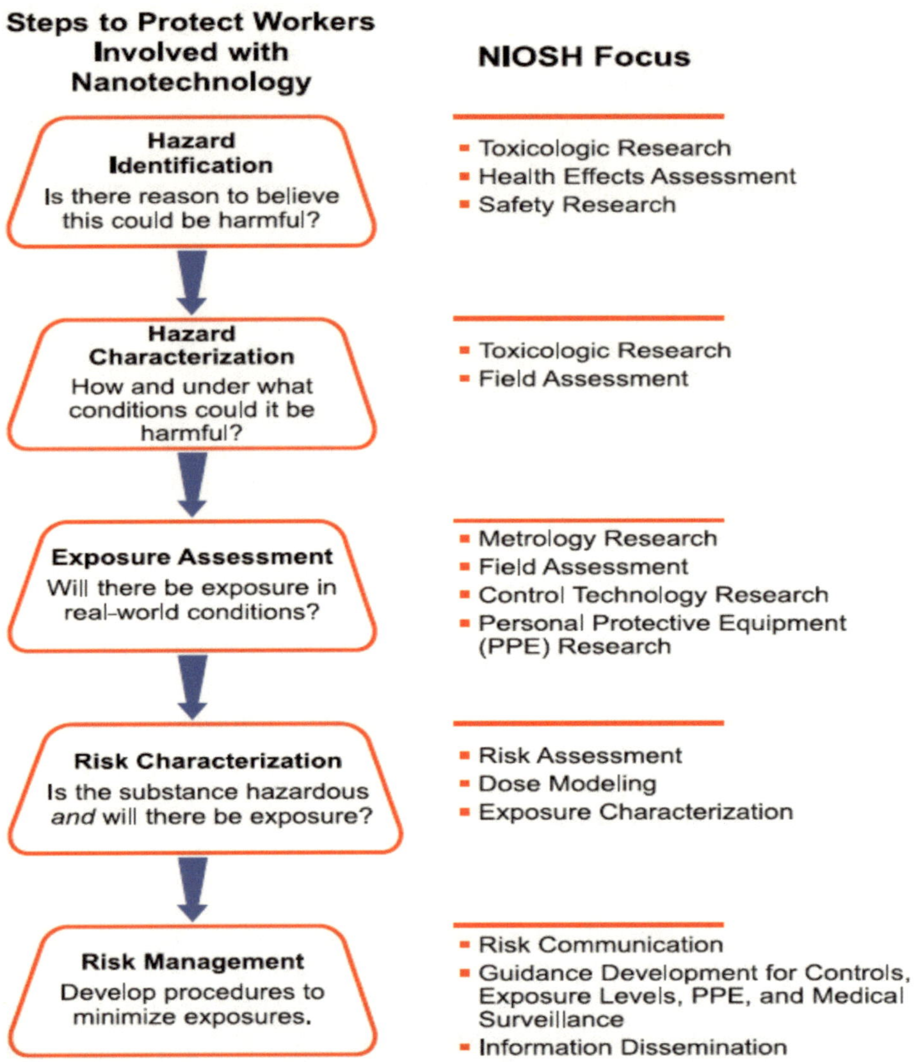

Fig. 5. Steps of NIOSH for workers/students involved in nanotechnology processes [5].

5. Conclusions

Although nanomaterials have superior properties for various applications, these materials could be more hazardous to human than their microscale equivalent if not properly handled or used. The nanomaterials mainly exposed through inhalation of suspended nanoscale particulates result in the inflammation of airways, bronchitis, asthma, emphysema, lung cancer, neurodegenerative diseases, and cardiovascular effects. Toxicity of nanomaterials has not been completely identified yet, and most studies have focused primarily on acute liver toxicity. The long-term toxicity of nanomaterials and examination of chronic exposure to these materials must be studied in detail to understand their toxicology mechanisms in the lungs and other organs. Even though several factors are involved in the toxicity of nanomaterials, more efforts and time are needed to study nanoproducts, their properties, and processing. Thus, students, scientists, engineers, doctors, policymakers, and regulators working in the field should take all the necessary precautions to protect themselves during the production, handling, and consumption of nanomaterials.

6. Acknowledgment

The author gratefully acknowledges Wichita State University for the support of this work.

7. References

[1] Rogers, B., Pennathur, S., and Adams, J., *Nanotechnology Understanding Small Systems,* CRC Press, 2008.

[2] Poole, C.P., *Introduction to Nanotechnology*, Wiley India Pvt. Ltd., 2009.

[3] Gogotsi, Y., *Nanomaterials Handbook*, CRC Press, 2006.

[4] Kumar, C., *Nanomaterials – Toxicity, Health and Environmental Issues*, Wiley-VCH, 2006.

[5] "Approaches to Safe Nanotechnology Managing the Health and Safety Concerns Associated with Engineered Nanomaterials," DHHS (NIOSH) Publication 2009-125.

[6] Karakoti, A.S., Hench, L.L., and Seal, S., "The Potential Toxicity of Nanomaterials—The Role of Surfaces," *JOM Journal of the Minerals, Metals and Materials Society*, Vol. 58, 2006, pp. 77-82.

[7] Brayner, R., "The Toxicological Impact of Nanoparticles," *Nanotoday*, Vol. 3, 2008, pp. 48-55.

[8] Asmatulu, R., Asmatulu, E., and Yourdkhani, A., "Toxicity of Nanomaterials and Recent Developments in the Protection Methods," SAMPE Fall Technical Conference, Wichita, KS, October 19-22, 2009, 12 pages.

[9] Asmatulu, R., Asmatulu, E., and Yourdkhani, A., "Importance of Nanosafety in Engineering Education," ASEE Midwest Conference, Lincoln, NB, September, 2009, 8 pages.

[10] Asmatulu, R., Khan, W.S., Asmatulu, E., and Ceylan, M., "Biotechnology and Bioethics in Engineering Education," ASEE Midwest Conference, Lawrence, KS, September 22-24, 2010, 10 pages.

[11] Asmatulu, R., Asmatulu, E., and Zhang, B., "Nanotechnology and Nanoethics in Engineering Education," ASEE Midwest Conference, Lawrence, KS, September 22-24, 2010, 11 pages.

[12] Navrotsky, A., "Nanomaterials in the Environment, Agriculture, and Technology (NEAT)," *Journal of Nanoparticle Research*, Vol. 2, 2000, pp. 321-323.

[13] Marchant, G.E., Sylvester, D.J., and Abbott, K.W., "Risk Management Principles for Nanotechnology," *Nanoethics*, Vol. 2, 2008, pp. 43-60.

[14] Osman, M.T., "Environmental, Health, and Safety Considerations for Producing Nanomaterials," *JOM Journal of the Minerals, Metals and Materials Society*, Vol. 60, 2008, pp. 14-17.

[15] O'Brien, N., and Cummins, E., "Development of a Three-Level Risk Assessment Strategy for Nanomaterials," *Nanomaterials: Risks and Benefits*, 2008, Springer, Netherlands, pp. 161-178.

[16] Singh, S., and Sing, H. N., "Nanotechnology and Health Safety-Toxicity and Risk Assessments of Nanostructured Materials on Human Health," *Journal of Nanoscience and Nanotechnology*, Vol.7, 2007, pp. 3048–3070.
[17] Oberdörster, G., Oberdörster, E., and Oberdörster, J., "Nanotoxicology: An Emerging Discipline Evolving from Studies of Ultrafine Particles," *Environmental Health Perspectives*, Vol. 113, 2005, No. 7, pp. 823–839.
[18] Maynard, A.D., "Safe Handling of Nanotechnology," *Nature*, Vol. 444, 2006, pp. 267–269.
[19] Casals, E., Vázquez-Campos, S., Bastús, N.G., and Puntes, V., "Distribution and Potential Toxicity of Engineered Inorganic Nanoparticles and Carbon Nanostructures in Biological Systems," *TrAC Trends in Analytical Chemistry*, Vol. 27, 2008, pp. 672–683.
[20] Morse, J., "Economic Impact of Nanomanufacturing Initiatives," *National Nanomanufacturing*, Vol. 2, Issue 3, March, 2009, 3 pages.
[21] Pacheco, K., Schwenz, R.W., and Jones, W.E., *Nanotechnology in Undergraduate Education*, Oxford University Press, Inc., 2010.
[22] Allhoff, F., Lin, P., Moor, J., and Weckert, J., *Nanoethics: The Ethical and Social Implications of Nanotechnology*, Wiley, 2007.
[23] Asmatulu, R., Khan, W. S., Asmatulu, E., and Ceylan, M., "Biotechnology and Bioethics in Engineering Education," ASEE Midwest Conference, Lawrence, KS, September 22–24, 2010, 10 pages.
[24] Asmatulu, R., Asmatulu, E., and Zhang, B., "Nanotechnology and Nanoethics in Engineering Education," ASEE Midwest Conference, Lawrence, KS, September 22–24, 2010, 11 pages.
[25] Colvin, V.L., "The Potential Environmental Impact of Engineered Nanomaterials," *Nature Biotechnology*, Vol. 21, 2003, pp. 1166–1170.
[26] U.S. Environmental Protection Agency, 2007 (www.epc.gov).
[27] Yavuz, C.T., Mayo, J. T., Yu, W.Y., Prakash, A., Falkner, J.C., Yen, S., Cong, L., Shipley, J.H., Kan, A., Tomson, M., Natelson, D., and Colvin, V.L. ,"Low-Field Magnetic Separation of Monodisperse Fe3O4 Nanocrystals," *Science*, Vol. 314, 2006, pp. 964–967.
[28] Hussain, S.M., Braydich-Stolle, L., Schrand, A.M., Murdock, R.C., Yu, K.O., Mattie, D.M., Schlager, J.J., and Terrones, M., "Toxicity Evaluation for Safe Use of Nanomaterials: Recent Achievements and Technical Challenges," *Advanced Materials*, Vol. 21, 2009, pp. 1549–1559.
[29] Gatti, A.M., and Montanari, S., "Nanoparticles and Nanosafety," University of Modena and Reggio Emilia, Laboratory of Biomaterials, European Commission, ICNT 2005, San Francisco.
[30] Gatti, A.M., Montanari, S., Monari, E., Gambarelli, A., Capitani, F., and Parisini, B., "Detection of Micro- and Nano-Sized Biocompatible Particles in the Blood," *Journal of Materials Science: Materials in Medicine*, Vol. 15, 2004, pp. 469–472.
[31] Gatti, A., Montanari, S., Gambarelli, A., Capitani, F., and Salvatori, R., "In-vivo Short- and Long-Term Evaluation of the Interaction Material-Blood," *Journal of Materials Science: Materials in Medicine*, Vol. 16, No. 12, 2005, pp. 1213–1219.
[32] Monteiro-Riviere, N.A., and Inman, A.O., "Challenges for Assessing Carbon Nanomaterial Toxicity to the Skin," *Carbon*, Vol. 44, 2006, pp. 1070–1078.

[33] Grabinski, C., Hussain, S., Lafdi, K., Braydich-Stolle, L., and Schlager, J., "Effect of Particle Dimension on Biocompatibility of Carbon Nanomaterials," *Carbon*, Vol. 45, 2007, pp. 2828-2835.

[34] Hurt, R.H., Monthioux, M., and Kane, A., "Toxicology of Carbon Nanomaterials: Status, Trends, and Perspectives on the Special Issue," *Carbon*, Vol. 44, 2006, pp. 1028-1033.

[35] Borisenko, V.E., and Ossicini, S. *What is What in the Nanoworld: A Handbook on Nanoscience and Nanotechnology*, Weinheim, Wiley-VCH, 2005.

[36] Buzea, C., Pacheco, I.I., and Robbie, K., "Nanomaterials and Nanoparticles: Sources and Toxicity," *Biointerphases*, Vol. 2, 2007, 55 pages.

[37] Brayner, R., Ferrari-Iliou, R., Brivois, N., Djediat, S., Benedetti, M.F., and Fiévet, F., "Toxicological Impact Studies Based on Escherichia Coli Bacteria in Ultrafine ZnO Nanoparticles Colloidal Medium," *Nano Letters*, Vol. 6, 2006, pp. 866-870.

[38] http://www.cdc.gov/niosh/, accessed March 15, 2011.

[39] Ramesh, K.T., *Nanomaterials: Mechanics and Mechanisms*, New York, Springer, 2009.

[40] Kashiwada, S., "Distribution of Nanoparticles in the See-through Medaka (Oryzias latipes)," *Environmental Health Perspectives*, Vol. 114, No. 11, 2006, pp. 1697-1702.

[41] Braydich-Stolle, L., Hussain, S., Schlager, J.J., and Hofmann, M.C., "*In Vitro* Cytotoxicity of Nanoparticles in Mammalian Germline Stem Cells," *Toxicological Sciences*, Vol. 88, 2005, pp. 412-419.

[42] Jia, G., Wang, H., Yan, L., Wang, X., Pei, R., and Yan, T., "Cytotoxicity of Carbon Nanomaterials: Single-Wall Nanotube, Multi-Wall Nanotube, and Fullerene," *Environmental Science and Technology*, Vol. 39, 2005, pp. 1378-1383.

[43] Nel, A., Xia, T., Madler, L., and Li, N., "Toxic Potential of Materials at the Nanolevel," *Science*, Vol. 311, 2006, pp. 622-627.

[44] Service, R.F., "Calls Rise for More Research on Toxicology of Nanomaterials," *Science*, Vol. 310, 2005, pp. 1609.

[45] Limbach, L.K., Bereiter,R., Müller, R., Krebs, R., Gälli, R., and Stark, W.J., "Removal of Oxide Nano-particles in a Model Waste-water Treatment Plant: Influence of Agglomeration and Surfactants on Clearing Efficiency," *Environmental Science and Technology*, Vol. 42, No. 15, 2008, pp. 5828-5833.

[46] Wu, M., Gordon, R.E., Herbert, R., Padilla, M., Moline, J., Mendelson, D., Litle, V., Travis, W.D., and Gil, J., "Case Report: Lung Disease in World Trade Center Responders Exposed to Dust and Smoke: Carbon Nanotubes Found in the Lungs of World Trade Center Patients and Dust Samples," *Environmental Health Perspectives*, Vol. 118, No. 4, 2010, pp. 499-504.

[47] Florito, S., Serafino, A., Andreola, F., Togna, A., and Togna, G., "Toxicity and Biocompatability of Carbon Nanoparticles," *Journal of Nanoscience and Nanotechnology*, Vol. 6, No. 3, 2006, pp. 591-599.

[48] Lam, C., James, J.T., McKluskey, R., Arepalli, S., and Hunter, R., "A Review of Carbon Toxicity and Assessment of Potential Occupational and Environmental Health Risks," *Critical Reviews in Toxicology*, Vol. 36, No. 3, 2006, pp. 189-217.

[49] Lam, C.W., James, J.T., McCluskey, R., and Hunter, R.L., "Pulmonary Toxicity of Single-wall Carbon Nanotubes in Mice 7 and 90 Days after Intratracheal Instillation," *Toxicological Sciences*, Vol. 77, 2004, pp. 126-134.

[50] Keenan, C.R., Goth-Goldstein, R., Lucas, D., and Sedlak, D.L., "Oxidative Stress Induced by Zero-Valent Iron Nanoparticles and Fe(II) in Human Bronchial Epithelial Cells," *Environmental Science and Technology*, Vol. 43, No. 12, 2009, pp. 4555–4560.

[51] Wang, B., Feng, W., Zhao, Y., Xing, G., Chai, Z., Wang, H., and Jia, G., "Status of Study on Biological and Toxicological Effects of Nanoscale Materials," *Science in China Series B: Chemistry*, Vol. 48, 2005, pp. 385–394.

[52] Hosokawa, M., Nogi, K., Naito, M., and Yokoyama, T., *Nanoparticles Technology Handbook*, Elsevier, 2007.

[53] Seaton, A., Tran, L., Aitken, R., and Donaldson, K., "Nanoparticles, Human Health Hazard and Regulation," *Journal of the Royal Society Interface*, Vol. 7, 2010, pp. S119–S129.

Part 2

Diagnosis and Treatment

7

Ventilator Associated Tracheobronchitis

Ignacio Martin-Loeches[1], Sara Rosich[2], Elisabeth Papiol[2], Pau Castell[3], Angel Pobo[2] and Alejandro Rodriguez[2]
[1]*Critical Care Center, Hospital de Sabadell, CIBER Enfermedades Respiratorias, Sabadell,*
[2]*Critical Care Department. Joan XXIII University Hospital, University Rovira i Virgili, IISPV, CIBER Enfermedades Respiratorias (CIBERes), Tarragona,*
[3]*Primary Care Center of Torreforta-La Granja, Tarragona,*
Spain

1. Introduction

Mechanical ventilation (MV), while life saving, also carries significant risks and complications. There is a huge information regarding ventilator-associated pneumonia (VAP) in terms of diagnosis, treatment and impact on the outcome of critically ill patients[1,2,3]. However, nosocomial tracheobronchitis, and specifically Ventilator associated Tracheobronchitis (VAT) in the ICU is a definition with a difficult and complicated diagnosis[4,5,6]. VAT represents an entity with several definitions and different treatment options up to different authors, without knowing exactly the impact on the outcome of critically ill patients. VAT is "microbiologically confirmed" when a patient with clinically diagnosed tracheobronchitis yields culture specimens that identify a causative pathogen. When a patient lacks fever or leukocytosis (or if culture specimens reveal few organisms) the differentiation between colonization and infection is difficult and controversial. Furthermore, the significance of tracheobronchial colonization as a risk factor for subsequent lower respiratory tract infection remains unclear[7]. This review attempts to summarize the current knowledge on VAT with special interest in the following questions: 1) What is the most appropriate definition of VAT? 2) How is the diagnosis performed in VAT? 3) When a VAT requires antibiotic treatment? and finally 4) What antibiotic treatment options might be considered?

2. Definition

The incidence of VAT varies widely in the literature[8,9,10,11]. Malacarne et al[7] in a recent multicenter study found, in more than 9000 patients included, an incidence of 15.5% tracheobronchitis, which is the third most common infection after pneumonia (47%) and tract urinary infection (26%). Another study[8] showed an incidence of VAT of 10.6%, with a prevalence significantly higher in surgical (15.3%) compared to medical patients (9.9%. P = 0.01). However, the true prevalence of VAT is difficult to compare between studies because of the different definitions being used for diagnosis[12,13]. For the CDC (Centers for Disease Control)[6] the definition of VAT in adult patients must meet the radiological criteria of absence of pneumonia in the X-ray and at least 2 of the following findings: 1) fever (> 38 ° C)

2) cough, 3) new or increased production of sputum, 4) rhonchi and wheezing and 5) bronchospasm. In addition, a positive culture of bronchial secretions obtained by endotracheal aspirate (ETA) or bronchoscopic technique should be positive.
Recent studies[7,8,14] have used a more updated definition that includes some changes from the CDC criteria (Table 1). The VAT is "microbiologically" confirmed if a patient with clinical suspicion of VAT has a growth of a potentially pathogenic microorganism with a number of colony-forming units (cfu) above the cut-off points for those used in a lower respiratory sample[4,5,7,11,12,13]. However, the definition of VAT has not been validated by studies using a comparable diagnosis techniques as a "gold standard." In patients in whom some of the items of the definition (fever or leukocytosis) are not present or the number of colony-forming units (cfu/ml) are below the suggested cutoff points, the differentiation between VAT (infection) and colonization might be difficult.

Criteria frequently used for diagnosis
• Fever (Temperature > 38ºC)
• New or increased sputum production.
• Leukocytosis.
• Absence of new pulmonary infiltrates in X-ray.

Table 1. Criteria for Nosocomial tracheobronchitis.

Another point to consider in diagnosis refers to the absence of pulmonary infiltrates, which remains a controversial issue. In intubated patients admitted to ICU, the clinical condition and the technical difficulties in carrying out a portable X-ray make the diagnosis of absence of "new thoracic infiltrates", which is required for the diagnosis of VAT, difficult to assure and has a marked character of subjectivity. Several authors[4,5,11,12,13] have also suggested the need to confirm or to rule out the existence of new thoracic infiltrates by chest computerized tomography (CT). However, this procedure is not always possible or routinely indicated in all ventilated patients when suspected VAT and its cost-benefit needs to be clarified. Therefore, it is necessary to assume a broad definition for this entity to identify patients at risk for VAT in order to identify those who must confirm the diagnosis by using complementary techniques and to decide whether or not starting antibiotic treatment.

3. Immune system interactions

The upper and lower airways can become colonized independently of each other[15], the lower respiratory tract becoming colonized as a primary event and does not necessary need an initial colonization of the oropharynx, particularly when Gram negative bacilli such as *Pseudomonas sp* are present.
In mechanically ventilated patients suggest a similar dichotomy between upper and lower airway colonization patterns. The upper airways contact with pathogenic microbes, therefore immune recognition principles have to be tightly controlled. Nuclear factor (NF)-kB is an important and highly inducible transcriptional factor activated by a variety of microbial components that signal through innate immune toll-like-receptors (TLR) and with a pivotal role in the transcription of genes involved in inflammatory response[7]. Cytokines are important mediators in both tracheal defense and inflammation. A constitutive secretion

of TGF-β (Transforming Growth Factor) by bronchial and tracheal epithelial showed a direct inhibitory effect on T lymphocyte proliferation[16].

Recent studies have demonstrated that bronchial/tracheal epithelial (BEC) cells are functionally different and represents a first step of injury[17]. BEAS-2B bronchial epithelial cells are able to inhibit the secretion of the pro-inflammatory cytokines such as TNF- and IL-12 by monocytes, macrophages and dendritic cells.

Moreover, epithelial cell-conditioned T lymphocytes showed increased differentiation towards IL-10-producing Tr1 cells[18]. Bronchial epithelial cells induce a non-inflammatory microenvironment that regulates local immune homeostasis. These include transforming growth factor (TGF)- /TGF receptor (TGFR) 1, TNF- /TNFR1, and Fas/Fas ligand (FasL)[7]

Human bronchial/tracheal epithelial cells are more sensitive than small airway epithelial cells to induced apoptosis apparently due to a Fas response by apoptosis (caspase-8 activation) stimulation via an amplification loop involving several elements of the caspase (-8, -9, -3 and -6 in BEC, but not in SAEC). Again several pathways have been reported to be involved in inducing apoptosis of T cells[19,7].

4. Diagnosis

As mentioned above, there is a lack of agreement for definition but also no consensus on how to make a diagnosis of VAT. Several ways of diagnosis have been used and are mainly differentiated on the need for laboratory confirmation and the value assigned to the cutoff points of the isolates[4,5,6,9,10].

Typically, the diagnosis of VAT it is considered when a patient under invasive mechanical ventilation stars with fever and increased mucus production by endotracheal tube and an absence of new radiographic infiltrates, but always after having ruled out other possible foci of infection. However, this case scenario is not uncommon in critically ill patients and the mere fact of making a diagnosis of VAT may be associated with an unnecessary antibiotic treatment resulting in selection pressure on pathogens. Additional information may help to accurate the diagnosis of VAT. With the use of a bronchoscopy, the characteristics of secretions might be evaluated and also by obtaining a deeper sample is a relatively simple procedure that can help in diagnosis[13]. If during the procedure purulent secretions come from the deep portions of the lung, the possibility of VAT diagnosis is increased[13].

Obtaining a sample of respiratory secretions for subsequent quantitative culture is mandatory in all patients with suspected VAT. Performing a Gram stain technique in respiratory sample allows assessing the degree of inflammation based on the number of PML and quickly guiding the antibiotic therapy used. The discovery of a potentially pathogenic microorganism in number of 10^5, 10^4 or 10^3 CFU for BAS, BAL and protected brush respectively can also help in minimizing antibiotic overtreatment. According to some authors[4,5,6,11,14],infection can be differentiated from airway colonization and therefore stop antibiotic therapy initiated if microbial growth is below the cut-off points mentioned. However, due to the complexity of the mechanically ventilated critical patients, it is often difficult to distinguish clearly to whom antimicrobial therapy may be discontinued based on the cutoff points and a more comprehensive therapeutic approach is needed in order to evaluate whether to continue antibiotic treatment.

Inflammatory biomarkers such as C-reactive protein (CRP) and procalcitonin (PCT) have been used for the diagnosis of VAP[20,21,22] and may also help in the diagnosis of VAT. Sierra et al[15] showed that CRP may be a good indicator of infection in patients with inflammatory response syndrome. In addition, while Lisboa et al.[16] showed a good correlation between bacterial load measured as CFU/ml on quantitative culture of respiratory secretions and serum CRP, Povoa et al[17] showed that the evolution of serum CRP could be related to the recognition and development of VAP. Finally, despite of there is a lack of evidence for VAT diagnosis based on CRP, high levels of PCT and CRP (> 30 U / L) probably suggest a high bacterial load and a greater inflammatory response secondary more evident when a VAP is present.

Whereas VAP and VAT present similar clinical features, VAT does not involve lung parenchyma manifested by thoracic infiltrates in X-ray, therefore to make a differential diagnosis remains difficult in critically ill patients. The VAT may represent an intermediate process between the colonization of the lower airway and the VAP and should probably be interpreted as a continuum and dynamic process between bronchitis and pulmonary parenchymal infection[5,13]. Figure 1. It Therefore, VAT might be considered as "a particular clinical entity" that in certain patients may require specific treatment, rather than requiring a rigid and uniform definition.

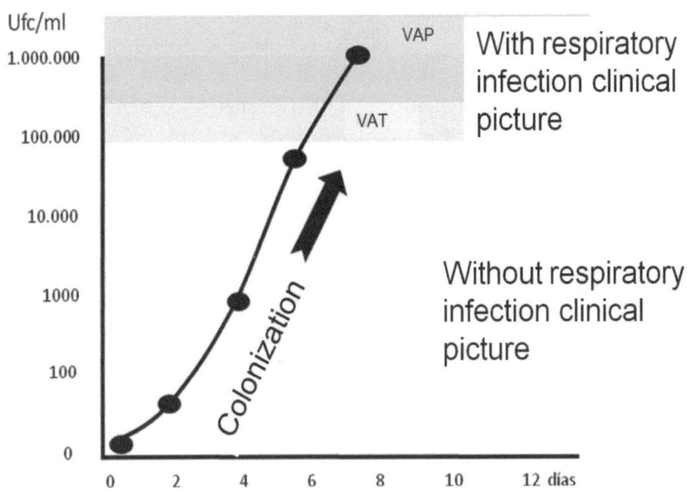

Fig. 1. Changes of tracheal colonization on mechanical ventilation patients in accordance to endotracheal bronchial aspirate. Note that colonization occurs without clinical signs of respiratory infection, Respiratory infection is present when colonization levels (CFU / ml) exceed 105. The difference between pneumonia (VAP) and tracheobronchitis (VAT) would be determined only by the lack of involvement of lung parenchyma in the VAT (Modified from reference 5).

5. Prevention and treatment

In an attempt to prevent bacterial colonization several strategies might be taken into account. Coated ETTs induced a nonsignificant reduction of the tracheal colonization, reduced bacterial colonization of the ETT and ventilator circuits, and prevented lung bacterial colonization[23].

In addition the role of tracheostomy in mechanically ventilated patients remains controversial. A patient who has a colonized airway and who undergoes percutaneous tracheotomy has an increased risk of VAP in the week following the procedure[24,7]. The presence of a plastic device always causes a low grade of local mucocutaneous inflammation. Microorganisms show an affinity for the tracheotomy rather than the oropharynx as the site of acquisition. In addition, introduction of microorganisms directly into the lower airways via the tracheotomy as a result of repeated suctioning and manipulation of the trachea represents an important exogenous pathway. Recently, Nseir et al[25] reported that tracheotomy was independently associated with a decreased risk of VAP due to the fact that liberation of the vocal cords, resulting in a reduced risk of aspiration of contaminated oropharyngeal secretions into the lung and the reduction in bacterial biofilm formation associated with regular changing of the tracheotomy cannula, but rates of tracheobronchitis were not reported. The role of tracheostomy in development of tracheobronchitis has not been studied and future research should be performed.

Prevention of lower respiratory infection in patients under MV is cornerstone in preventing the development of VAT. Different prevention strategies may also help to avoid the development of VAT and VAP subsequently which must be implemented systematically in every patient (Figure 2).

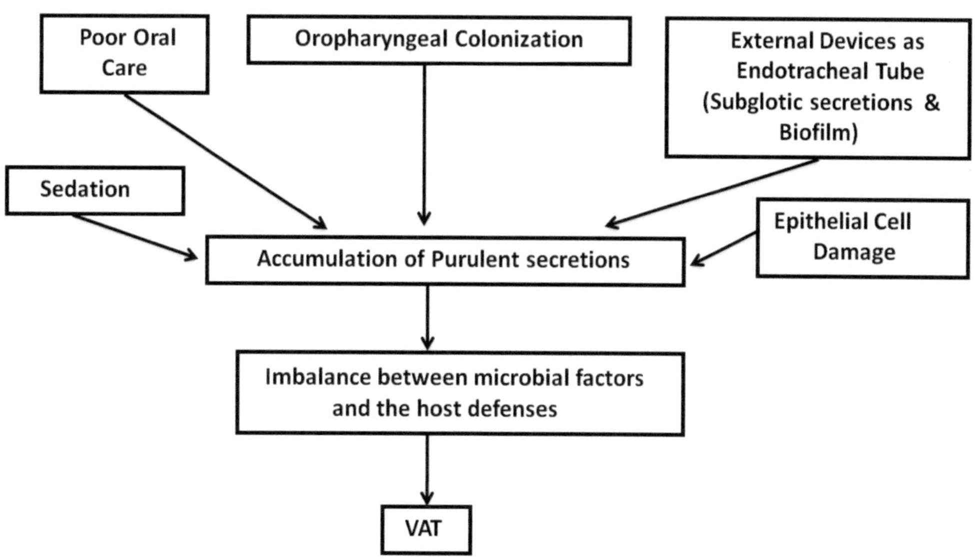

Fig. 2. Ventilator Associated Tracheobronchitis Pathophysiology

Antibiotic treatment, timing to start antimicrobial and route of administration when a patients is affected by a VAT is a subject of ongoing controversy[4,5,13].There is little doubt to start promptly intravenous antibiotic in a hemodynamically unstable patient under MV with fever when VAT is a reasonable diagnosis, and after rolling out other sources of infection. However, there are many critically ill patients presenting VAT without hemodynamic compromise. In these cases, antimicrobial therapy is questionable. The use of antibiotics in VAT has been evaluated in 2 recent Randomized Controlled Trials (RCT). Palmer et al[26] conducted a double-blind, placebo-control RCT in ICU. Patients were assigned to receive antibiotics (ATB) nebulized (gentamicin and / or vancomycin) for 14 days or until extubation or to receive placebo (saline). Patients assigned to receive nebulized

ATB had a lower incidence of VAP, faster weaning and less use of systemic ATB. These results should be interpreted with caution, since the administration of systemic ATB was not standardized and based on the attending physician. Moreover, quantitative culture of respiratory secretions was not performed. In the other hand, Nseir et al[14] conducted a prospective, multicenter randomized study in intubated patients based on surveillance quantitative culture of tracheal aspirates obtained after intubation. Patients were randomized to receive or not intravenous ATB for 8 days after performing the diagnosis of VAT by a quantitative culture of bronchial secretions with> 10^6 CFU / ml and a growth of a new pathogen not present on admission. The main findings were that the group treated with ATB had a lower mortality rate, more VM free-days and lower incidence of VAP. While these results are interesting, some important limitations of this study make to consider the findings very carefully. The study included only 34 patients after 2 years of study but had to be interrupted by the low recruitment and showed lower mortality in the interim analysis with a non pre-defined number of patients. In addition, the increased mortality in the untreated group might be due to higher incidence of *Pseudomonas aeruginosa* VAP and not directly related to the VAT.

The results of these prospective studies, although inconclusive, are attractive and open the debate regarding when patients affected by VAT should be treated or not with ATB. In our opinion, if the patient has clinical signs of VAT with fever, leukocytosis, and purulent secretions, a short course of ATB (5-7 days) should be initiated after obtaining a respiratory specimen for culture. The administration of aerosolized ATB / nebulized in patients with uncomplicated VAT is also a attractive idea, but new well-designed prospective studies are warranted in order to implement future therapeutic decisions

6. Conclusions

VAT is a relatively common entity in ventilated patients admitted to an ICU. Differential diagnosis with VAP is difficult and might require additional information based on biomarkers such as CRP or PCT. The development of VAT seems to be associated with an increase development of VAP, a longer time under MV, longer hospital stay and possibly increased mortality with probably. Recent studies seem to suggest that ATB treatment of VAT is associated with lower mortality and a reduction of days of mechanical ventilation. Nevertheless and based on the limitations suggested for previous studies conducted, the indication to start antibiotic therapy as well as the most effective route of administration should be defined by future RCT.

Until these results are published, the most appropriate behavior in a patient with symptoms of VAT seems to correspond to the administration of a short course of systemic ATB.

7. References

[1] Vidaur L, Sirgo G, Rodríguez A, Rello J. Clinical approach to the patients with suspected ventilador-associated pnuemonia. Respir Care 2005; 50:965-74

[2] Agbaht K, Lisboa T, Pobo A et al. Management of ventilator-associated pneumonia in a multidisciplinary intensive care unit: does trauma make a difference?. Intensive Care Med 2007;33:1387-95

[3] Garnacho-Montero J, Sa-Borges M, Solé-Violán J et al. Optimal management therapy for *Pseudomonas aeruginosa* ventilator-associated pneumonia: An observational,

multicenter sutdy comparing monotherapy with combination antibiotic therapy. Crit Care 2007; 35:1888-95
[4] Nseir S, Ader F, Marquette CH. Nosocomial tracheobronchitis. Curr Opin Infect Dis 2009; 22: 148-153
[5] Craven DE, Chroneou A, Zias K, Hijalmarson KI. Ventilator-associated tracheobronchitis. The impac of target antibiotic therapy on patient outcomes. Chest 2009;135:521-28
[6] Garner JS, Jarvis WR, Emori TG, Horan TC, Hughes JM. CDC definitions for nosocomial infectons, 1988. Am J Infect Control 1988;16:128-40
[7] Martín-Loeches I, Pobo A. What is new in ventilador-associated tracheobronchitis? Clin Pulm Med 2009 (in press)
[8] Malacarne P. Langer M, Nascimben E et al. Building a continuous multicenter infections surveillance system in the intensive care unit: finding from initial date set of 9493 patients from 71 Italian intensive care units. Crit Care Med 2008;36;1105-13.
[9] Nseir S, Di Pompeo C, Pronnier P et al. Nosocomial tracheobronchitis in mechanically ventilated patients: incidence aetiology and outcome. Eur Respr J 2002;20:1483-89
[10] Rouby JJ, De Lassale E, Poete P, et al. Nosocomial bronchopneumonia in the critically ill. Histologic and bacteriologic aspects. Am Rev Respir Dis 1992; 146:1059-66
[11] Rello J, Ausina V, Castella J et al. Nosocomial respiratory tract infections in multiple trauma patients : influence of level of consciousness with implications for therapy. Chest 1992; 102:525-29.
[12] Craven DE. Ventilator-associated tracheobronchitis (VAT): questions, answers, and a new paradigm?. Crit Care 2008;12:157
[13] Torres A, Valencia M. Does ventilator-associated tracheobrochitis need antibiotic treat?. Crit Care 2005;9:255
[14] Nseir S, Favory R, Jozefowicz E et al. Antimicrobial treatment for ventilator-associated tracheobronchitis: a randomized, controlled, multicenter study. Crit Care 2008;12:R62.
[15] Niederman MS, Ferranti RD. Ziegler A, Merrill WW, Reynolds HY. Respiratory infection complicating long-term tracheostomy: the implication of persistent gram-negative tracheobronchial colonization. Chest 1984; 85:39-44
[16] Ward PA, Lentsch AB Endogenous regulation of the acute inflammatory response. Mol Cell Biochem 2002 234–235: 225–228
[17] Mayer AK, Bartz H, Fey F, Schmidt LM, Dalpke AH Airway epithelial cells modify immune responses by inducing an anti-inflammatory microenvironment. Eur J Immunol. 2008 Jun;38(6):1689-99.
[18] Sillett HK, Cruickshank SM, Southgate J, and Trejdosiewicz LK. Transforming growth factor-beta promotes `death by neglect' in post-activated human T cells. Immunology 2001 102: 310–316.
[19] R. Ray, B. Keyser, D. Andres, S. Hauck, B. Benton, C. Carpin, A. Daher, C. Simbulan-Rosenthal, and D. Rosenthal Human bronchial/tracheal epithelial cells (BEC) are more sensitive than small airway epithelial cells (SAEC) to sulfur mustard-induced apoptosis apparently due to a Fas (death receptor) response amplification loop FASEB J. 22: 648.6
[20] Sierra R, Rello J, Bailén MA et al. C-reactive protein used as an early indicator of infection in patients with systemic inflammatory response syndrome. Intensive Care Med 2004; 30:2038-45

[21] Lisboa T, Seligman R, Díaz E et al. C-reactive protein correlatos with bacterial load and appropriate antibiotic therapy in suspected ventilator-associated pneumonia. Crit Care Med 2008; 36:166-171

[22] Povoa P, Coelho L, Almeida E et al. C-reactive protein as a marker of ventilador-associatedpneumonia. Eur Respir J 2005;25:804-12

[23] Kollef MH, Afessa B, Anzueto A, Veremakis C, Kerr KM, Margolis BD, Craven DE, Roberts PR, Arroliga AC, Hubmayr RD, Restrepo MI, Auger WR, Schinner R; NASCENT Investigation Group. Silver-coated endotracheal tubes and incidence of ventilator-associated pneumonia: the NASCENT randomized trial.JAMA. 2008 Aug 20;300(7):805-13

[24] Daniel T, Blandine M, Claude R,etal: Risk and routes for ventilator associated pneumonia with Pseudomonas aeruginosa. Am J Respir Crit Care Med 1998; 157:978-984

[25] Nseir S, Di Pompeo C, Jozefowicz E, et al. Relationship between tracheotomy and ventilator-associated pneumonia: a case–control study. Eur Respir J 2007; 30: 314–320

[26] Palmer LB, Smaldone GC, Chen JJ et al. Aerosolized antibiotics and venilator-associated tracheobronchitis in the intensive care unit. Crit Care Med 2008;36:2008-13

8

Recurrent Respiratory Infections in Children – Definition, Diagnostic Approach, Treatment and Prevention

Milos Jesenak[1], Miriam Ciljakova[1], Zuzana Rennerova[2], Eva Babusikova[3] and Peter Banovcin[1]
[1]*Department of Paediatrics, Comenius University in Bratislava, Jessenius Faculty of Medicine, Martin*
[2]*Pneumo-Alergo Centrum, Bratislava*
[3]*Department of Medical Biochemistry, Comenius University in Bratislava, Jessenius Faculty of Medicine, Martin*
Slovak Republic

1. Introduction

Paediatric respiratory tract infections are one of the most common reasons for physician visits and hospitalisation, and are associated with significant morbidity and mortality. Respiratory infections are common and frequent diseases and present one of the major complaints in children and adolescents. The role of physicians and other healthcare providers has expanded from merely treating disease to implementing measures aimed at health maintenance and disease prevention (Bellanti, 1997). Respiratory infections (RI), mainly involving the upper airways, are common in children and their recurrence constitutes a demanding challenge for the paediatricians. There are many children suffering from so-called recurrent respiratory infections (RRI). The child with recurrent respiratory infections presents a difficult diagnostic challenge. It is necessary to discriminate between those with simply-managed cause for their symptoms such as recurrent viral infections or asthma, from the children with more serious underlying pathology such as bronchiectasis or immune dysfunction. Many different disorders present this way, including cystic fibrosis, various immunodeficiency syndromes, congenital anomalies of respiratory tract, but in some children lung damage could follow a single severe pneumonia or can be the consequence of the inhalation of food or foreign body (Couriel, 2002). According to the epidemiological studies it was estimated that around 6% of the children younger than 6 years of age present RRI. In developed countries, up to 25% of children aged < 1 year and 18% of children aged 1-4 years experience RRI (Bellanti, 1997). Moreover, ENT infections represent the most frequent pathologies in children aged from 6 months to 6 years. Although the etiologic agents responsible for RRI are not always readily identifiable, viral agents are typically the main cause. The real task for the paediatricians is to discriminate the normal children with high respiratory infections frequency related to an augmented exposure to environmental risk factors from the children affected by other underlying pathological conditions (immunological or not), predisposing to infectious respiratory diseases (de Martino & Ballotti, 1981). Usually, the children with RRI are not affected by severe alterations and RRI represent essentially the consequence of an increased exposure to infectious agents due to environmental factors during the first years of life (Arden et al., 2006).

In the clinical practice, most of the children suffer from the recurrent infections of the upper airways, but in approximately 10-30%, the lower tract is also affected. There are two peaks of the incidence of RRI (Couriel, 2002):

- 6-12 months of age → after consumption of the maternal passively transferred immunoglobulins with concomitant postponed synthesis of own antibodies,
- the involvement of the child in to the group of children at nursery or school.

Upper respiratory infections are common but are unlikely to indicate an underlying medical condition when they occur in isolation (Wood, 2009). When evaluating the patients with recurrent infections, it is reasonable to use acronym **SPUR** (**s**evere, **p**ersistent, **u**nusual, **r**ecurrent) to prompt appropriate investigations for underlying causes. Children with RRI have the course of the airway infections (feature, severity and duration) similar to those presented by children with "normal" incidence of respiratory infections. The frequency of RI in children with RRI shows typical seasonality with the highest rate during autumn and winter (Arden et al., 2006). Typically, these children are not affected by the recurrent infections of the other systems (gastrointestinal tract, central nervous system, uro-genital tract or skin). While most children with recurrent infection have a normal immunity, it is important to recognize the child with an underlying primary immunodeficiency and investigate and treat appropriately and not over-investigate normal children (Slatter & Gennery, 2008).

RRI are a common problem mainly in preschool age, usually due to the presence of unfavourable environmental conditions, including early socialization, as well as the immaturity and inexperience of the immune system (Dellepiante et al., 2009). In infancy and early childhood the immune system encounters antigens for the first time, mounting immune responses and acquiring memory. Young children mix with other children in families or nursery and are exposed to many pathogens and therefore there are more vulnerable to infection and recurrent infections are common (Slatter & Gennery, 2008). Many of the children are simply having the repeated viral upper respiratory tract infections that are a normal part of growing up. In others, the symptoms are the first manifestations of asthma. If there is a history of persistent or recurrent pneumonia with or without chronic sputum production, it is indicating more severe pathology (Couriel, 2002). RRI initially occur as a viral respiratory tract infection, but bacterial growth is demonstrated in 60% of patients with symptoms of an upper respiratory tract infection of at least 10 days duration (Kowalska et al., 2003; Salami et al., 2008). The children with prolonged or recurrent respiratory illnesses most often have a series of infections rather than persistent infection with one virus strain (Jartti et al., 2008). Some children experience considerable morbidity as a result of RRI and receive repeated courses of antibacterials that are not effective against viral infectious agents and can increase bacterial resistance (Bousquet & Fiocchi, 2006).

2. Recurrent respiratory infections – definition

Definition of RRI is problematic and clear consensus does not exist. In case of otitis media, a reference standard for occurrence is three episodes within 6 months or four episodes within 12 months. Recurrent infectious rhinitis is usually defined as more than five episodes per year and recurrent pharyngitis or tonsillitis more than three episodes within 12 months

(Bellanti, 1997; Graham, 1990; Teele et al., 1989). Every definition of RRI is arbitrary and too generic and restrictive. Rather then defining if a child has recurrent infections with an objective numeric evaluation, it is better to know (Don et al., 2007):

- if the child generally feels good,
- if there are conditions that could be diagnosed and treated as a true disease,
- if the findings on the history and physical examination are suggestive of an immunodeficiency.

It is evident, that only a few appropriate tests are enough helpful to discriminate between a "well-being" child and a patient with immune dysfunction (Woroniecka & Ballow, 2000).
It has been proposed that to diagnose RRI at least one of the following criteria has to be present (Gruppo di Studio di Immunologia della Societá Italiana di Pediatria, 1988):

- $\geq$ 6 respiratory infections per annum,
- $\geq$ 1 respiratory infections per month involving the upper airways from September to April,
- $\geq$ 3 respiratory infections per annum involving the lower airways.

3. "Physiological" respiratory morbidity

Most children with RRI do not have any serious underlying immunological or non-immunological pathology, it is possible to talk about "physiologic" respiratory in children. It means that certain number of respiratory infections can be considered as physiological due to the development of immature immune system in these children. The normal frequency of the respiratory tract is six to eight episodes during the autumn and winter in infancy (in children aged 1-5 years) and two to four episodes in older children (aged 6-12 years). Even the higher frequency of respiratory infections can be a source of great worry of the parents or paediatricians, most of the children with RRI are practically not ill and we are not able to detect any serious underlying illness or disturbance of immune system (de Vries, 2001).

4. Immunology of recurrent respiratory infections

The recurrent respiratory infections in infants and children are among the most common causes of counselling and admission to the hospital. They are responsible for significant morbidity measured by school days lost. Many factors can play an important role in the genesis of the episodes of RRI that can act alone or together. In some children, it is possible to detect also transient or permanent immune system deficiencies (Bellanti, 1997). It should be pointed, that a true immunodeficiency is rare and the first cause of RRI is the childhood itself (Wheeler, 1996), because both humoral and phagocytic immunity reach their best efficacy during the first fifth or sixth years of age (Wheeler & Steiner, 1992; Yang & Hill, 1991). Typically, children with RRI are usually not affected by severe alterations of the immune system functions. The majority of these children do not have recognised immunodeficiencies, but some may have low levels of some laboratory parameters, usually of immunoglobulin isotypes or rarely other immunological parameters such as phagocytosis. Some of the observed immunological alterations are of questionable significance and not convincingly related to an increased susceptibility to respiratory infections (Litzman et al., 1999). Most children with RRI do not have an immunodeficiency. If they do, this is often due to an antibody deficiency. Finocchi et al. (2002) evaluated humoral immune defects in apparently 67 non-atopic patients with recurrent infections and in 55% a humoral defect was diagnosed.

According to the literature, several alterations in immune system and its function have been observed among children suffering from RRI (Atkinson et al., 2004; Bossuyt et al., 2007; Day et al., 2004; de Martino & Ballotti, 2007; Don et al., 2007; Finocchi et al., 2002; Gomi et al., 2004; Ianni et al., 2001; Kvestad et al., 2006; Li Volti et al., 2003; Ottenhoff et al., 2002; Pryjma et al., 1999):

- defects of Fcγ receptor IIIa (CD16) on natural killer cells,
- defect of interleukin receptor-associate kinase 4 (IRAK4),
- reduction in IL-12 production,
- polymorphisms in genes *CCR2*, *CCR5* and mannose-binding lectin gene,
- mutations in TLR-4 encoding sequences,
- defective removal of the apoptotic neutrophils by alveolar macrophages,
- pathologic phagocytosis and production of reactive oxygen intermediates from polymorphonuclear cells,
- decrease neutrophil chemotaxis,
- mild decrease in the number of $CD4^+$, $CD8^+$, $CD19^+$ and NK-cells,
- alterations in the cytokine production by lymphocytes (↑ IL-4, ↑ IL-10, ↓ IFN-γ, ↓ IL-2),
- decreases IgM, IgA, IgG subclasses, mannose-binding lectin, L-ficolin,
- defects in the production post-infectious specific antibodies.

The children with estimated diagnosis of RRI usually have no significant alteration of the immune system and its functions. Coexistence of two or more partial mild immune deteriorations in children with RRI, which was observed by several authors, confirms the secondary post-infective nature of these changes (Bossuyt et al., 2007). It is probable, that all the observed non-specific deteriorations of immunity are rather the consequence of repeated viral infections than the predisposing factor leading to RRI. Various infections (especially viral) can influence immune reaction, cytokine responses and phagocytosis. The combination of RRI and viral infection can lead to the deeper virus-induced immune dysfunction which can favour the recurrence of further respiratory infections (de Martino & Ballotti, 2007; Li Volti et al., 2003).

5. Recurrent respiratory infections as a warning sign of primary immunodeficiencies

Primary immunodeficiencies (PID) are generally the results of genetic defects that interfere with a component of the immune system. In general, these disorders are rare with some exceptions such as selective IgA deficiency or mannose-binding lectin deficiency. The most frequent PID are usually asymptomatic or have only mild clinical symptoms.

An underlying immunodeficiency is more likely when some of the following "warning" symptoms or signs occur (Champi et al., 2002; Slatter & Gennery, 2008):

- eight or more new ear infections (otitis media) within 12 months,
- two or more serious sinus infections within 12 months,
- two or more episodes of pneumonia within 12 months,
- two or more invasive infections in the history (meningitis, cellulitis, osteomyelitis, septicaemia),
- failure of an infant to gain weight or grow normally ± chronic diarrhoea,
- recurrent deep skin or organ abscesses,
- persistent superficial candidiasis after age 1 year,
- two or more months on antibiotics with little or no effect,

- need for intravenous antibiotics to clear infections,
- a family history of primary immunodeficiency.

A pattern of recurrent or persistent infection is the major manifestation of primary immunodeficiencies. While most children with RRI have normal immunity, it is essential to recognise the child with underlying PID and investigate and treat appropriately. Prompt, accurate diagnosis of PID helps to direct the most appropriate treatment, predict prognosis and facilitate genetic counselling for the family.

6. Risk factors for recurrent respiratory infections

The increased prevalence of RRI in younger children could be attributed to the several factors (de Martino & Ballotti, 2007):

- increased exposure to infectious agents during the first years of life, especially when the child is attending a group of children at preschool- or school facilities,
- general immaturity of the immune system of younger children,
- social and environmental factors e.g. day-care attendance, family size, air pollution, parental smoking, home dampness.

To the risk factors contributing to the increased frequency of respiratory infections in children with RRI belong (Ballow, 2008; Bellanti, 1997; Bloomberg, 2011; Bousquet & Fiocchi, 2007; de Martino & Ballotti, 2007, Don et al., 2007; Karmaus et al., 2008; Wheeler, 1996):

- day-care attendance,
- early socialization,
- large family size, overcrowding,
- positive family history on atopic diseases,
- school-aged siblings,
- praematurity,
- low bodyweight infants,
- reduction of breast-feeding,
- climate and environmental factors (indoor and outdoor pollutions exposure),
- home dampness,
- pets at home (especially cats and dogs),
- parental smoking and smoking in pregnancy,
- anatomic or functional alterations of the upper or lower airways,
- allergy/atopy,
- gastroesophageal reflux,
- male gender,
- poor socio-economic conditions with malnutrition,
- intense training and physical stress,
- missed vaccination.

6.1 Day-care attendance

Comparing the children in day-care centres with those cared at home, the first one have substantially higher risk of acute respiratory infections. Approximately 70% of the children with RRI attend day-care centres and about 75% of them start to suffer from RRI during their first year at child-care facilities (Celedon et al., 1999). Early enrolment can although on one side accelerate the acquisition of immunological experiences, but on the other hand this requires the cost on the disease because of the naivety of the immune system. The younger the child, the greater risk of developing of symptomatic infection and therefore the postponed enrolment of children at day-care centres may prevent this excess risk of acute respiratory illness (de Martino & Balloti, 2007; Kamper-Jorgensen et al., 2006). It is known, that children attending day care outside home are more likely to have infections than children in home care. Early recurrent infections in early life are associated with asthma and reduced lung functions (Shaheen et al., 1994), although it has also been suggested that such infections may have a protective effect on later asthma (Cookson & Moffatt, 1997). It was confirmed that also the number of the children in collective have influence on the incidence of RRI (Marbury et al., 1997).

6.2 Indoor pollution and climate

It was showed that dose-response relation between the number of cigarettes smoked in the home and RI in children exists (Jaakkola et al., 2006; Stick, 2006). Maternal smoking during the pregnancy can influence the development of the immune system of the infants (Noakes et al., 2006). Passive smoking, allergic inflammation and predisposing anatomic variants play an important role in RRI (Arrieta et al., 2004). The exposure to home dampness and moulds (especially early in life), increased the risk of the development of atopic diseases and common respiratory infections.

6.3 Outdoor pollutions

It has been observed the relation between the outdoor pollutions (e.g. SO_2, NO_2) and the augmented respiratory symptoms, reduced expiratory flow rates, incidence of chronic cough or the increased risk of hospitalization due to respiratory infections (Colley, 1975; Chauhan & Johnston, 2003).

6.4 Physical stress

The association between increased psychical and physical stress and the frequency of respiratory infections was suggested by several studies. Highly trained athletes present a higher risk of RRI incidence. During the extreme physical stress several deterioration in the immune system have been reported (e.g. transitory decrease in serum IgA levels, reduction of phagocytosis, decrease of NK-cells) (Bergendiova et al., 2011; Nieman et al., 2002; Tiollier et al., 2005) and also possible prevention of these changes with some immunomodulators such as beta-glucans has been achieved (Bergendiova et al., 2011). It was also observed, that infants attending swimming pool during the first year of life have higher frequency of RRI and otitis media (Nystad et al., 2003).

6.5 Positive family history on atopic diseases

Positive family history on atopic and allergic respiratory diseases is significantly associated with increased risk of recurrent wheezing in children (Chong & Neto, 2010). On the other hand, the recurrent respiratory infections do not protect these children from the development of the atopic diseases of the airways (Balemans et al., 2006; Ciprandi et al., 2006). The children of parents with atopy have higher risk of respiratory tract infections (Nystad et al., 2003).

6.6 Atopy

Non-recognised allergy could lead to the similar clinical picture as RRI or could make the airways more susceptible to the infectious agents, esp. viruses. The relation between atopy and RRI has been evaluated in several studies, but the results were inconclusive. It was documented, that atopy is a frequent condition among the children with RRI and it is likely that atopy is a favouring factor for RRI (Dellepiante et al., 2009). Atopy affects 15-20% of children and causes chronic inflammation of the airways that can mimic recurrent of chronic upper respiratory infections. Atopy can also facilitate the adherence of pathogens to the respiratory epithelium and thus promote infections (Ballow, 2008). Allergic children have more numerous and severe respiratory infections than non-allergic children (Ciprandi et al., 2006).

7. Diagnostic approach to the child with recurrent respiratory infections

The assessment of the children with RRI is demanding: it requires close attention to the history and examination, and in the selected cases, extensive investigations. Early and accurate diagnosis is essential to ensure that optimal treatment is given and to minimize the risk of progressive or irreversible lung damage. The challenge for the physicians is to distinguish between the child with self-limiting or minor problems and the child with serious, perhaps progressive lung disease. The most common and frequent symptoms of recurrent respiratory infections is chronic cough.

Diagnostic algorithm should be aimed on the exclusion of the underlying severe illness. The diagnosis of RRI is very probable if:

- milder respiratory infection with the similar characteristics as the respiratory infections in children with normal respiratory "morbidity" (severity, duration, absence of complications, good response to the conventional symptomatic therapy and empirical antibiotic therapy),
- the absence of severe and invasive systemic infections,
- absence of failure to thrive,
- negative family history for immune disorders.

To the diagnostic algorithm of RRI belongs the investigation of the possible causes of chronic cough, such as allergy, asthma, α1-antitrypsin deficiency, primary or secondary ciliary dyskinesias, congenital anomalies, gastroesophageal reflux (GER), recurrent pulmonary aspiration of post-nasal drip syndrome (the most frequent cause of chronic cough in children) (de Martino & Ballotti, 2007). The recurrence of the infections in the same specific site should be aimed the attention to the possible congenital developmental anomalies of the respiratory tract or the presence of foreign aspirated body. Recurrent or chronic infections can be associated with anatomic defects that characteristically involve one organ system (Panigada et al., 2009). Foreign body should be considered when the infections are chronic and localized to one anatomical sire, e.g. one ear canal or one nostril. Recurrent symptoms in small children accompanied by malabsorption or nasal polyps should be re-evaluated for possible cystic fibrosis (CF), also despite negative neonatal screening. The incidence of CF is in some countries more common when compared with an incidence of PID. Therefore, the combination of above mentioned symptoms is indication to perform sweat test with the following genetic analysis. RRI can be also the sign of repeated aspiration of gastric content in GER, swallow dysfunction, under-diagnosed bronchial asthma or immotile cilia syndrome (Vaughan & Katkin, 2002). Recurrent otitis media is associated with Eustachian tube dysfunction secondary to atopy (Ghezzi et al., 2011). GER is usually associated with asthma symptoms, but sometimes can be confused with bronchitis or lead to aspiration and recurrent pneumonias. GER can be also factor involved in the pathogenesis of recurrent otitis media and sinusitis. Children who develop recurrent pneumonia from aspiration in association with GER tend to be younger than 2 years of age. Children who have a history of nocturnal cough or wheeze with exercise or protracted coughing after upper respiratory illnesses should undergo spirometry and assessment of bronchodilator responsiveness (Panitch et al., 2005). Recurrent sino-pulmonary infections with *situs viscerum inversus* may indicate immotile cilia syndrome (primary ciliary dyskinesia, Kartagener syndrome) (Ballow, 2008; Skeik & Jabr, 2011).

The evaluation of the frequency of respiratory infections is usually less important, that the assessment of other characteristics of RRI such as:

- the course of the infections,
- alteration of the general health status,
- duration,
- accompanying fever,
- possible complications,
- response to the standard symptomatic therapy,
- response to the empiric antibiotic treatment,
- causal isolated pathogen.

The diagnostic algorithm for children with RRI contains (de Vries, 2001; Slatter & Gennery, 2008):

- ENT examination with exclusion of adenoidal hypertrophy,
- chest X-ray,
- determination of specific IgE or the performance of skin prick test with common inhalant and food allergens,
- measurement of total IgE levels in serum,
- determination of the levels of IgG, IgA and IgM in serum,
- blood cell count together with absolute count of lymphocytes, neutrophil and eosinophil granulocytes,
- bacteriological cultivation and serological tests,
- viral serological tests,
- in selected patients:
  - levels of IgG-subclasses,
  - production of specific post-vaccination antibodies against *Streptococcus pneumoniae, Haemophilus influenzae type b,* tetanus and diphtheria toxoids taken 4 weeks after vaccination of not previously exposed to vaccine antigens,
  - levels of C3 and C4 components of complement, mannose-binding lectin and functional tests of complement system (CH_{50}, AP_{50}).

8. Treatment and prevention of recurrent respiratory infections

The children with RRI represent a great challenge for the paediatricians, from both therapeutic and preventive standpoints. It is necessary to determine whether these RRI are because of host-derived factors or are the result of increased environmental exposure. Host derived factors may be non-immunological and immunological (related to host immunodeficiency.

In recent years, following the increase in the incidence of antibiotic resistance, interest in preventive treatment has intensified. Such treatment should contribute to the prevention of

RRI, thus reducing the usage and excessive consumption of antibiotics (Marseglia et al., 2007). A diagnosis of viral infection does not justify prescription of antibiotics.
Recent approach in the prevention of RRI includes the encouragement of breastfeeding, the use of intravenous or subcutaneous immunoglobulins and respiratory syncytial virus immune globulin, as well as methods of stimulating immunity, such as bacterial lysates or various nature-based products (Bellanti, 1997).

8.1 Bacterial extracts (lysates)

Since the 1970s, when using of bacteria-derived immune modulators started, several products were developed and their using becomes very popular around the world. Currently more than 8 million patients are treated with bacterial extracts every year and approximately 150 million patients have been treated since their licensing (Bousquet & Fiocchi, 2006).
Bacterial extracts are made from different bacterial species most frequent responsible for recurrent respiratory or urinary tract infections. The most often included species are: *Staphylococcus aureus, Streptococcus viridans, Streptococcus pneumoniae, Streptococcus pyogenes, Klebsiella pneumoniae, Klebsiella ozenae, Moraxella catarrhalis, Hemophilus influenzae.* Bacterial extracts are usually administered orally, although subcutaneous or intranasal forms were tested sooner (Braido et al., 2007; Matricardi et al., 2003).
Bacterial immune modulators could be divided into two-generation preparations:

1. First generation products are bacterial extracts containing killed bacteria or their lysate.
2. Second generation products contain the most immunogenic components of bacteria (e.g. ribosomes, proteoglycans).

Bacterial extracts stimulate both non-specific and specific immunity mechanisms through naturally evoked immune response. The intrusion of pathogen in the human body leads first to non-specific response and consequently to specific response for the epitopes of the pathogen. Bacteria recognition and response takes place in mucosal associated lymphoid tissue (MALT). Typically bacterial extracts are administered orally and absorbed in the intestine, triggering Payer's patches in gut associated lymphoid tissue (GALT). M-cells in Payer's patches are responsible to bacterial recognition. Toll-like receptors (TLR) and other receptors recognize components common to a range of bacteria (e.g. lipopolysaccharide, peptidoglycan, lipoteichoic acid, lipoarabinomannan, un-methylated DNA with CpG motif and bacterial lipoproteins), so-called pathogen-associated molecular patterns (PAMPs). Interactions between PAMPs and TLR result in the activation of dendritic cells, macrophages, NK cells with cytokines and chemokines production, activation of phagocytosis and early pathogens destruction. Enhanced innate immune response also stimulates adaptive immune response. Antigen-specific T and B cells are generated in the Payer's patches as well as a considerable number of lymphoblasts, mostly IgA+ precursors of the IgA producing plasmocytes. Lymphocytes and lymphoblasts maturate in mesenteric lymph node and subsequently migrate into mucosal associated lymphoid tissue in different organs. The protective effect of bacteria-derived immune modulators is particularly related to memory cells and antigen-defined induction of immunoglobulin synthesis, mostly IgA, with quick and specific immune response after future contact with the same antigen (Braido et al., 2007; Del-Rio-Navarro et al., 2006; Rozy & Chorostowska-Wynimko, 2008).
In vitro studies showed that the action of OM-85 BV is mediated, at least in part, by the activation of TLR2 and TLR4 (Alyanakian et al., 2006). Proteoglycans from cell membrane of

Klebsiella pneumoniae strain has been described as a potential TLR-2 inducer (Bellanti et al., 2003). Bacterial extracts enhance natural killer cells activity, increase production of proinflamatory cytokines, increase the expression of adhesion molecules in phagocytes, inhibit serum induced IL-12 expression in peripheral blood lymphocytes (Rozy & Chorostowska-Wynimko, 2008; Matricardi et al., 2003). Bacterial extracts up-regulated oxidative metabolism, superoxide anion and nitric oxide production (Manuel et al., 1989). Bacterial immune modulators induce maturation of dendritic cells; enhanced expression of CD83, CD86 and HLA II molecules - markers of dendritic cells maturation has been observed following bacterial extracts application. Dendritic cells might be important for preferential triggering of T_H1 response (Boccaccio et al, 2002; Zelle-Rieser et al., 2001). In newborn animals bacterial extracts increase IFN-γ and decrease IL-4 productions, which contribute to preferential development of the T_H1 immunity (Bowman & Holt, 2001).

Various clinical trials with children, both young (< 6 yrs) as well as school children, have demonstrated positive effect of bacterial extracts mostly on frequency, duration of the infection episodes and less antibiotic requirements. Recently, reduction of rate and duration of wheezing attacks and improvement of atopic dermatitis after treatment with bacterial extracts in children has been described (Brunetti et al., 2005; Razi et al., 2010). On the other hand, some studies have not demonstrated preventive effect of bacterial immunotherapy (Saracho-Weber et al., 2001; Vautel et al., 1993).

Findings from different clinical trials have been evaluated and summarized with some review and meta-analysis. However, due to heterogeneity and often the poor quality of the trials, the results should be interpreted with caution. Cochrane meta-analysis from 2008 evaluated the effect of all used immune modulators to acute respiratory tract infections in children. 34 placebo-controlled trials were included (24 with bacterial extracts). This review showed that immunostimulants reduce the incidence of acute respiratory infections in children, by 40% on average. The subgroup analysis of bacterial extracts studies produced similar results, with lower heterogeneity (Del-Rio-Navarro et al., 2006). In review performed by Braido et al. (2007) both in children and adults protective effect of bacterial extracts was found such as general reduction of infection rates, reduction of their duration, beneficial effect on symptoms, and reduction of the use of antibiotics. Bousquet & Fiocchi (2006) review demonstrated that ribosomal immunotherapy reduces number, duration, and severity of infectious episodes, reduce antibacterial use and the likelihood of consequent development of bacterial resistance. Other favorable results included a reduction in antibacterial treatments, shorter duration of recurrent episodes, reduced need for other medications, smaller number of lost school days or parent absenteeism from work, less fever, and reduced hearing loss (Bousquet & Fiocchi, 2006). In other review the effect of OM-85 BV to acute respiratory infections in children were examined. 13 included trials were of low or moderate quality. There was a trend for fewer and shorter infections and a reduction of antibiotic use in group treated by bacterial extract versus placebo, but with weak evidence (Steuer- Stey et al., 2007). Recently, other meta-analysis with OM-85 BV has been published. This meta-analysis includes 8 randomized controlled trials and shows significant decrease of recurrent respiratory tract infections frequency. The effect seems to be greater in patients at increased risk of RRI (Schaad, 2010).

Safety and tolerance of bacterial extracts in all paediatric trials were good. Adverse events occurred occasionally and were mild and transitory with rapid resolution. The majority of adverse events were gastrointestinal or cutaneous findings. Reported adverse effects included eczema, urticaria, diarrhoea, abdominal pain, headache, rhinitis, and cough. No serious adverse events in relation with bacterial extracts treatment have been reported in the literature (Del-Rio-Navarro et al., 2006; Olivieri et al., 2009; Schaad, 2010). No casual association between bacterial extracts and autoimmunity disease has been reported in literature (Olivieri et al., 2009).

8.2 Biologically active polysaccharides (glucans)

Metabolites and components of fungi have been used in medicine for many centuries in order to exploit the properties of several of their active compounds. Many of these substances naturally contained in fungi have demonstrable effects on different components of the immune system. The most important groups of these immunomodulating substances include: polysaccharides (glucans in particular), polysaccharide peptides, polysaccharide proteins and proteins. The main mechanism is their mitogenic and activating effect on different populations of immunocompetent cells, such as hemopoietic stem cells, lymphocytes, macrophages, dendritic cells and NK cells, and subsequent production of several cytokines with complex effects. Besides typical immune system cells, glucans also have demonstrable effects on other cell populations, such as fibroblasts, keratinocytes, or other connective tissue cells. This is why many clinical and experimental studies have focused on the effects of these substances on the prevention and treatment of acute and recurring infectious diseases, congenital and acquired immune disorders, oncologic, autoimmune and allergic diseases (Lull et al., 2005; Vetvicka & Vetvickova, 2009).
Glucans are polysaccharides of natural origin, naturally appearing in fungi, plants and some bacteria. In fungi, they represent the main component of cell walls, and are composed of glucose molecules bound with two types of bonds: β-(1→3) in the main linear chain and β-(1→6), which binds side chains of variable length to the main polysaccharide chain. Immunomodulating effects of various extracts from fungi have been known for a long time, but recently, the attention has been focused mainly on glucans, which occur in nature as a typical structural element of fungal cell walls. They represent a large group of natural substances with immunomodulating effects, and the structure and mechanism of action of many of them have been described in detail. Particular glucans differ in the intensity of their immunostimulating/immunomodulating effect. Imunoglucan - pleuran (*Pleurotus ostreatus*, Oyster mushroom), Schizophyllan (*Schizophyllum commune*, Split gill) and Lentinan (*Lentinus edodes*, Shiitake mushroom) are considered the most effective ones (Lull et al., 2005).
There are several possible mechanisms of action of glucans on the immune system. The activation of human immune system is enhanced through a system of receptors that are able to recognize the so called molecular patterns of microorganism pathogenicity (PAMPs, *pathogen-associated molecular patterns*). Receptors able to identify these PAMPs include mostly those that are involved in recognizing extracellular pathogens - Toll-like receptors and C-type lectin receptors. On the other hand, the activation of these receptors triggers a cascade of inflammatory response associated with subsequent release of many cytokines, chemokines and other soluble factors that lead to the activation of several populations of immunocompetent cells of both specific and non-specific part of the immune system, and the development of antigen-specific immunity (Vetvicka & Vetvickova, 2009). The ability of glucans to activate various components of the immune system and thus modulate the immune response depends on the length of their chain, level of branching, as well as on their tertiary structure (Bohn & Bemiller, 1995). The ability of glucans to modulate the immune response has many potential applications in both clinical and experimental medicine in order to provide an effective defence against negative influences from both

external (e.g. microorganisms) and internal environment (e.g. tumour or damaged cells). Many studies focused on the effects of parenterally administered glucans, although the research has confirmed that they are also active and effective when administered orally (Hong et al., 2004). Among all the glucan receptors (dectin-1, Toll-like receptors, complement receptor 3, so called scavenger receptors, lactosylceramide, etc.), the most important is dectin-1, which is a primary receptor for glucans at least on the surface of leukocytes and plays an essential role in immunomodulation mediated through glucans (Brown & Gordon, 2003; Chen & Seviour, 2007). Whether particular glucans show immunostimulating or immunosuppressive effects in different phases of the immune response depends on the dosage, method of application, frequency of administration, as well as on the overall state of the organism' immune system.

Glucans act on the immune system on many levels. Among all the known mechanisms, the following should be highlighted in particular (Chen & Seviour, 2007; Kodama et al., 2002; Lehne et al., 2006; Lesourd, 1997; Wasser, 2002):

- ↑ metabolic and functional activity of immunocompetent cells (specific and non-specific immunity),
- ↑ proliferation and differentiation of both T and B lymphocytes,
- ↑ content of secretory IgA antibodies in saliva, thus increasing local defence of mucous membranes,
- ↑ phagocytosis → ↑ effectiveness of immune response to both endogenous and exogenous stimulus,
- ↑ bactericidal activity of monocytes and neutrophils,
- they activate complement cascade through both classic and alternative pathways with subsequent formation of many compounds with direct or indirect immunomodulating effect,
- stimulating effect on NK cells → ↑ defence against intracellular viral, bacterial and parasitic infections,
- ↑ phenotypic and functional maturation of dendritic cells (DC), they potentiate the stimulating effect of DC on the proliferation of T lymphocytes and increase the expression of several differentiating marks on the surface of DC (e.g. MHC I, MHC II, CD-86, CD-80, etc.) → more effective presentation of foreign antigens,
- ↑ release and activity of many enzymes (such as lysozyme, elastase, collagenase, nitric oxide synthase), complement components, cytokines (IL-1β, IL-10, IL-12, IL-18, TNF-α, IFN-γ, GM-CSF), other signal molecules (nitric oxide and other nitro-compounds) → proliferation of immunocompetent cells, their migration, ↑ bactericidal and cytocidal effect,
- they have a regulatory effect on the differentiation of T_H1/T_H2 lymphocytes → ↑ Th1 immune response → ↑ IL-10, IL-2, IL-18 → reduction of the symptoms of allergic diseases and prevention of the development of atopy,
- ↑ T_H1 cytokine response with simultaneous suppression of Th2 response → potential use in diseases and states associated with Th1 response insufficiency (e.g. type II diabetes mellitus, ageing), as well as in diseases with inadequate stimulation of T_H2 response (e.g. allergic diseases).

One of the most important indications of glucans application in children are recurring infections of upper and lower respiratory tract, primary and secondary immunodeficiencies of different etiology, as well as repeated administration of antibiotics. Semberova et al. (2009) observed a significant decrease in the volume of adenoid vegetation in children after 40-days treatment using a product containing glucan.

The effect of imunoglucan (Imunoglukan P4H® syrup) on the course and frequency of recurrent infections of upper respiratory tract has shown also multi-centric study. A positive response to the treatment, i.e. ≥50% reduction of the frequency of recurrent respiratory infections, was observed in 153 children (71.2%). The average annual incidence of respiratory infections in children with a positive response to the syrup was 3.6 and was significantly lower compared to that in unresponsive patients (3.6 vs. 8.9, $p<0.001$). The therapy did not show statistically significant effect on the frequency of febrile episodes, need for antibiotics or duration of infection. No adverse effects of Imunoglukan P4H® were reported, with the therapy being very well tolerated. This study proved the therapeutic and preventive effects of biologically active polysaccharides on the frequency of recurrent respiratory infections in children (Jesenak et al., 2010).

8.3 Systemic enzyme therapy

A therapeutic method consisting of a systemic peroral administration of special combined mixtures of enzymes has been gradually developed since the middle of the 20th century. This method was named systemic enzyme therapy (SET). Initially, SET was applied only empirically. Currently, there are a number of relevant data about a biological availability of active substances, their complex activities as well about their favourable clinical effects in many inflammatory diseases (Honzikova et al., 2004). Originally, an empirical treatment of mainly inflammatory diseases due to the many controlled clinical studies was changed to a method which optimizes and modulates several immune functions disrupted in many pathological states. SET is predestinate to using in many indications by their targeted intervention into regulatory and biochemical pathways. The basic pharmacological effects of SET include anti-oedematous, fibrinolytic, anti-inflammatory and immunomodulatory activities (Biziulevicius, 1998; Kleine, 1998). Enzymes bind to the blood antiproteases after resorption through the mucosa of gastrointestinal tract and then they are distributed to sites of inflammation where they modulate and restore the imbalance in immune responses. They are involved in the activation as non-specific as specific immunity mechanisms (Biziulevicius, 1998; Desser et al., 2001; Douwe, 2005; Manhart et al., 2002; Targoni et al., 1999; Zavadova et al., 1995; Zavadova & Desser, 1997). Enzyme therapy can change the expression of adhesion molecules and receptors on the surface of T lymphocytes, reduce the activation of many populations of immunocompetent cells and they increase the activation threshold of autoaggressive T-lymphocytes in the mechanism of specific immunity (Biziulevicius, 1998; Desser et al., 2001; Douwe, 2005; Lauer et al., 2001; Manhart et al., 2002; Targoni et al., 1999; Zavadova et al., 1995; Zavadova & Desser, 1997). Generally, we can say that SET is involved in the regulation of both acute and chronic inflammatory processes, as well as in the activation of individual components of the immune system.

Many respiratory disease of infectious or allergic etiology became an important indication for the using of SET. SET has only additional importance in the case of allergic diseases and it normalizes disrupted functions of immune system. SET appears to be a good adjuvant treatment of atopic dermatitis and asthma. SET reduces the number of febrile states, helps to reach a compensation of disease and reduces the dose of inhaled corticosteroids in asthmatic patients. Many studies have demonstrated the effect of SET in recurrent respiratory infections. The Czech post-multicenter study compared the effect of SET (preparation Wobenzym ®) and the bacterial immunomodulators (BIM) on the course and recurrence of respiratory infections in a cohort of 468 children aged 3-18 years. In both groups, there was a statistically significant decrease in the average number of respiratory tract inflammation (by 59% in SET and 32% for BIM) and the average number of related antibiotic treatments (68% in SET and 35% for BIM). The positive results achieved by the administration of SET can be explained by favourable immunomodulatory effects of these preparations (Honzikova et al., 2004). Similar effects were also observed other authors (Helms and Miller, 2006; Lanchava et al., 2005; Zavadova et al., 1995). Interesting finding was also the observed improvement in spirometric lung function indices following the application of SET in children with recurrent obstructive bronchitis (Lanchava et al., 2005). SET administration is also effective in the treatment of acute or chronic sinusitis, tonsillitis, acute and recurrent laryngitis and chronic secretory otitis media (Vegh & Vegh, 2009). In patients with elevated IgE, the application of SET can result in the decline or even normalization of their levels.

8.4 Isoprinosine

Isoprinosine (inosiplex, inosine pranobex) is a synthetic immunomodulating agent with pluripotent effects on the immune system. It possesses T-lymphocyte and phagocyte function enhancing immuno-modulating effect similar to those of another synthetic drug, levamisole. Isoprinosine was developed as an anti-viral agent, but in reality, the action of Isoprinosine in viral infections has been attributed to immunomodulatory rather than direct anti-viral effects. *In vitro*, Isoprinosine enhances T-lymphocyte function, stimulates NK cell activity, macrophages and neutrophils. It increases IL-1, IL-2 and interferon gamma production and up-regulates interleukin-2 receptor expression. The data on the effect of this agent on the frequency a re-occurrence of RRI are conflicting. The study of Litzman et al. (1999) does not support the continued use of Isoprinosine in the prevention of RRI in children with normal immune systems. The use of Isoprinosine in the patients with mild but clearly defined immunodeficiencies is probably effective (Litzman et al., 1999).

8.5 Transfer factors

Transfer factors (TFs) present a complex of low-molecular biologically active substances with possible effect of normalization of the disturbances in humoral and cellular immunity. Transfer factors are small proteins that "transfer" the ability to express cell-mediated immunity from immune donors to non-immune recipients. We developed a process for purifying specific transfer factors to apparent homogeneity. This allowed us to separate individual transfer factors from mixtures containing several transfer factors and to demonstrate the antigen-specificity of transfer factors (Kirkpatrick, 2000). The treatment with TFs is an active immunotherapy, which is based on the application of the substance with the capacity to influence the reactivity of the organism to different immunogenic impulses. TFs act as an antigen-dependent, antigen-specific micromolecular polypeptide cytokine. There are two possible sources of TFs: the extract from the peripheral bovine or human leucocytes. The mechanism of TFs action consists from the influence of both specific and non-specific immunity (Barnet et al., 1996; Bystron et al., 1996).

Several studies have demonstrated the effect of TFs in the treatment and prevention of recurrent respiratory or urinary infections in children and also in adults (Anttila et al., 1977; Grohn, 1977; Jose & Ford, 1976). TFs can be used also in the prevention of recurrent herpetic infections, in different secondary immunodeficiencies (especially of cellular immunity) or as a complementary therapy of psoriasis vulgaris, atopic eczema, sepsis or chronic fatigue syndrome. It is also possible to apply Tfs in the cases without confirmed immunodeficiency (Jones et al., 1981; Meduri et al., 1996; Pizza et al., 1996).

8.6 Thymus hormones

On the market there are available preparations containing extract of thymus from different animals. These products are generally recommended as a dietary supplement to restore and strengthen the immune system. They are polypeptide complexes: peptides and signalling factors designed to optimize intercellular communication between cells of the immune system and for maturation, proliferation and activation of T-lymphocytes. Extracts of thymus contain complex mixture of peptides with a stimulating effect on T-lymphocytes and they are called thymus hormones. They have immuno-normalizing effect, so do not affect normal immune function, but reduced functions return to the normal state. Among the indications of using of these products are included acute, chronic and recurrent respiratory infections. They are non-toxic, with minimum side effects. This preparations are contraindicated for pregnant and breastfeeding women and patients taking immunosuppressants. Nowadays their production is stopped and it is tested the production of synthetic analogs (Ambrogi et al., 1983; de Mattia et al., 1993; Longo et al., 1988).

8.7 Vitamins and minerals

Vitamins and minerals are necessary for normal immune system function. Low levels of vitamins and minerals, caused mainly by malnutrition, lead - besides other complications - to increase of infection rate. It is questionable if prophylactic treatments in "healthy" subjects can influence frequency and duration of respiratory tract infections.
Numerous studies have evaluated effect of vitamin C supplementation to prevention of respiratory tract infections with various results. Preventive treatment with vitamin C reduced cold duration and severity of symptoms (Douglas et al., 2004).
Several trials and meta-analysis have examined prophylactic use of zinc for respiratory tract infections with mixed results (Aggarwal et al., 2007; Mathew, 2010). In some children studies decrease incidence of upper or lower respiratory infections has been observed (McElroy & Miller, 2002; Roth et al., 2008).
Also clinical trials examining effect of routine vitamin A supplementation to prevention and treatment of respiratory infections have yielded contradictory results; no significant effect in children has been observed (Roth et al., 2008).

8.8 Prebiotics, probiotics & nucleotides

Breastfeeding is associated with a significant decrease incidence of respiratory infections. Breast milk contains variety of substance with antimicrobial, anti-inflammatory and immunomodulatory activity. High concentration of oligosaccharides in breast milk induces accurate colonization of infant neonatal tract, predominantly with *Bifidobacteria* and *Lactobacili*. Healthy gut flora protect against infection via a number of mechanisms including competitive inhibition of epithelial binding by enteropathogenic bacteria and effects on tight junctions. Accurate colonization plays also important role in the development of mucosal and systemic immune system, and tolerance to non-pathogenic antigens (Jones et al., 2010).
Nonhuman milk oligosaccharides - prebiotics, such as small-chain galacto-oligosaccharides and long-chain fructo-oligosaccharides are used to substitute these functions in formula-fed infants. Supplementation with neutral oligosaccharides leads to optimalized colonization like in breast-feeding infants, but the clinical outcomes are not conclusive yet. Reduced incidence of atopic diseases has been described (Arslanoglu et al., 2008; Moro et al. 2006). Some studies confirmed positive effect of oligosaccharides supplementations in infant formula to incidence of respiratory infections (Arslanoglu et al., 2007).

Breast milk is also rich in nucleotides with immunomodulatory activity. Beneficial effect of nucleotides supplementations in formula-fed infants on various components of the immune system has been reported. Nucleotides added to infant formula augment infantile NK-cell activity and humoral response and my have limited protection against diarrhoea (Jones et al. 2007, Pickering et. al, 1998).

Probiotics are defined as "live microorganisms which when administered in adequate amounts confer a health benefit on the host" (FAO/WHO). The most common bacteria in this group include *Bifidobacteria* and *Lactobacili.* Use of probiotics early in life could favour correct maturation of the immune system, and reduce development of allergy. Effects of probiotics include competitive inhibition with pathogenic bacteria, immunomodulation of local immunity (maintains gut wall integrity) and systemic immunity (enhances non-specific and specific response) (Singh & Das, 2010). The most documented efficacy of probiotics is in the treatment and prevention of infectious and antibiotic-associated diarrhoea. Probiotics are generally regarded as safe, but caution must be given in immunocompromised patients. Only a limited number of trials have evaluated the potential effect of probiotics in reducing the risk respiratory tract infections with inconsistent results. Studies differed in the probiotic strains evaluated, indications for use, dosing or study design. Review of 14 performed trials showed, that probiotics may have a beneficial effect on the severity and duration of symptoms, but do not appear to reduce the incidence of RRI (Vouloumanou et al., 2009).

8.9 *Echinacea* extracts

Non-prescriptional natural therapeutics are used widely and their popularity continue to increase, including children's treatment. Usually these products are well tolerated and believed to be safe, but the true safety is often unknown. Usually there are limited data about efficacy, mechanism of action, active components, and potential drugs - herbal interactions. Well-controlled trials with reliable data about different products are often missing.

Echinacea extracts are one of the most frequent used herbal preparations, especially in North America. Traditionally these herbs were used by indigenous peoples for the treatment of many illnesses (colds and other respiratory diseases, wound healing, candidiasis). Nowadays *Echinacea* extracts are predominantly used for treating and preventing respiratory tract infections, mainly common cold and influenza.

The photochemical composition of *Echinacea* preparations may differ widely both between and within species. *Echinacea* products contain variable amounts of ingredients with pharmacological activity, such as polysaccharides, flavorous, chicory acid glycosides, essential oils, oxyacetylene and alkyl amides (Gunning, 1999). The biological activities of *Echinacea* appear to be the result of a combined action of its components rather that of one single group.

Several studies have shown *in vitro* and *in vivo* effects on immunological parameters, but until now the clear immunomodulatory mechanism has not been identified. *Echinacea* appears to affect mainly non-specific immune response. Macrophage activation, enhanced neutrophil phagocytosis and cytokine expression has been reported (Melchart et al., 1995; Synching et al., 2006). Stimulation of the cannabin receptor (CB2) by alamedas present in *Echinacea* could also play a role in immunomodulatory activity (Rudner et al., 2006). Bactericidal effect against some of the bacteria (*Streptococcus pyogenes, Homophiles influenzae, Legion Ella pneumophilla*) and direct antiviral effects have been also described (Fusco et al., 2010; Sharma et al., 2010).

Many clinical trials with different *Echinacea* preparations have been conducted with variable results on reduction, duration and severity of symptoms associated with respiratory infection. Majority of studies have been performed in adults for assessment the effect of *Echinacea* extracts in the treatment of acute infection, mainly common cold. Some studies have reported decrease frequency, duration and severity of respiratory tract infection, but some did not find any positive effect of *Echinacea* treatment (Barrett et al., 2010; Goel et al., 2004; Melchart et al., 1998; O'Neil et al., 2008; Sperber et al., 2004). In children's study was found no effect on duration of illness or severity of symptoms. Treatment with *Echinacea* was associated with increased risk of rash compared with placebo group (Taylor et al., 2003). In other study treatment with extract of *Echinacea*, vitamin C and propolis reduced significantly number and duration of illness episodes in children when compared with placebo treated group (Cohen et al., 2004). Several meta-analysis were performed with great heterogeneity of trials and results suggest that *Echinacea* extracts might have beneficial effect in the early treatment of common colds, but the there was insufficient evidence to suggest an effect on prevention (Gilles et al., 2000; Linde et al., 2006; Shah et al., 2007). On the other hand, in other meta-analysis *Echinacea* extracts were effective in prevention of the common cold after clinical inoculation (Schoop et al., 2006).

Echinacea products apart from allergic reactions and increased incidence of rash are reported to be generally safe (Mullins, 1998; Mullins & Heddle, 2002). *Echinacea* preparation should not be used by patients with allergy to other members of the Asteraceae family due to possible cross-reactivity. *Echinacea* extracts should be avoided by patients with progressive immune diseases, on treatment with corticosteroids and immunosuppressants. *Echinacea* should not be taken orally for more than 8 weeks because of the potential for decreased immune response after a long-term application (Gunning, 1999).

8.10 Ginseng

Ginseng is composed of a number of different species, which belong to the same plant family, the Araliaceae. Korean, Japanese and American ginseng belong to the genus Panax, whereas Siberian ginseng is of the genus Eleutherococcus (Vohra et al., 2008). Polysaccharide and oligosaccharide fractions are responsible for the immunomodulating effects of North American ginseng (Panax quinquefolium L., Fam. Araliaceae), glykosides called eleutherosides for effects of Siberian ginseng (Mc Elhaney et al., 2004; Roxas et al., 2007).

Ginseng products *in vitro* induce the production of INF-γ, TNF-α, IL-1, IL-2, IL-6, stimulate natural killer cell activity, increase phagocytosis. B-cell proliferation in the spleen with increased circulating immunoglobulin G levels has also been demonstrated (Jie et al., 1984; Kim et al., 1990; Wang et al., 2001). Subjects who took extract of Siberian ginseng for one months have had a significant increase in total lymphocyte, T helper, T suppressor, natural killer and B lymphocyte cells counts compared to placebo. *In vitro* liquid extract of the Siberian ginseng root inhibits replication of RNA viruses (Glatthaar-Saalmuller et al., 2001). Extracts appear to have cytotoxic effects on a wide range of tumour cell lines.

Clinical studies performed mainly in adults showed variable results (Mc Elhaney et al., 2004; Preddy et al., 2005). In the reviews of 5 trials with North American ginseng there was insufficient evidence to conclude that ginseng reduces the incidence or severity of common colds. It appears to be effective in shortening the duration of cold or acute respiratory infections (Seida et al., 2009). In one trial with Siberian Ginseng decrease frequency of respiratory infections in children was observed (Vohra et al., 2008).

8.11 Astralagus

Astralagus membranaceus is rich in polysaccharides, flavonoids, multiple trace minerals and amino acids, all of them contribute to Astragalus's complex immunomodulatory properties. Astralagus demonstrated activation and proliferation of immune cells, particularly $CD8^+$ and $CD4^+$ T lymphocytes compared to placebo. In one trial with small number of children treatment with Astralagus extract reduced incidence of respiratory tract infections (Roxas & Jurenka, 2007).

8.12 Viscum album

Viscum album extracts were shown to have immunomodulatory functions, especially on NK cell functions (Braedel-Ruoff, 2010). *Viscum album* is widely used in complementary medicine for the treatment of cancer. The effects on frequency of recurrent respiratory infections were examined in one trial in children living in areas exposed to the radioactive fallout from Chernobyl. Preparations were effective in reducing frequency of infections and reducing clinical symptoms (Chernyshov et al., 2000).

8.13 Propolis

Propolis, the bee's product, has highly variable composition, depending on geographic location, plant species and the season of collection. Biological activity is mainly due to flavonoids, terpens, caffeic, ferulis and cumaric acids and esters. Anti-microbial and anti-inflammatory properties of propolis documented in some *in vitro* studies may be useful for prevention of upper respiratory tract infections (de Vecchi & Drago, 2007). In children with recurrent acute otitis media suspension of propolis and zinc significantly reduce the risk of new acute otitis media episodes (Marchisio et al., 2010). Because of pollen containing in propolis suspension there is a risk of allergic reactions and sensitisation and preventive treatment with propolis should not be recommended in general for children.

8.14 Other natural products

Different natural products declare to have immunomodulating properties or be assigned to treatment and prevention of acute respiratory disease (e.g. elderberry, garlic, larch arabinogalactans - polysaccharides from *Larix occidentalis*, olive leaf extracts, tea tree oil, colostrum). Until now insufficient number of trials with these preparations have been done, frequently only *in vitro* studies, or with small number of participants (rarely with children) and questionable quality, so it is difficult to make any conclusions regarding use of these preparations in prevention of acute respiratory tract infections.

9. Follow-up and education

When a diagnosis of RRI has been formulated, parents or care-givers should be reassured about the benign and transient nature of this condition. Accurate environmental prophylaxis and regimen changes are crucial. When RRI diagnosis has been formulated, removal of environmental risk factors (e.g. precocious day-care attendance, reducing the smoking in the household) must first be suggested. In some cases, the postponed enrolment of children at day-care centres could be the solution for the prevention and decrease number of RRI. Optimal day-care centres enrol only a limited number of children, have large clean rooms with a good ventilation to guarantee the removal of the air suspended microbial agents and are located in modern buildings in areas with less air pollution (de Martino & Ballotti, 2007;

Uhari et al., 1999). Prophylactic antibiotic treatment is neither indicated nor useful, even could interfere with normal development of the mucosal microflora and immune system functions. In the selected children, adenoidectomy and tonsillectomy should be recommended according to the validated guidelines (Frohna, 2005). Children with RRI are "immunologically normal" and therefore intensive impacts into the developing immune system can be harmful and contra-productive.

10. Conclusion

Respiratory diseases belong to the most frequent and common disorders in clinical praxis of every paediatrician. Recurrent viral infections are part of the growing up process of any child. Especially in children we can observe some which suffer from recurrent upper or lower respiratory tract infections. In general, a thriving child with recurrent respiratory infections does not suffer from a serious underlying disease. Most of the children do not have an immunodeficiency, but if they do, this often concerns an antibody deficiency. It there positive history for immunodeficiency, detailed immunological investigation is mandatory. In other children, immunological examination should be performed after the exclusion of other, more frequent causes of RRI such as gastroesophageal reflux, allergy or ENT focal infection (adenoidal hypertrophy). Treatment and prevention of these infections has its own rules and should consist of early, aimed antibiotic therapy acute attacks of infection, long and appropriate reconvalescence, elimination of all possible focuses and origins of infection and complete examination of the child's immunostatus. There are several possibilities of immunomodulating therapy. Many clinical and experimental trials have confirmed their efficacy and pharmacological safety. The prescription and application of each immunomodulation agent should be performed in correct manner only in indicated cases with individual approach to each child taking into account all the rules of immunomodulation therapy.

11. Acknowledgement

This work was supported by project "**MEASUREMENT OF CILIARY KINETICS OF THE RESPIRATORY TRACT**" co-financed from EU sources and European Regional Development Fund.

12. References

Adams, E.L., Rice, P.J., Graves, B., Ensley, H.E., Yu, H., Brown, G.D., Gordon, S., Monteiro, M.A., Papp-Szabo, E., Lowman, D.W., Power, T.D., Wempe, M.F., & Williams. D.L. (2008). Differential high affinity interaction of Dectin-1 with natural or synthetic glucans is dependent upon primary structure and is influenced by polymer chain length and side chain branching. *The Journal of Pharmacology and Experimental Therapeutics*, Vol. 325, No. 1, (April 2008), pp. 115-123.

Aggarwal, R., Sentz, J., & Miller, M.A. (2007). Role of zinc administration in prevention of childhood diarrhea and respiratory illnesses: a meta-analysis. *Pediatrics,* Vol. 119, No. 6, (June, 2007), pp. 1120-1130.

Akramiene, D., Kondrotas, A., Didziapetriene, J., & Kevelaitis, E. (2007). Effects of β-glucans on the immune system. *Medicina (Kaunas)*, Vol. 43, No. 8, pp. 597-606.

Alyanakian, M.A., Grela, F., Aumeunier, A., Chiavaroli, C., Gouarin, C., Bardel, E., Normier, G., Chatenoud, L., Thieblemont, N., & Bach, J.F. (2006). Transforming growth factor-{beta} and natural killer T-cells are involved in the protective effect of a bacterial extract on type 1 diabetes. *Diabetes,* Vol. 55, No. 1, (January, 2006), pp. 179–185.

Ambrogi, F., Petrini, M., Caracciolo, F., Azzara, A., & Carulli, G. (1983). Effect of thymostimulin on human lymphocytes adenosine deaminase and purine nucleotide phosphorylase activities: physiological and therapeutic effects. *Advances in Experimental Medicine and Biology,* Vol. 166, pp. 101-104.

Antilla, R., Grohn, P., & Krohn, K. (1977). Transfer factor and cellular response in urinary infections in children. *Acta Paediatrics Scandinavica,* Vol. 66, No. 2, (March 1977), pp. 219-224.

Arden, K.E., McErlean, P., Nissen, M.D., Sloots, T.P., & Mackay, I.M. (2006). Frequent detection of human rhinoviruses, paramyxoviruses, coronaviruses and bocavirus during acute respiratory tract infections. *Journal of Medical Virology,* Vol. 78, No. 9, (September 2006), pp. 1232-1240.

Arrieta, A., & Singh, J. (2004). Management of recurrent and persistent acute otitis media: new option with familiar antibiotics. *Pediatric Infectious Diseases Journal,* Vol. 23, Suppl. 2, (February 2004), pp. 115-124.

Arslanoglu, S., Moro, G.E., & Boehm, G. (2007). Early supplementation of prebiotic oligosaccharides protects formula fed infants against infections during the first 6 months of life. *The Journal of Nutrition,* Vol.137, No. 11, (November 2007), pp. 2420-2424.

Arslanoglu, S., Moro, G.E., Schmitt, J., Tandoi, L., Rizzardi, S., & Boehm, G. (2008). Early dietary intervention with a mixture of prebiotic oligosaccharides reduces the incidence of allergic manifestations and infections during the first two years of life. *The Journal of Nutrition,* Vol. 138, No. 6, (June 2008), pp. 1091-1095.

Atkinson, A.P. M., Cedzynski, M., Szemraj, J., Swierzko, A. St., Bak-Romaniszyn, L., Banasik, M., Zeman, K., Matsushita, M., Turner, M.L., & Kilpatrick, D.C. (2004). L-ficolin in children with recurrent respiratory infections. *Clinical and Experimental Immunology,* Vol. 138, No. 3, (December 2004), pp. 517-520.

Balemans, W.A., Rovers, M.M., Schildern, A.G., Sanders, E.A., Kimpen, J.L., Zielhuis, G.A., & Ent, C.K. (2006). Recurrent childhood upper respiratory tract infections do not reduce the risk of adult atopic disease. *Clinical & Experimental Allergy,* Vol. 36, No. 2, (February 2006), pp. 198-203.

Ballow, M. (2008). Approach to the patient with recurrent infections. *Clinical Review in Allergy and Immunology,* Vol. 34, No. 2, (April 2008), pp. 129-140.

Barnet, K., Vacek, A., Cech, K., & Pekarek, J. (1996). The effect of DLE-fractions on GM-progenitors on haemopoetic stem cells in vitro. *Biotherapy,* Vol. 9, No. 1-3, pp. 171-174.

Barrett, B., Brown, R., Rakel, D., Mundt, M., Bone, K., Phyto, D., Barlow, S., & Ewers, T. (2010). Echinacea for Treating the Common Cold. A Randomized Trial. *Annals of International Medicine,* Vol. 153, No. 12, (December, 2010), pp. 769-777.

Bellanti, J., Olivieri, D., & Serrano E. (2003). Ribosomal immunostimulation: assessment of studies evaluating its clinical relevance in the prevention of upper and lower respiratory tract infections in children and adults. *BioDrugs,* Vol. 17, No. 5, pp. 355–367.

Bellanti, J.A. (1997). Recurrent respiratory tract infection in paediatric patients. *Drugs,* Vol. 54, Suppl. 1., pp. 1-4.

Bergendiova, K., Tibenska, E., & Majtan, J. (2011). Pleuran (β-glucan from *Pleurotonus ostreatus*) supplementation, cellular response and respiratory tract infections in athletes. *European Journal of Applied Physiology,*

Bhave, S.Y. (2001). Approach to recurrent respiratory infections. *Indian Journal of Pediatrics,* Vol. 68, Suppl. 2, (April 2001), pp. 26-32.

Biziulevicius, G.A. (2006). Where do the immunostimulatory effects of oral proteolytic enzymes (‚systemic enzyme therapy') come from? Microbial proteolysis as a possible starting point. *Medical Hypotheses,* Vol. 67, No. 6, (July 2006), pp. 1386-1388.

Bloomberg, G.R. (2011). The influence of environment, as represented by diet and air pollution, upon incidence and prevalence of wheezing illnesses in young children. *Current Opinion in Allergy and Clinical Immunology,* Vol. 11, No. 2, (April 2011), pp. 144-149.

Boccaccio, C., Jacod, S., Kaiser, A., Boyer, A., Abastado, J.P., & Nardin, A. (2002). Identification of a clinical-grade maturation factor for dendritic cells. *Journal of Immunotherapy,* Vol. 25, No. 1, (January-February 2002), pp. 88-96.

Bohn, J.A., & BeMiller, J.N. (1995). (1 → 3)-beta-D-glucans as biological response modifiers: a review of structure-functional activity relationships. *Carbohydrate Polymers,* Vol. 28, pp. 3-14.

Bossuyt, X., Moens, L., Van Hoeyveld, E., Jeurissen, A., Bogaert, G., Sauer, K., Proesmans, M., Raes, M., & De Boeck, K. (2007). Coexistence of (partial) immune defects and risk of recurrent respiratory infections. *Clinical Chemistry,* Vol. 53, No. 1, (January 2007), pp. 124-130.

Bousquet, J., & Fiocchi, A. (2006). Prevention of recurrent respiratory tract infections in children using a ribosomal immunotherapeutic agent. A clinical review. *Pediatric Drugs,* Vol. 8, No. 4, (December 2006), pp. 235-243.

Bowman, L.M., & Holt, P.G. (2001). Selective enhancement of systemic Th1 immunity in immunologically immature rats with an orally administered bacterial extract. *Infection and Immun*ity, Vol. 69, No. 6, (Jun 2001), pp. 3719–3727.

Braedel-Ruoff, S. (2010). Immunomodulatory effects of Viscum album extracts on natural killer cells: review of clinical trials. *Forsch Komplementmedicine,* Vol. 17, No. 2, (April, 2010), pp. 63-73.

Braido, F., Tarantini, F., Ghiglione, V., Meliolli, G., & Canonica, G.W. (2007). Bacterial lysate in the prevention of acute exacerbation of COPD and in respiratory recurrent infections. *International Journal of Chronic Obstructive Pulmonary Disease,* Vol. 2, No. 3, (September 2007), pp. 335–345.

Brown, G.D. (2006). Dectin-1: a signalling non-TLR pattern-recognition receptor. *Nature Reviews Immunology,* Vol. 6, No. 1, (January 2006), pp. 33-43.

Brown, G.D., & Gordon, S. (2003). Fungal beta-glucans and mammalian immunity. *Immunity,* Vol. 19, No. 3, (September 2003), pp. 311-315.

Brown, G.D., & Gordon, S. (2005). Immune recognition of fungal β-glucans. *Cellular Microbiology,* Vol. 7, No. 4, (April 2005), pp. 471-479.

Brunetti, L., Francavilla, R., Tesse, R., Fiermonte, P., Dambra, P., Massagli, M., Loria, M.P., & Armenio, L. (2005). Effects of oral bacterial immunotherapy in children with atopic eczema/dermatitis syndrome: A pilot study. *BioDrugs,* Vol. 19, No. 6, (2005), pp. 393-399.

Bystron, J., Cech, K., Pekarek, J., & Jilkova, J. (1996). Effect of anti-herpes specific transfer factor. *Biotherapy,* Vol. 9, pp. 73-75.

Celedon, J.C., Litonjua, A.A., Weiss, S.T., & Gold, D.R. (1999). Day care attendance in the first year of life and illness of the upper and lower respiratory tract in children with a familial history of atopy. *Pediatrics*, Vol. 104, No. 3, (September 1999), pp. 495-500.

Champi, C. (2002). Primary immunodeficiency disorders in children: prompt diagnosis can lead to lifesaving treatment. *Journal of Pediatrics Health Care*, Vol. 16, No. 1, (January-February 2002), pp. 16-21.

Chauhan, A.J., & Johnston, S.L. (2003). Air pollution and infection in respiratory illness. *British Medical Bulletin*, Vol. 68, No. 1, (December 2003), pp. 95-112.

Chen, J., & Seviour, R. (2007). Medicinal importance of fungal beta-(1 → 3), (1 → 6)-glucans. *Mycological Research*, Vol. 111, No. 6, (June 2007), pp. 635-652.

Chernyshov, V.P., Heusser, P., Omelcheno, L.I., Chernyshova, L.I., Vodyanik, M.A., Vykhovanets, E.V., Galazyuk, L.V., Pochinok, T.V., Gaiday, N.V., Gumenyuk, M.E., Chong Neto, H.J., Rossario, N., Solé, D. & Mallol, J. (2010). Associated factors for recurrent wheezing in infancy. *Allergy*, Vol. 65, No. 3, (March 2010), pp. 406-407.

Ciprandi, G., Tosca, M.A., & Fasce, L. (2006). Allergic children have more numerous and severe respiratory infections than non-allergic children. *Pediatric Allergy and Immunology*, Vol. 17, No. 5, (August 2006), pp. 389-391.

Cohen, H.A., Varsano, I., Kahan, E., Sarrell, E.M., & Uziel, Y. (2004). Effectiveness of an herbal preparation containing echinacea, propolis, and vitamin C in preventing respiratory tract infections in children: a randomized, double-blind, placebo-controlled multi-center study. *Archives of Pediatrics and Adolescent Medicine*, Vol. 158, No. 3, (March, 2004), pp 217-221.

Colley, J.R. (1975). Air pollution and respiratory disease in children and young adults. *Community Health (Bristol)*, Vol. 7, No. 1, (July-August 1975), pp. 28-31.

Cookson, W.O.C.M., & Moffatt, M.F. (1997). Asthma: an epidemic in the absence of infections? *Science*, Vol. 275, No. 5296, (January 1997), pp. 41-42.

Couriel, J. (2002). Assessment of the child with recurrent chest infections. *British Medical Bulletin*, Vol. 61, No. 1, (March 2002), pp. 115-132.

Day, N., Tangisinmankong, N., Ochs, H., Rucker, R., Picard, C., Casanova, J.L., Haraguchi, S., & Good, R. (2004). Interleukin receptor-associated kinase (IRAK-4) deficiency associated with bacterial infections and failure to sustain antibody response. *Journal of Pediatrics*, Vol. 144, No. 4, (April 2004), pp. 524-526.

de Martino, M., & Balloti, S. (2007). The child with recurrent respiratory infections: normal or not? *Pediatric Allergy and Immunology*, Vol. 18, Suppl. 18, (November 2007), pp. 13-18, ISSN 0905-6157.

de Martino, M., Galli, L., & Vierucci, A. (1989). The child with recurrent respiratory infections. In: *Pathogenesis and Control of Viral Infections*, Aiuti F., eds., pp. 225-231, Raven Press, ISBN-13: 9780881675085, New York.

de Martino, M., Rossi, M.E., Muccioli, A.T., & Vierucci, A. (1984). T lymphocytes in children with recurrent respiratory infections: effect of the use of thymostimulin on the alterations of T-cell subsets. *International Journal of Tissue Reactions*, Vol. 6, No. 3, pp. 223-228.

de Mattia, D., Decandia, P., Ferrante, P., Pace, D., Martire, B., Ciccarelli, M., Caradonna, L., Ribaud, M.R., Jirillo, E., & Schettini, F. (1993). Effectiveness of thymostimulin and study of lymphocyte-dependent antibacterial activity in children with recurrent respiratory infections. *Immunopharmacology and Immunotoxicology*, Vol. 15, No. 4, (August 1993), pp. 447-459.

de Vecchi, E., & Drago, L. (2007). Propolis antimicrobial activity: what's new? *Le infezioni in Medicina*, Vol. 15, No. 1, (March, 2007), pp.7-15.

de Vries, E. (2001). Immunological investigations in children with recurrent respiratory infections. *Paediatric Respiratory Reviews*, Vol. 2, No. 1, (March 2001), pp. 32-36.

Dellepiane, R.M., Pavesi, P., Patria, M.F., Laicini, E., Di Landro, G., & Pietrogrande, M.C. (2009). Atopy in preschool Italian children with recurrent respiratory infections. *La Pediatrica Medica e Chirurgica*, Vol. 31, No. 4, (July-August 2009), pp. 161-164.

Del-Rio-Navarro, B.E., Espinosa-Rosales, F.J., Flenady, V., & Sienra-Monge, J.J.L. (2006). Immunostimulants for preventing respiratory tract infection in children. *Cochrane Database of Systematic Reviews*, Vol. 18, No. 4, (October 2006), CD004974.

Desser, L., Holomanova, D., Zavadova, E., Pavelka, K., Mohr, T., & Herbacek, I. (2001). Oral therapy with proteolytic enzymes decreases excessive TGF-β levels in human blood. *Cancer Chemother Pharmacol*, 47, 2001. s. 10-15.

Don, M., Fasoli, L., Gregorutti, V., Pisa, F., Valent, F., Prodan, M., & Canciani, M. (2007). Recurrent respiratory infections and phagocytosis in childhood. *Pediatrics International*, Vol. 49, No. 1, (February 2007), pp. 40-47.

Engwerda, C.R., Andrew, D., Ladhams, A., & Mynott, T.L. (2001). Bromelain modulates T cell and B cell immune responses *in vitro* and *in vivo*. *Cellular Immunology*, Vol. 210, No. 1, (May 2001), pp. 66-75.

Finocchi, A., Angelini, F., Chini, L., Di Cesare, S., Cancrini, C., Rossi, P., &Moschese, V.(2002). Evaluation of the relevance of humoral immunodeficiencies in a pediatric population affected by recurrent infections. *Pediatric Allergy and Immunology*, Vol. 13, No. 6, (December 2002), pp. 443-447.

Frohna, J.G. (2005). Effectiveness of adenotonsillectomy in children with mild symptoms of throat infections of adenotonsillar hypertrophy: open, randomized controlled trial. *Journal of Pediatrics*, Vol. 146, No. 3, (March 2005), pp. 435-436.

Fusco, D., Liub, X., Savagec, C., Taurb, Y., Xiaoe, W., Kennellye, E., Yuanf, J., Cassilethg, B., Salvatorea, M., & Papanicolaoub, G.A. (2010). *Echinacea purpurea* aerial extract alters course of influenza infection in mice. *Vaccine*, Vol. 28, No. 23, (May, 2010), pp. 3956–3962.

Ghezzi, M., Silvestri, M., Guida, E., Pistorio, A., Sacco, O., Mattioli, G., Jasonni, V. & Rossi, G.A. (2011). Acid and weakly acid gastroesophageal refluxes and type of respiratory symptoms in children. *Respiratory Medicine*, ahead of print.

Giles, J.T., Palat, C.T.III, Chien, S.H., Chang, Z.G., & Kennedy, D.T. (2000). Evaluation of Echinacea for treatment of the common cold. *Pharmacotherapy*, Vol. 20, No. 6, (June, 2000), pp.690-697.

Ginseng C.A. Meyer in the mouse. *Agents and Actions*, Vol. 15, No. 3-4, (October, 1984), pp. 386–391.

Glatthaar-Saalmuller, B., Sacher F., & Esperester A. (2001). Antiviral activity of an extract derived from roots of *Eleutherococcus senticosus*. *Antiviral Research*, Vol. 50, No. 3, (June, 2001), pp. 223-228.

Goel, V., Lovlin, R., Barton, R., Lyon, M.R., Bauer, R., Lee, T.D., & Basu, T.K. (2004). Efficacy of a standardized echinacea preparation (Echinilin) for the treatment of the common cold: a randomized, double-blind, placebo-controlled trial. *Journal of Clinical Pharmacy and Ther*apeutics, Vol. 29, No. 1, (February, 2004), pp. 75-83.

Gomi, K., Tokue, Y., Kobayashi, T., Takahashi, H., Watanabe, A., Fujita, T., & Nukiwa, T. (2004). Mannose-binding lectin gene polymorphism is a modulating factor in repeated respiratory infections. *Chest*, Vol. 126, No. 1, (July 2004), pp. 95-99.

Graham, M.H. (1990). The epidemiology of acute respiratory infections in children and adults: a global perspective. *Epidemiologic Reviews*, Vol. 12, No. 1, pp. 149-178.

Grohn, P. (1977). Transfer factor in chronic and recurrent respiratory tract infections in children. *Acta Paediatrica Scandinavica*, Vol. 66, No. 2, (March 1977), pp. 211-217.

Gruppo di Studio di Immunologia della Società Italiana di Pediatria. (1988). Le infezioni ricorrenti nel bambino: definizione ed approccio diagnostico. *Rivista di Immunolgia ed Allergologia Pediatrica*, Vol. 2, pp. 127-134.

Gunning, K. (1999). Echinacea in the treatment and prevention of upper respiratory tract infections. *The Western Journal of Medicine*, Vol. 171, No. 3, (September, 1999), pp. 198-200.

Helms, S., & Miller, A.L. (2006). Natural treatment of chronic rhinosinusitis. *Alternative Medicine Review*, Vol. 11, No. 3, (September 2006), pp. 196-207.

Hong, F., Yan, J., Baran, J.T., Allendorf, D.J., Hansen, R.D., Ostroff, G.R., Xing, P.X., Cheung, N.K., & Ross, G.D. (2004). Mechanism by which orally administered beta-1,3-glucans enhance the tumoricidal activity of antitumor Monoclonal antibodies in murine tumor models. *Journal of Immunology*, Vol. 173, No. 2, (July 2004), pp.797-806.

Honzikova, M. (2004). Systémová enzymoterapie v komplexní léčbě recidivujících zánětů dýchacích cest u dětí - postregistrační retrospektivní multicentrické hodnocení. *Česko-slovenská Pediatrie*, Vol. 59, pp. 513-521.

Ianni, A., Majore, S., Arzani, D., Carboni, I., Corbo, G.M., & Romano-Spica, V. (2001). CCR2 and CCR5 gene polymorphisms in children with recurrent respiratory infections. *Respiratory Medicine*, Vol. 95, No. 5, (May 2001), pp. 430-432.

Jaakkola, J.J., Kosheleva, A.A., Katsnelson, B.A., Kuzmin, S.V., Privalova, K.I., & Spengler, J.D. (2006). Prenatal and postnatal tobacco smoke exposure and respiratory health in Russian children. *Respiratory Research*, Vol. 7, No. 48, (March 2006), pp. 1-9.

Jartti, T., Lee, W.M., Pappas, T., Evans, M., Lemanske, R.F., & Gern, J.E. (2008). Serial viral infections in infants with recurrent respiratory illnesses. *European Respiratory Journal*, Vol. 32, No. 2, (August 2008), pp. 314-320.

Jesenak, M., Sanislo, L., Kuniakova, R., Rennerova, Z., Buchanec, J., & Banovcin, P. (2010). Imunoglukan P4H® in the prevention of recurrent respiratory infections in childhood. *Cesko-Slovenska Pediatrie*, Vol. 65, No. 11, pp. 639-647.

Jones, K.D.J., Berkley, J.A., & Warner, J.O. (2010). Perinatal nutrition and immunity to infection. *Pediatric Allergy and Immunology*, Vol. 21, No. 4p1, (Jun 2010), pp.564–576.

Jones, J.F., Minnich, L.L., Jeter, W.S., Pritchett, R.F., Fulginiti, V.A., & Wedgwood, R.J. (1981). Treatment of childhood Epstein-Barr virus/cytomegalovirus infection with oral bovine transfer factor. *Lancet*, Vol. 2, No. 8238, (July 1981), pp. 122-124.

Jose, D.G., & Ford, G.W. (1976). Therapy with parent´s lymphocyte transfer factor in children with infection and malnutrition. *Lancet*, Vol. 1, No. 7954, (February 1976), pp. 263-266.

Kamper-Jorgensen, M., Wohlfahrt, J., Simonsen, J., Gronbaek, M., & Benn, C.S. (2006). Population-based study of the impact of childcare attendance on hospitalizations for acute respiratory infections. *Pediatrics*, Vol. 118, No. 4, (October 2006), pp. 1439-1446.

Karmaus, W., Dobai, A.L., Ogbuanu, I., Arshard, S.H., Matthews, S., & Ewart, S. (2008). Long-term effects of breastfeeding, maternal smoking during pregnancy, and recurrent lower respiratory tract infections on asthma in children. *Journal of Asthma*, Vol. 45, No. 8, (October 2008), pp. 688-695.

Kirkpatrick, C.H. (2000). Transfer factors: identification of conserved sequences in transfer factor molecules. *Molecular Medicine*, Vol. 6, No. 4, pp. 332-341.

Kodama, N., Komuta, K., Sakai, N., & Nanba, H. (2002). Effects of D-fraction, a polysaccharide from Grifola frondosa on tumor growth involve activation of NK cells. *Biological & Pharmaceutical Bulletin*, Vol. 25, No. 12, (December 2002), pp. 1647-1650.

Kowalska, M., Kowalska, H., Zawadzka-Glos, L., Debska, M., Szerszen, E., Chmielik, M., & Wasik, M. (2003). Dysfunction of peripheral blood granulocyte oxidative metabolism in children with recurrent upper respiratory tract infections. *International Journal of Pediatric Otorhinolaryngology*, Vol. 67, No. 4, (April 2003), pp. 365-371.

Kvestad, E., Kvaerner, K.J., Roysamb, E., Tambs, K., Harris, J.R., & Magnus, P. (2006). Recurrent otitis media and tonsillitis: common disease predisposition. *International Journal of Pediatric Otorhinolaryngology*, Vol. 70, No. 9, (September 2006), pp. 1561-1568.

Lanchava, N., Nemsadze, K., Chkhaidze, I., Kandelaki, E., & Nareklishvili, N. (2005). Wobenzym in treatment of recurrent obstructive bronchitis in children. *Georgian Medical News*, Vol. 127, (October 2005), pp. 50-53.

Lehne, G., Haneberg, B., Gaustad, P., Johansen, P.W., Preus, H., & Abrahamsen, T.G. (2006). Oral administration of a new soluble branched beta-1,3-D-glucan is well tolerated and can lead to increased salivary concentrations of immunoglobulin A in healthy volunteers. *Clinical and Experimental Immunology*, Vol. 143, No. 1, (January 2006), pp. 65-69.

Lesourd, B.M. (1997). Nutrition and immunity in the elderly: modification of immune responses with nutritional treatments. *The American Journal of Clinical Nutrition*, Vol. 66, No. 2, (August 1997), pp. 478S-484S.

Li Volti, G., Malaponte, G., Bevelacqua, V., Messina, A., Bianca, S., Mazzarino, M.C., & Li Volti, S. (2003). Persistent high plasma levels of interleukin 18 and 4 in children with recurrent infections of the upper respiratory tract. *Transplantation Proceeding*, Vol. 35, No. 8, (December 2003), pp. 2911-2915.

Linde, K., Barrett, B., Wölkart, K., Bauer, R., & Melchart, D. (2006). Echinacea for preventing and treating the common cold. *Cochrane Database of Systematic Reviews*, Vol. 1, No. CD000530, (January, 2006).

Litzman, J., Lokaj, J., Krejčí, M., Pešák, S., & Morgan, G. (1999). Isoprinosine does not protect against frequent respiratory tract infections in childhood. *European Journal of Pediatrics*, Vol. 158, No. 1, (January 1999), pp. 32-37.

Longo, F., Lepore, L., Agosti, E., & Panizon, F. (1988). Evaluation of the effectiveness of thymomodulin in children with recurrent respiratory infections. *Pediatria Medica a Chirgica*, Vol. 10, No. 6, (December 1988), pp. 603-607.

Lull, C., Wichers, J., & Savelkoul, H.F. (2005). Antiinflammatory and immunomodulating properties of fungal metabolites. *Mediators of Inflammation*, Vol. 2005, No. 2, (June 2005), pp. 63-80.

Malaponte, G., Bevelacqua, V., Li Volti, G., Petrina, M., Nicotra, G., Sapuppo, V., Li Volti, S., Travali, S., & Mazzarino, M.C. (2004). Soluble adhesion molecules and cytokines in children affected by recurrent infections of the upper respiratory tract. *Pediatric Research*, Vol. 55, No. 4, (April 2004), pp. 666-673.

Manhart, N., Akomeah, R., Bergmeister, H., Spittler, A., Ploner, M., & Roth, E. (2002). Administration of proteolytic enzymes bromelain and trypsin diminish the number of CD4+ cells and the interferon-gamma response in Peyer´s patches and spleen in endotoxemic balb/c mice. *Cellular Immunology*, Vol. 215, No. 2, (February 2002), pp. 113-119.

Marbury, M.C., Maldonado, G., & Waller, L. (1997). Lower respiratory illness, recurrent wheezing and day care attendance. *American Journal of Respiratory Critical Care Medicine,* Vol. 155, No. 1, (January 1997), pp. 156-161.

Marchisio, P., Esposito, S., Bianchini, S., Desantis, C., Galeone, C., Nazzari, E., Pignataro L., & Principi, N. (2010). Effectiveness of a propolis and zinc solution in preventing acute otitis media in children with a history of recurrent acute otitis media. *International Journal of Immunopathology and Pharmacology,* Vol. 23, No. 2, (April-June, 2010), pp. 567-575.

Marseglia, G.L., Tosca, M., Cirillo, I., Licari, A., Leone, M., Larseglia, A., Castellazzin, A.M., & Ciprandi, G. (2007). Efficacy of *Bacillus clausii* spores in the prevention of recurrent respiratory infections in children: a pilot study. *Therapeutics and Clinical Risk Management,* Vol. 3, No. 1, (March 2007), pp. 13-17.

Mathew, J.L. (2010). Zinc Supplementation for Prevention or Treatment of Childhood Pneumonia: A Systematic Review of Randomized Controlled Trials. *Indian Pediatrics,* Vol. 47, No. 1, (January, 2010), pp. 61-66.

Matricardi, P.M., Bjorksten, B., Bonini, S., Bousquet, J., Djukanovic, R., Dreborg, S., Gereda, J., Malling, H.J., Popov, T., Raz, E., Renz, H., & Wold, A. for EAACI Task Force 7. (2003). Microbial products in allergy prevention and therapy. *Allergy,* Vol. 58, No. 6, (June, 2003), pp. 461-471.

Mauel, J., Van Pham, T., Kreis, B., & Bauer J. (1989). Stimulation by a bacterial extract (Broncho-Vaxom) of the metabolic and functional activities of murine macrophages. *International Journal of Immunopharmacol*ogy, Vol. 11, No. 6, pp. 637–645.

McElroy, B.H., & Miller, S.P. (2002). Effectiveness of zinc gluconate glycine lozenges (Cold-Eeze) against the common cold in school-aged subjects: a retrospective chart review. *American Journal of Therapeutics,* Vol. 9, No. 6, (November-December, 2002), pp. 472-475.

Meduri, R., Campos, E., Scorolli, L., De Vinci, C., Pizza, G., & Viza, D. (1996). Efficacy of transfer factor in treating patients with recurrent ocular herpes infections. *Biotherapy,* Vol. 9, No. 1-3, pp. 61-66.

Melchart, D., Linde, K., Worku F, Sarkady, L., Holzmann, M., Jurcic, K., & Wagner, H. (1995). Results of five randomized studies on the immunomodulatory activity of preparations of Echinacea. *Journal of Alternative and Complementary Med*icine, Vol. 1, No. 2, (Summer, 1995), pp. 145-160.

Melchart, D., Walther, E., Linde, K., Brandmaier, R., & Lersch, Ch. (1998). Echinacea root extracts for prevention of upper respiratory tract infections. *Archives of Family Medicine,* Vol. 7, No. 6, (November-December, 1998), pp.541-545.

Moro, G., Arslanoglu, S., Stahl, B., Jelinek, J., Wahn, U., Boehm, G. (2006). A mixture of prebiotic oligosaccharides reduces the incidence of atopic dermatitis during the first six months of age. *Archives of Disease in Childhood,* Vol. 91, No. 10, (October 2006), pp. 814-819.

Mullins, R.J. (1998). Echinacea associated anaphylaxis. *The Medical Journal of Australia,* Vol. 168, No. 4, (February,1998), pp. 170-171.

Mullins, R.J., & Heddle, R. (2002). Adverse reactions associated with echinacea: the Australian experience. *Annals of Allergy, Asthma and Immunology,* Vol. 88, No. 1, (January, 2002), pp. 42-51.

Nieman, D.C., Henson, D.A., Fagoaga, O.R., Utter, A.C., Vinci, D.M., Davis, J.M., & Nehlsen-Cannarella, S.L. (2002). Change in salivary IgA following a competitive marathon race. *Internal Journal of Sports Medicine,* Vol. 23, No. 1, (January 2002), pp. 69-75.

Noakes, P.S., Hale, J., Thomas, R., Lane, C., Devadason, S.G., & Prescott, S.L. (2006). Maternal smoking is associated with impaired neonatal toll-like-receptor-mediated immune responses. *European Respiratory Journal*, Vol. 28, No. 4, (October 2006), pp. 721-729.

Nystad, W., Nja, F., Magnus, P., & Nafstad, P. (2003). Baby swimming increases the risk of recurrent respiratory tract infections and otitis media. *Acta Paediatrica*, Vol. 92, No. 8, (August 2003), pp. 905-909.

Nystad, W., Skrondal, A., & Magnus, P. (1999). Day care attendance, recurrent respiratory tract infections and asthma. *International Journal of Epidemiology*, Vol. 28, No. 5, (October 1999), pp. 882-887.

O'Neil, J., Hughes, S., Lourie, A., & Zweifler, J. (2008). Effects of Echinacea on the frequency of upper respiratory tract symptoms: a randomized, double-blind, placebo-controlled trial. *Annals of Allergy, Asthma and Immunology*, Vol. 100, No. 4, (April, 2008), pp. 384-388.

Olinder-Nielsen, A.M., Granert, C., Forsberg, P., Friman, V., Vietorisz, A., & Bjorkander, J. (2007). Immunoglobulin prophylaxis in 350 with IgG subclass deficiency and recurrent respiratory tract infections: a long-term follow-up. *Scandinavian Journal of Infectious Diseases*, Vol. 39, No. 1, (January 2007), pp. 44-50.

Olivieri, D., Fiocchi, A., Pregliasco, F., Veehof, S., & Cantoni, V. (2009). Safety and tolerability of ribosome-component immune modulator in adults and children. *Allergy and Asthma Proceedings*, Vol. 30, Suppl. 1, (July-August 2009), pp.S33-S36.

Ottenhoff, T.H., Verreck, F.A., Lichtenauer-Kaligis, E.G., Hoeve, M.A., Sanal, O., & Van Dissel, J.T. (2002). Genetics, cytokines and human infectious disease: lessons from weakly pathogenic mycobacteria and samlonellae. *Nature Genetics*, Vol. 32, No. 1, (September 2002), pp. 97-105.

Panigada, S., Sacco, O., Girosi, D., Toma, P., & Rossi, G.A. (2009). Recurrent severe lower respiratory tract infections in a child with abnormal tracheal morphology. *Pediatric Pulmonology*, Vol. 44, No. 2, (February 2009), pp. 192-194.

Pickering, L.K., Granoff, D.M., Erickson, J.R., Masor, M.L., Cordle, C.T., Schaller, J.P., Winship, T.R., Paule, C.L., & Hilty, M.D. (1998). Modulation of the immune system by human milk and infant formula containing nucleotides. *Pediatrics*, Vol. 101, No. 2, (February 1998), pp. 242-249.

Pizza, G., De Vinci, C., Fornarola, V., Palareti, A., Baricordi, O., & Viza, D. (1996). In vitro studies during long-term oral administration of specific transfer factor. *Biotherapy*, Vol. 9, No. 1-3, pp. 175-185.

Predy, G.N., Goel, V., Lovlin, R., Donner, A., Stitt, L., & Basu, T.K. (2005). Efficacy of an extract of North American ginseng containing poly-furanosyl-pyranosyl-saccharides for preventing upper respiratory tract infections: a randomized controlled trial. *Canadian Medical Association Journal*, Vol. 173, No. 9, (October, 2005), pp.1043-1048.

Pryjma, J., Kaszuba-Zwoinska, J., Pawlik, J., Pogorzelski, A., Lis, G., Baran, J., & Zebrak, J. (1999). Alveolar macrophages of children suffering from recurrent infections of respiratory tract are less efficient in eliminating apoptotic neutrophils. *Pediatric Pulmonology*, Vol. 27, No. 3, (March 1999), pp. 167-173.

Raduner, S., Majewska, A., Chen, J.Z., Xie, X.Q., Hamon, J., Faller, B., Altmann, K.H., & Gertsch, J. (2006). Alkylamides from Echinacea are a new class of cannabinomimetics – Cannabinoid type 2 receptor-dependent and -independent immunomodulatory effects. *Journal of Biological Chemistry*, Vol. 281, No. 20, (May 2006), pp. 14192-14206.

Razi C.H., Harmanci, K., Abaci, A., Őzdemir, O., Hizli, S., Renda, R., & Keskin, F. (2010). The immunostimulant OM-85 BV prevents wheezing attacks in preschool children. *The Journal of Allergy and Clinical Immunology,* Vol. 126, No. 4, (October 2010), pp. 763-769.

Roth, D.E., Caulfield, L.E., Ezzatib, M., & Blacka, R.E. (2008). Acute lower respiratory infections in childhood: opportunities for reducing the global burden through nutritional interventions. *Bulletin of the World Health Organization,* Vol. 86, No. 5, (May, 2008), pp.356–364.

Roxas, M., & Jurenka, J. (2007). Colds and Influenza: A review of diagnosis and conventional, botanical, and nutritional considerations. *Alternative Medicine Review,* Vol. 12, No. 1, (March, 2007), pp.25-48.

Rozy, A., & Chorostowska-Wynimko, J. (2008). Bacterial immunostimulants – mechanism of action and clinical application in respiratory diseases. *Pneumonologia i Alergologia Pol*ska, Vol. 76, No. 5, pp. 353–359.

Salami, A., Dellepiante, M., Crippa, B., Mora, F., Guastini, L., Jankowska, B., & Mora, R. (2008). Sulphurous water inhalations in the prophylaxis of recurrent upper respiratory tract infections. *International Journal of Pediatric Otorhinolaryngology,* Vol. 72, No.11, (November 2008), pp. 1717-1722.

Schaad, U.B. (2010). OM-85 BV, an immunostimulant in pediatric recurrent respiratory tract infections: a systematic review. *World Journal of Pediatrics,* Vol. 6, No. 1, (February 2010), pp. 5-12.

Schoop, R., Klein, P., Suter, A., & Johnston, S.L. (2006). *Echinacea* in the Prevention of Induced Rhinovirus Colds: A Meta-Analysis. *Clinical Therapeutics, Vol.* 28, No. 2, (February, 2006), pp. 174-183.

Seida, J.K., Durec, T., & Kuhle, S. (2009). North American (Panax quinquefolius) and Asian Ginseng (Panax ginseng) Preparations for Prevention of the Common Cold in Healthy Adults: A Systematic Review. *Evidence- Based Complementary and Alternative Medicine,* Vol. 2011, 1-7

Šemberová, J., Paulovičová, E., Jelemenská, A., & Jakubíková, J. (2009). Indukcia TNF-α imunomodulačnou liečbou s obsahom β-glukánu u detských pacientov so zväčšenou nosohltanovou mandlou. *Klinická Imunológia a Alergológia,* Vol. 19, pp.15-17.

Senchina, D.S., Flagel, L.E., Wendel, J.F., & Kohut, M.L. (2006). Phenetic comparison of seven Echinacea species based on immunomodulatory characteristics. *Economic Botany,* Vol. 60, No. 3, (September, 2006), pp. 205-211.

Shah, S.A., Sander, S., White, C.M., Rinaldi, M., & Colemn, C.I. (2007). Evaluation of echinacea for the prevention and treatment of the common cold: a meta-analysis. *The Lancet Infection Disease,* Vol. 7, No. 7, (July, 2007), pp. 473–480.

Shaheen, S.O., Barker, J.P., Shiell, A.W., Crocker, F.J., Wield, G.A., & Holgate, S.T. (1994). The relationship between pneumonia in early childhood and impaired lung function in late adult life. *American Journal of Respiratory Critical Care Medicine,* Vol. 149, No. 3, (March 1994), pp. 616-619.

Sharma, S.M., Anderson, M., Schoop, S.R., & Hudson, J.B. (2010). Bactericidal and anti-inflammatory properties of a standardized Echinacea extract (Echinaforces): Dual actions against respiratory bacteria. *Phytomedicine,* Vol. 17, No. 8-9, (Jul, 2010), pp. 563–568.

Skeik, N. , & Jabr, F.I. (2011). Kartagener syndrome. *International Journal of Genetic Medicine,* Vol. 4, No. 1, (January 2011). pp. 41-43.

Slatter, M.A. & Gennery, A.R. (2008). Clinical Immunology Review Series: An approach to the patient with recurrent infections in childhood. *Clinical and Experimental Immunology*, Vol. 152, No. 3, (June 2008), pp. 389-396.

Sperber, S.J., Shah, L.P., Gilbert, R.D., Ritchey T.W., & Monto, A.S. (2004). *Echinacea purpurea* for prevention of experimental rhinovirus colds. *Clinical Infection Dis*ease, Vol. 38, No. 10, (May, 2004), pp. 1367-1371.

Steurer-Stey, C., Lagler, L., Straub, D.A., Steurer, J., & Bachmann, L.A. (2007). Oral purified bacterial extracts in acute respiratory tract infections in childhood: a systematic quantitative review. *European Journal of Pediatr*ics, Vol. 166, No. 4, (April 2007), pp. 365–376.

Stick, S. (2006). The effects of in-utero tobacco-toxin exposure on the respiratory system in children. *Current Opinion in Allergy and Clinical Immunology*, Vol. 6, No. 5, (October 2006), pp. 312-316.

Stimpel, M., Proksch, A., Wagner H., & Lohman-Matthes, M.L. (1984). Macrophage activation and induction of macrophage cytotoxicity by purified polysaccharide fractions from the plant *Echinacea purpurea. Infection and Immun*ity, Vol. 46, No. 3, (December, 1984), pp. 845-849.

Targoni, O.S., Tary-Lehmann, M., & Lehmann, P.V. (1999). Prevention of murine EAE by oral hydrolytic enzyme treatment. *Journal of Autoimmunity*, Vol. 12, No. 3, (May 1999), pp. 191-198.

Taylor, J.A., Weber, W., Standish, L., Quinn, H., Goesling, J., McGann, M., & Calabrese, C. (2003). Efficacy and Safety of Echinacea in Treating Upper Respiratory Tract Infections in Children. A Randomized Controlled Trial. *The Journal of American Medical Association*, Vol. 290, No. 21, (December, 2003), pp. 2824-2830.

Teele, D.W., Klein, J.O., & Rosner, B. (1989). Epidemiology of otitis media during the first seven years of life in children in greater Boston: a prospective, cohort study. *Journal of Infectious Diseases*, Vol. 160, No. 1, (July 1989), pp. 83-94.

Tiollier, E., Gomez-Merino, D., Burnat, P., Jouanin, J.C., Bourrilhon, C., Filaire, E., Guezennec, C.Y., & Chennaoui, M. (2005). Intense training: mucosal immunity and incidence of respiratory infections. *European Journal of Applied Physiology*, Vol. 93, No. 4, (January 2005), pp. 421-428.

Tsoni, S.V., & Brown, G.D. (2008). Beta-Glucans and Dectin-1. *Annals of the New York Academy of Sciences*, Vol. 1143, (November 2008), pp. 45-60.

Tzianabos, A.O. (2000). Polysaccharide immunomodulators as therapeutic agents: structural aspects and biologic function. *Clinical Microbiology Reviews*, Vol. 13, No. 4, (October 2000), pp. 523-533.

Uhari, M., & Mottonen, M. (1999). An open randomized controlled trial of infection prevention in children day-care centers. *Pediatric Infectious Diseases Journal*, Vol. 18, No. 8, (August 1999), pp. 672-677.

Vaughan, D., & Katkin, J.P. (2002). Chronic and recurrent pneumonias in children. *Seminars in Respiratory Infectections*, Vol. 17, No. 1, (March 2002), pp. 72-84.

Vautel, J.M., Cauquil, J., Perruchet, A.M., & Thomas, AM. (1993). Prevention of recurrent ear, nose, and throat infections in young children with Ribomunyl, double-blind, placebo-controlled study. *Current Therapeutic Research, Clinical and Experimental*, Vol. 53, No. 6, (June 1993), pp. 722–729.

Vegh, V., & Vegh, T. (2009). Přehled doplňkové imunomodulace v pediatrii. *Pediatrická prax*, Vol. 10, pp. 28-31.

Vetvicka, V., & Vetvickova, J. (2009). Beta-glucan-indomethacin combination produces no lethal effects. *Biomedical Papers of the Medical Faculty of the University Palacky Olomouc Czech Republic*, Vol. 153, No. 2, (June 2009), pp. 111-116.

Vohra, S., Johnston, B.C., Laycock, K.L., Midodzi, W.K., Dhunnoo, I., Harris E., & Baydala., L. (2008). Safety and Tolerability of North American Ginseng Extract in the Treatment of Pediatric Upper Respiratory Tract Infection: A Phase II Randomized, Controlled Trial of 2 Dosing Schedules. *Pediatrics,* Vol. 122, No. 2, (August, 2008), pp. e402-e410, ISSN: 1098-4275

Vouloumanou, E.K., Makris, G.C., Karageorgopoulos, D.E., & Falagas, M.E. (2009). Probiotics for the prevention of respiratory tract infections: a systematic review. *International Journal of Antimicrobial Agents,* Vol. 34, No. 3, (September 2009), pp.197.e1-10.

Wang, M., Guilbert, L.J., Ling, L., Li, J., Wu, Y., Xu, S., Pang, P., & Shan, J.J. (2001). Immunomodulating activity of CVT-E002, a proprietary extract from North American ginseng (Panax quinquefolium). *The Journal of Pharmacy and Pharmacology,* Vol. 53, No. 11, (November, 2001), pp. 1515–1523.

Wheeler, J.G. (1996). Evaluating the child with recurrent infections. *American Family Physician*, Vol. 54, No. 7, (November 1996), pp. 2276-2282.

Wheeler, J.G., & Steiner, D. (1992). Evaluation of humoral responsiveness in children. *Pediatric Infectious Diseases Journal*, Vol. 11, No. 4, (April 1992), pp. 304-310.

Woroniecka, M., & Ballow, M. (2000). Office evaluation of children with recurrent infection. *Pediatric Clinics of North America*, Vol. 47, No. 6, (December 200), pp. 1211-1224.

Yang, K.D., & Hill, H.R. (1991). Neutrophil function disorders: pathophysiology, prevention, and therapy. *Journal of Pediatrics*, Vol. 119, No. 3, (September 1992), pp. 343-354.

Zavadova, E., & Desser, L. (1997). Proteolytic enzymes stimulates the cytotoxic activity of human granulocytes in vitro and in vivo. *International Journal of Immunotherapy*, Vol. 13, pp. 147-151.

Zavadova, E., Desser, L., & Mohr, T. (1995). Stimulation of reactive oxygen species production and cytotoxicity in human neutrophils in vitro and after oral administration of a polyenzyme preparation. *Cancer Biotherapy,* Vol. 10, No. 2, (Summer 1995), pp. 147-152.

Zelinsky, G.M., Schaefermeyer, H., & Schaefermeyer, G. (2000). Immunomodulatory and clinical effects of Viscum album (Iscador M and Iscador P) in children with recurrent respiratory infections as a result of the Chernobyl nuclear accident. *American Journal of Therapeutics,* Vol. 7, No. 3, (May, 2000), pp.195-203.

Zelle-Rieser, C., Ramoner, R., Bartsch, G., & Thurnher, M. A. (2001). clinically approved oral vaccine against pneumotropic bacteria induces the terminal maturation of CD83+ immunostimulatory dendritic cells. *Immunology Lett*ers, Vol. 76, No. 1, (February 2001), pp. 63–67.

9

High Resolution Computed Tomography and Chronic Obstructive Pulmonary Disease

Prem Parkash Gupta
*Department of Respiratory Medicine and COPD Clinic,
Postgraduate Institute of Medical Sciences,
University of Health Sciences, Rohtak,
India*

1. Introduction

Chronic obstructive pulmonary disease (COPD) is a preventable and treatable respiratory disease with some significant extrapulmonary effects that may contribute to the severity in individual patients. Its pulmonary components are characterized by airflow limitation that is not fully reversible. COPD is a leading cause of morbidity and mortality worldwide. The economic and social burdens due to it are substantial and anticipated to increase in the coming decades due to continued exposure to COPD risk factors and the changing age profile of the world's population. COPD mortality trends generally track several decades behind smoking trends. In US in 2000, more women than men died of COPD or its related complications.
COPD comprise of a heterogeneous group of disorders conventionally including emphysema, chronic bronchitis, peripheral airways disease and pulmonary vascular disease. It is a disease state that has seen significant changes in defining and excluding criteria over past 50 years. Spirometry, the most frequently used tool to diagnose COPD and to assess response to treatment in these patients, can provide only functional assessment. In contrast to spirometry, radiological imaging allows for regional assessment of the various compartments involved i.e. airways, parenchyma and vasculature. High-resolution computed tomography (HRCT) is recommended for the non-invasive and sensitive assessment of morphological changes in emphysema and has been shown to correlate well with pathology. With the advent of new imaging techniques like multi-detector row CT (MDCT), contrast-enhanced CT methods, spirometric controlled MDCT, use of Xenon gas to assess regional ventilation of the lungs, magnetic resonance imaging (MRI) of the lung developing its own arsenal like hyperpolarized He-3 MRI - new avenues are being opened up which are now increasingly supplemented with advanced and dedicated softwares.

2. Advantages of high resolution computed tomography

At present the diagnostic criteria recommended by the Global Strategy for the Diagnosis, Management and Prevention of Chronic Obstructive Lung Disease (GOLD guidelines) do not consider CT findings during initial diagnostic assessment (Pauwels & Buist 2001) and principally rely on spirometry. However, enough scientific literature suggests that HRCT is an important and indispensable tool for evaluation of COPD. Some of the uses of HRCT are described below in next sections.

2.1 Identifying causes of airway obstruction other than COPD

Chronic airflow obstruction may be caused by a wide variety of diseases like bronchiectasis, upper airway lesions, bronchiolar diseases, interstitial lung diseases etc that may often produce clinical symptoms inseparable those due to COPD. HRCT can clearly identify different causes of airflow obstruction. Kurashima et al (2005) showed in 516 consecutive patients whose postbronchodilator FEV1/FVC was less than 70%, HRCT was able to identify 12.7% of patients with pulmonary diseases other than COPD including sarcoidosis, diffuse panbronchiolitis and pneumoconiosis. The exact diagnosis of underlying pathology leading to air flow obstruction is essential in management and to predict response to treatment in these patients.

2.2 Identification of emphysema before appearance of clinical symptoms

HRCT can detect pulmonary emphysema even in asymptomatic smokers with normal lung functions. Recent GOLD guidelines have abolished stage 0 that included asymptomatic patients who were smokers and had normal lung functions; however, Sverzellati et al (2007) observed that 13/18 subjects with stage 0 had emphysema detected over HRCT scan. It reflects that HRCT is a sensitive tool to detect emphysema before it is manifesting clinically or with deranged pulmonary functions. Detection of early emphysema may be of enormous value to prevent its progression by smoking cessation and medical intervention (Morgan 1992).

2.3 Identifying and quantifying emphysema in patients with COPD

Emphysema, characterised by a parenchymal-predominant pathology in COPD and chronic bronchitis with an airway-predominant one are distinct phenotypes and might have evolved due to different responses to and pathogenesis related to smoking (Patel et al 2006). The emphysematous phenotype is conventionally associated with a more severe form of disease (Boschetto et al 2003, 2006). COPD patients with emphysema on HRCT have been observed to have higher BODE index (body mass index, airflow obstruction, dyspnoea, exercise performance) and a lower inspiratory capacity to total lung capacity ratio (IC/TLC) than those without emphysema. This suggests emphysematous patients have more extensive systemic involvements (Boschetto et al 2006). The ability to separate airway-predominant from parenchymal-predominant pathology in COPD may prove useful in applying specific therapies designed to prevent airway remodelling and parenchymal destruction (Grenier 2005).

HRCT often makes it possible to distinguish between different phenotypes of emphysema: smoking related phenotype, the centriacinar emphysema; and phenotype associated with α1-antitrypsin deficiency, panacinar emphysema. Moreover, HRCT can detect the coexistence of both panacinar and centriacinar emphysema in the same individual, as some patients with α1-antitrypsin deficiency may also be smokers (Copley et al 2002).

2.4 Detection of co-existing bronchiectasis

Presence of bronchiectasis in COPD patients on functional evaluation using spirometry is often not detected; this fact become appreciable when HRCT studies are done. One study observed that 29% of COPD patients who were having frequent exacerbations had bronchiectatic changes detected on HRCT (O'Brien et al 2000). Patel et al (2004) found that the extent of lower lobes bronchiectasis in these patients was related to colonization by the potential pathogens, increased inflammatory markers, and a longer time to symptom recovery after exacerbation.

The likely pathogenesis for typical structural abnormalities seen on HRCT include damaged muco-ciliary transport, localized or diffuse peripheral obliteration of the bronchial tree and lung tissue scarring - all these may be acting in concert in COPD.

2.5 Evaluation of large airways

Airway predominant pathology in COPD is significant and it is diagnosed conventionally based on clinical symptomatology of chronic or recurrent excess of mucus secretion in the bronchial tree (chronic was defined as occurring on most days of three months of a year, for at least two successive years), in whom other causes of chronic cough have been excluded (American thoracic society 1995). With the development of multidetector-row computed tomography (MDCT) understanding of the larger airway diseases has been improved dramatically. Volumetric thin-section CT scans are able to detect small pits or diverticulae along the inner surfaces of the large bronchi (Zompatori et al 2006). These pits are supposed to correspond to dilated bronchial gland ducts opening into the large airway lumen (Grenier et al 2004; Zompatori et al 2006).

2.6 Assessment of regional distribution of emphysema

HRCT scan can also provide details regarding regional distribution of emphysema. The role of distribution of emphysema on HRCT as a predictor of mortality is a hot topic. One study reported a greater proportion of emphysema in the lower lung versus the upper lung to be predictive of mortality; the authors speculated that lower-lobe emphysema may be either a marker of increased disease severity or, alternatively, a phenotypic or pathobiologic variant (Martinez et al 2006). Other studies explored the influence of the distribution pattern of emphysema on different lung function parameters. A higher percentage of emphysema in the core was associated with a more reduction in diffusion capacity (Aziz et al 2005). The contribution of emphysema at core to pulmonary dysfunction (with FEV1/ FVC %) may be larger than at periphery (Nakano et al 1999).

2.7 Essential for surgical interventions in COPD

Two surgical therapies, bullectomy and lung volume reduction surgery (LVRS), are sometimes recommended in COPD patients. A chest radiograph may suggest the presence of bullae, but accurate existence and extent of such lesions can only be assessed with chest CT scans (Martinez & Chang 2005). Similarly, the presence, extent, and distribution of emphysema can precisely be determined with a chest CT scan. The work over lung volume reduction surgery (LVRS) suggests more benefits in patients with upper lobe emphysema (Cooper et al 1995).
A chest CT scan is an important tool to determine patients who should not undergo LVRS (Group NETTR 2001). In NETT, LVRS was associated with a high risk of death (16% with LVRS compared with 0% in subjects treated medically) at 30 days in two types of subjects with emphysema: (1) those with FEV1 of less than or equal to 20% of predicted and non-upper lobe-predominant disease, and (2) subjects with FEV1 of less than or equal to 20% of predicted and a diffusing capacity less than or equal to 20% of predicted.

3. High resolution computed tomography: evolution with the time

During the last couple of decades, HRCT has been widely used to evaluate emphysematous and chronic bronchitis components of COPD. The initial work by Edinburg group was to use computed tomography to diagnose emphysema in living patients (Gould et al 1988). Since then, HRCT has been widely established to detect and quantify COPD and its subtypes. Several workers have studied the correlation of semi-quantitative scoring of COPD by HRCT, pathology, clinical features and pulmonary function tests (Sanders et al 1988; Gupta et al 2008, 2009). HRCT indices of emphysema reflect lung anatomy and represent the best way to assess emphysema severity in life (Newell et al 2004). The introduction of multidetector-row CT (MDCT) scanners has provided powerful tools to evaluate changes in both small and large airways. In addition, dynamic imaging via MDCT allows the assessment of perfusion and ventilation in the lung parenchyma. Therefore, CT is able to precisely define the pathological process by providing accurate anatomic informations as well as functional data from the area of interest.

The parameters that have been extensively used by different workers to detect and differentiate various diseases grouped under COPD, and to quantify these diseases are described in following sections.

4. Measurements of lung density

The digital data provided by HRCT can be analyzed to detect the presence and severity of emphysema by several means. The measurement of lung density for quantifying emphysema may be done by **visual estimation** or **automated techniques**, both of which have their proponents (Desai et al 2006). These methods demonstrated good correlation with pathological assessment of emphysema severity (Muller et al 1988; Gevenois et al 1996). The extent of the lung density representing the disease can be visually graded according to a categorical scale. A potential drawback of visual estimation is inter-observer variation, although observer disagreement in scoring the extent of emphysema has been an insignificant factor in many of previous studies (Desai et al 2006). The potential interobserver variation is balanced by the speed and the simplicity of the technique.

The extent of emphysema can be determined by using a **threshold technique** for image segmentation. This is accompanied by setting of lower threshold for normal lung attenuation. The total area of volume of lung is calculated first using the lower threshold value and amount of emphysematous lung is determined by calculating the percentage of lung that is less than threshold value (Muller et al 1988). This technique is called as "**density mask method**". Routinely, -910 HU is taken as threshold value. In a study, authors compared CT lung densitometry in 20 COPD patients and in control subjects (Lamers et at al 1994). They found that percentage of pixels with attenuation less than -910 HU correlated well with visual emphysema score. In another study, HRCT scans were obtained with 1 cm intervals in 38 subjects (Gevenois et al 1996). The percentage areas occupied by attenuation values inferior to thresholds ranging from -900 HU to -970 HU were calculated. Emphysema was microscopically quantified in resected lung specimen. The strongest correlation was found for -950 HU and pulmonary function tests also correlated with emphysema measured by density mask method. However, other workers tried to correlate relative areas occupied by attenuation values lower than eight thresholds ranging from -900 to -970 HU with macroscopic emphysema and observed that a standard can not be recommended for the measurement of emphysema. Using precise morphometric evaluation of resected lung tissue, Bankier et al (1999) showed that observers, regardless of their experience, tend to overestimate the extent of emphysema on CT, whereas CT densitometry correlates better with the morphometric reference. The density mask has been used to identify subgroups of patients who may show benefit from lung volume reduction surgery (Fishman et al 2003). The percentage of emphysema quantified by density mask is also predictive of survival in α1-antitrypsin-induced emphysema (Dawkins et al 2003).

Another objective way to measure emphysema on HRCT is assessment of **mean lung density** (Nowell 2002). CT density is expressed as a linear scale in HU (water = 0, air = -1000). In this range, lung density is a direct measure of physical density and is determined by the relative mix of air, blood and interstitial fluid in tissue. Emphysema will lead to decrease in mean lung density on CT. Several studies have assessed CT lung density in normal subjects. However, the range of normality remains to be standardized. In a study, authors assessed the progression of pulmonary emphysema in 23 patients by means of lung density (Zagiers et al 1996). Patients were scanned twice with a 1 year interval. Mean lung densities decreased within this duration and proved to be more sensitive than FEV1 and carbon monoxide diffusion.

The **image histogram curve** of CT lung density values can be obtained using softwares and measures of skewness can be looked at as another mean of detecting and assessing the presence of emphysema. Tail of high density value is produced by large vessels and airways and in emphysema, there is an increase in the numbers of low density pixels and the whole curve is shifted to the left (MacNee et al 1991). In a study, three groups of individuals, 20 with emphysema, 20 with chronic bronchitis and healthy individuals underwent CT and cut-off point in the histogram that defines the lowest 10th percentile of the histogram was derived (Lamers et al 1994). They observed that it is possible to classify lung disease using this parameter.

The softwares available in addtion with MDCT scanners make it possible to recognize and quantify emphysema faster than human evaluation; and it is now possible to apply techniques measuring lung density to volumetric data. The resolution achieved in thoracic HRCT allows the application of **high-precision 3D image analytic tools** to CT data (Kuhnigk et al 2005). The analyses allow a convenient regional assessment of CT parameters including total volume, mean density, pixel index, and emphysema type (Kuhnigk et al 2005).

A density-masking approach alone is not sufficient to accurately distinguish between normal and diseased lung, especially in the case of early or mixed pathologic processes (Uppaluri et al 1997, 1999; Hoffman et al 2006). Further, CT densitometry is known to be influenced by several factors (eg, age, weight, beam hardening from adjacent ribs etc.) and calibration must be performed in order to obtain reliable densitometry. Neither visual nor pure densitometric approaches to CT quantification of emphysema are, therefore, perfect.

In addition to assessment of percentage of voxels below a certain threshold, more sophisticated analytic softwares may analyse the CT scan data, contiguous emphysematous lesions can be clustered to obtain the volumes for small-sized, medium-sized, and large-sized emphysematous areas (**cluster distribution**) (Blechschmidt et al 2001; Zaporozhan et al 2005). A serial assessment of cluster distribution is useful in revealing the pattern of progression of emphysema. Uppaluri et al (1997, 1999) examined multiple features of the CT images and X-ray attenuation values to describe the lung and developed the **Adaptive Multiple-Feature Method** (AMFM), which can assess up to 22 independent textural features from HRCT scans to classify a tissue pattern. This is found to be useful to distinguish smokers from non-smokers in the absence of other disease (Hoffman et al 2006).

5. Mosaic attenuation pattern and air trapping

Abnormalities on HRCT that reflect small airways disease can be broadly categorized into indirect and direct signs: widespread scarring and obliteration of the bronchioles results in the indirect sign of patchy density differences of the lung parenchyma, representing areas of under-ventilated and under-perfused lung (**mosaic attenuation pattern**). The considerable thickening of the small airways walls by inflammatory infiltrate and/or luminal and surrounding exudate render the affected **small airways directly visible** (Hansell 2001). Air trapping or hyperinflation is a common manifestation of COPD (Stern & Frank 1994). Persistent aeration caused by collateral pathways, or hyperaeration from trapped air, produces the mosaic attenuation pattern which is characterized by nonhomogenous lung density, i.e. areas that remain relatively lucent interspersed with areas of normal higher lung density. The air trapping and mosaic attenuation pattern is more pronounced, on scans obtained at end-exhalation instead of the more conventional end-inspiration technique (Arakawa & Webb 1998). In a recent study, it was found that mosaic attenuation pattern in addition to other HRCT features is helpful in distinguishing different entities grouped under COPD (Copley et al 2002).

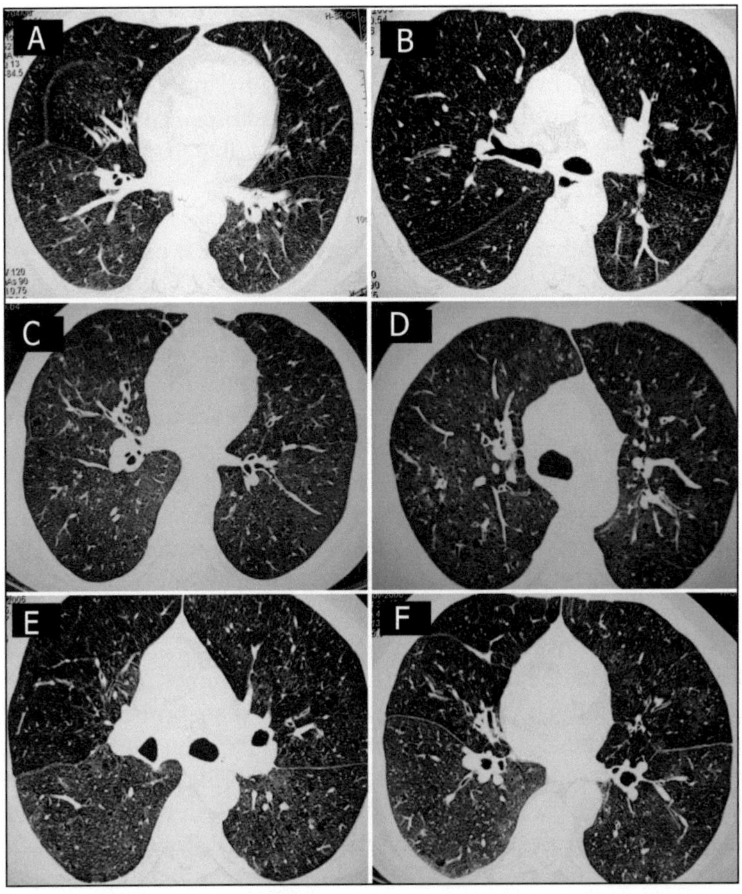

Fig. 1. HRCT scans showing non-homogenous lung density – a cardinal feature of mosaic attenuation pattern (A-F) observed on HRCT scan obtained from different COPD patients.

In our studies (Gupta et al 2008, 2009) including 40 COPD patients who were diagnosed based on GOLD criteria and who were evaluted for HRCT characteristics, 16/40 patients had classic mosaic attenuation pattern; the HRCT scans were undertaken during full inspiration. Some of these are shown in figure 1 (A to F).

6. Directly visible small airways

Several pathological studies have shown that the major site of airway obstruction in COPD is in airways with internal diameter lesser than 2 mm. The 2 mm airways are located between the fourth and the 14th generation of the tracheobronchial tree. These airways are not visible on HRCT scan in normal subjects. However, considerable thickening of the bronchiolar walls by inflammatory infiltrate and/or luminal and surrounding exudates render them directly visible (Hansell 2001). These diseased airways are visible on HRCT as dilated, air-filled, branching, tubular or ring-like structures in the lung periphery by wall thickening and dilation. When the airways are obliterated by submucosal or peribronchial fibrosis, nodular, linear, or branching peripheral opacities may be seen (Teel et al 1996). In our study, 36 out of 40 COPD patients showed directly visible small airways (figure 2).

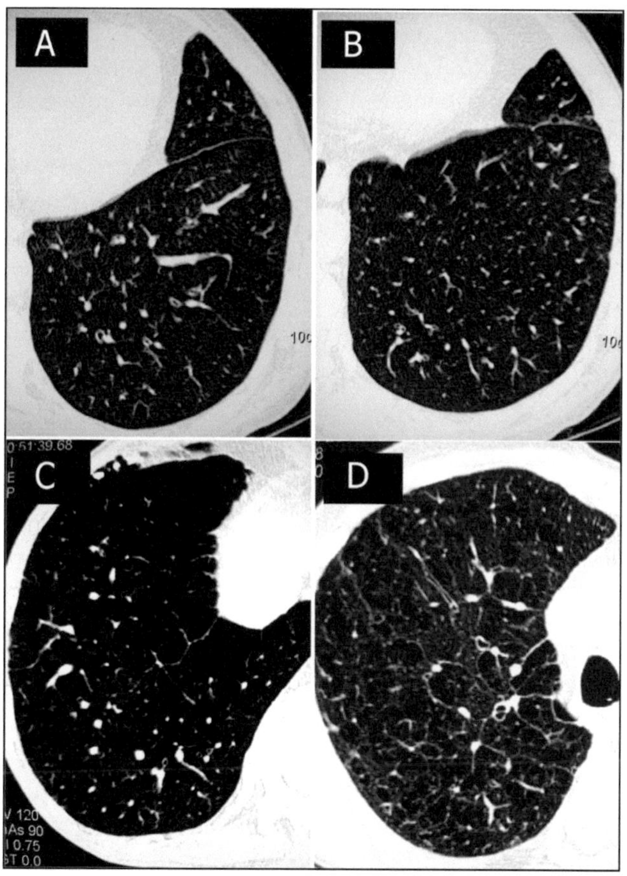

Fig. 2. HRCT axial scans showing directly visible small airways as (A-C) air filled ring like structures and (D) air filled branching tubular structures.

7. Measurements of airway wall thickness

It has been observed that the size of the large and intermediate airways reflect airway dimensions in the smaller airways (Nakano et al 2005). Due to the interobserver disagreement in the visual interpretation of bronchial wall thickness on CT scans (Muller and Coxson 2002), there has been considerable interest in the development of objective measurements of airway wall dimensions. The most frequently reported method for measuring the airway lumen and wall areas relies on the **"full-width-at-half-maximum" (or "half-max") technique**, in which the inner and outer airway wall boundaries are defined as the point corresponding to the half maximal intensity of the airway wall voxels (Nakano et al 2000; de Jong et al 2005). Using the half-max method, Nakano et al (2000) showed that an increased thickness of the apical right upper lobe bronchus over HRCT correlated with the severity of airflow obstruction in COPD patients. However, the measurements of airway lumen and wall area depends on the lung volume and angle between the airway central axis and the plane of section (Grenier et al 2004).

In 42 COPD patients, bronchi with external diameter of greater than 2 mm and maximum to minimum diameter ratio less than 1.5 were selected (Orlandi et al 2005). Thickness to diameter ratio (TDR) and the percentage wall area (PWA) of these bronchi were computed. For each patient, mean TDR and mean PWA were calculated. The combination of PWA, TDR and PWA normalized to body weight correlated significantly ($P < 0.05$) with FEV1/SVC ratio and DLco in patients with chronic bronchitis but not in patients without chronic bronchitis.

In another study, thickness to diameter ratio (TDR), and percentage of wall area (WA%) were calculated on HRCT in 4 groups of patients : group O - healthy non smokers, group I - healthy current smokers, group II - patients with moderate COPD and group III - those with severe COPD as per GOLD classification (Deveci et al 2004). Both groups II and III had higher T/D ratio and WA% than group I and group I had higher values than group O. Airway wall thickening was found to be inversely correlated with FEV1 and positively related to the quantum of smoking.

8. Low attenuation areas of emphysema

HRCT is a reliable tool for demonstrating even subtle changes in secondary pulmonary lobules. Low attenuation areas of emphysema are distinctly visible on HRCT scan. These focal areas of decreased attenuation present differently in different types of emphysema (Nowell 2002).

Centriacinar emphysema is the commonest type of pulmonary emphysema and is characterized by an enlargement of the centriacinar airspace, with the effect mainly occurring in proximal respiratory bronchioles, leaving normal distal alveolar ducts and sacs. In centriacinar emphysema, focal areas of decreased attenuation have no discernable wall and usually have a focal arteriole at or near the centre of lesion (Figure 3 A-F). Centriacinar abnormalities always have a distance of about 2.5 mm from the perilobular structure, including interlobular septum, pleura and large pulmonary vessels. Cigarette smoking and dust inhalation are the most important risk factors for the development of centriacinar emphysema. The disease is usually distributed to the upper lobe or the superior segment of the lower lobe. The inner zone is more severely affected than the outer zone, probably due

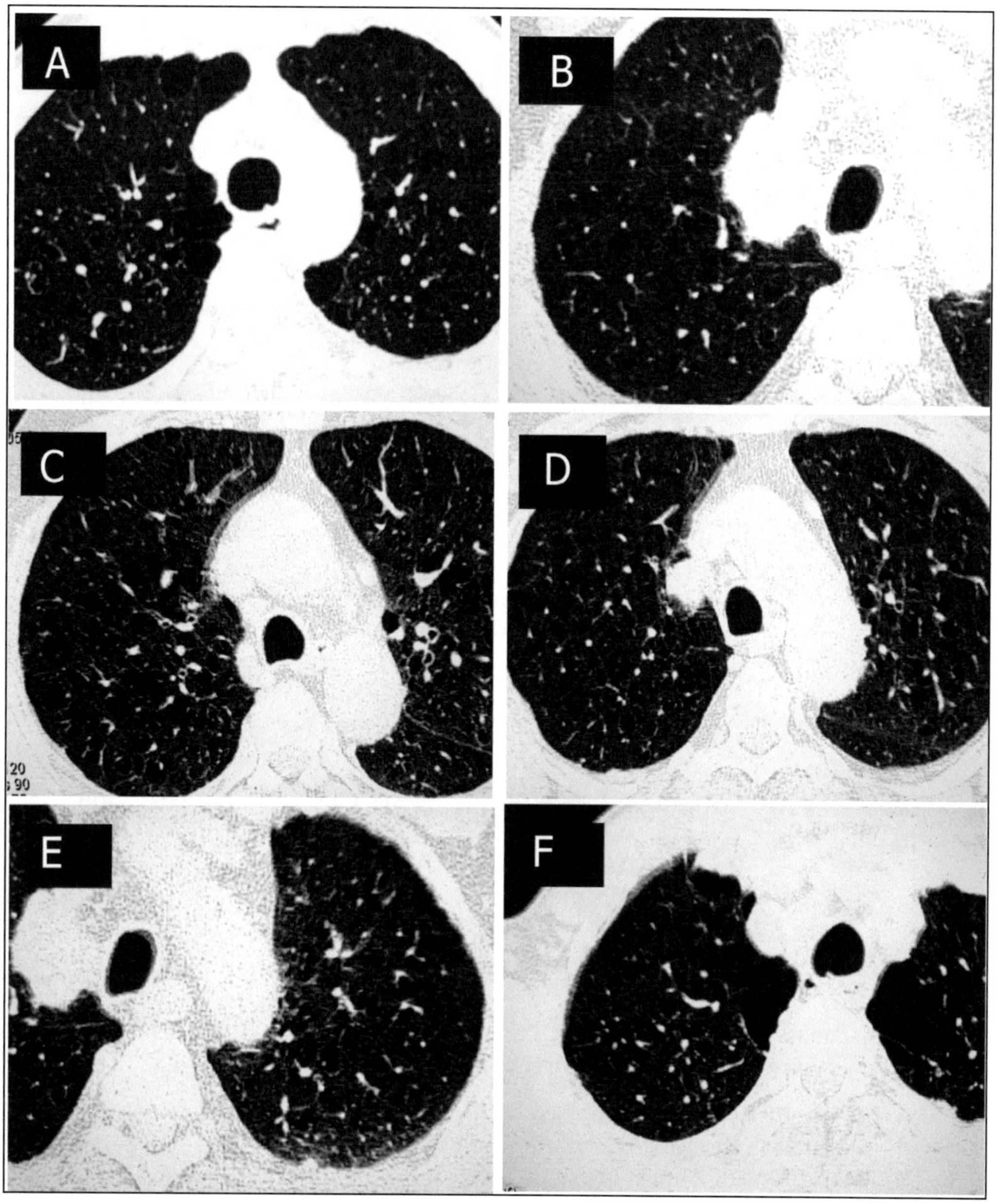

Fig. 3. HRCT scans in patients with centriacinar emphysema showing multiple, round lucent regions of various sizes surrounded by normal parenchyma (A-F).

to zonal differences in respiratory kinetics and lymph flow. HRCT in early centriacinar emphysema shows evenly distributed centrilobular tiny areas of low attenuation with ill-defined borders; with enlargement of the dilated airspace, the surrounding lung parenchyma is compressed and a clear border may be observed between the emphysematous area and normal lung.

Panacinar emphysema is characterized by a uniform dilatation of the air space from the respiratory bronchioles to the alveoli, leading to evenly distributed emphysematous changes within secondary lobules. Panacinar emphysema is characterized by large areas of decreased lung density or decreased attenuation on CT with poorly defined margins; the caliber of the vessels in the involved area is decreased due to overinflation of the air space [Figure 4 (A-D)]. Alpha 1-antitrypsin deficiency is thought to be a major cause of panacinar emphysema. Other rare etiologies, including Swyer-James syndrome and ritalin abuse, have been reported. The characteristics that distinguish panacinar emphysema from centriacinar emphysema are as follows: the disease is dominant in the lower lung field, the degree of lung inflation is greater than that in centriacinar emphysema; there is a tendency for the airway to be narrowed; and bullous formation is less frequently observed compared to centriacinar emphysema.

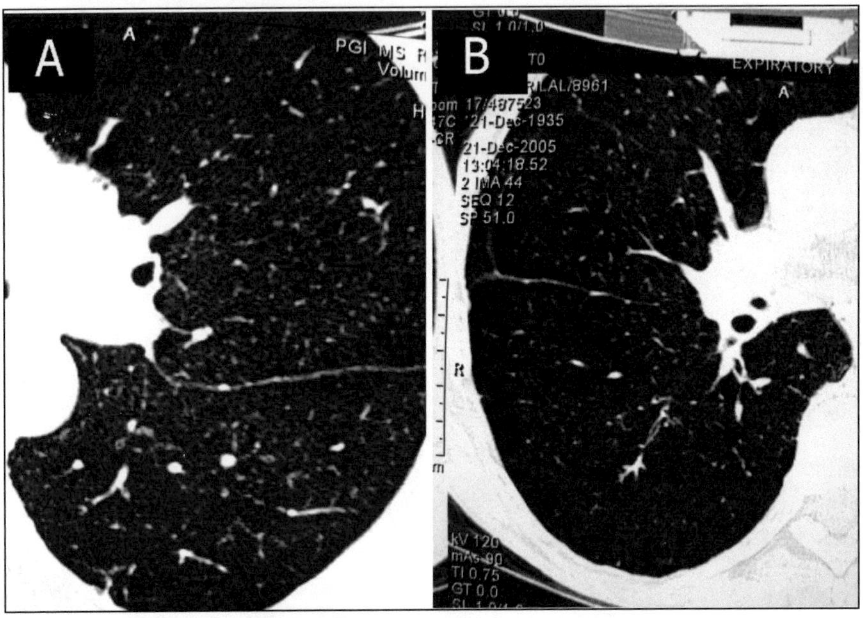

Fig. 4. (A-B): Panacinar emphysema: HRCT scans showing diffuse low attenuation lung parenchyma - typical of panacinar emphysema

Distal acinar emphysema is characterized by focal areas of subpleural emphysema. Distal acinar or paraseptal emphysema is characterized by an enlarged airspace at the periphery of acini. The lesion is usually limited in extent, occurs most commonly along the dorsal surface of the upper lung. The patients are usually asymptomatic, but distal acinar emphysema is considered to be a cause of pneumothorax in young adults.

The subtypes of emphysema can usually be determined in mild or moderate cases, but classification into anatomic subtypes becomes more difficult by HRCT and pathological examinations as emphysema becomes more severe, with even highly trained and experienced pathologists sometimes disagreeing on the classification. Centriacinar and panacinar emphysema may coexist in the same patient; for example, with centriacinar emphysema in the upper lobe and panacinar emphysema in the lower lobe.

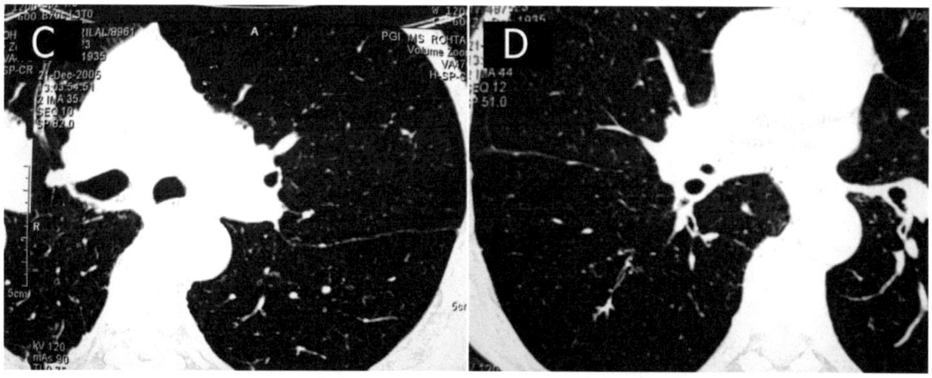

Fig. 4. (C-D): Some more HRCT scans showing panacinar emphysema

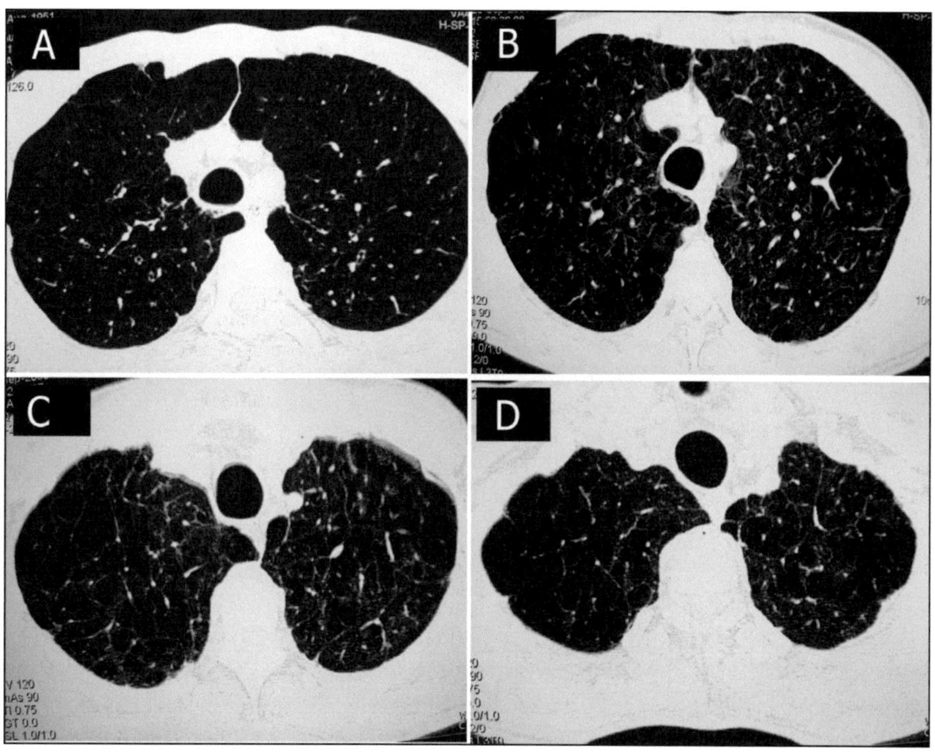

Fig. 5. (A-D): HRCT scans showing small subpleural areas of hyperlucency - characteristic of paraseptal emphysema.

Studies have been done to assess the accuracy of CT in diagnosis of emphysema by visual scoring of low attenuation areas. In a study, CT thorax was performed on 32 patients scheduled for elective thoracotomies for suspected lung tumours (Bergin et al 1986). Each slice was assessed and graded depending upon the percentage area showing emphysematous areas. Similarly, emphysema was graded on the resected lung specimens. It was found that compared to pulmonary function tests, CT was a better predictor of assessing the presence and severity of emphysema.

A retrospective study used HRCT scans for scoring the severity of emphysema (Klein et al 1992). Each of the six lung sections was evaluated and extent of emphysema multiplied by the severity was summed for the six sections. Concomitant chest radiographs and pulmonary function tests were reviewed. The severity of emphysema on HRCT correlated inversely with single breath carbon monoxide diffusion capacity. **HRCT allowed detection of emphysema in symptomatic patients when chest radiographs and pulmonary function tests were non-diagnostic.**

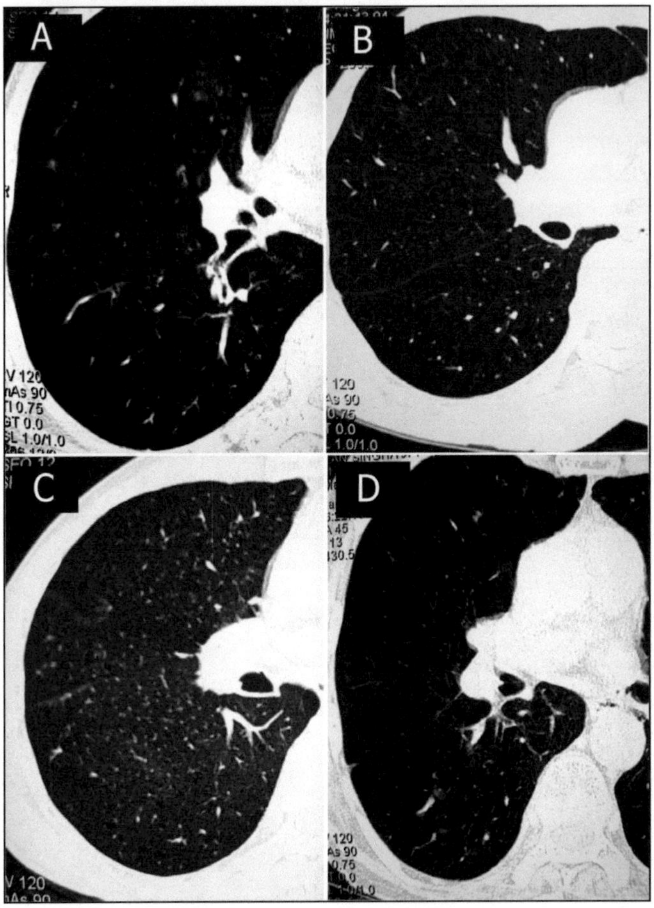

Fig. 6. (A-D) : HRCT scans of different COPD patients showing vascular attenuation characterized by thinning of pulmonary vessels at the peripheral lung field along with reduction in their number.

9. Vascular attenuation and vascular distortion

On HRCT of emphysema patients, low attenuation areas are frequently accompanied with vascular attenuation and distortion (Norwell 2002). **Vascular attenuation** is defined as thinning of pulmonary vessels and reduction in their number [figure 6 (A-D)]. **Vascular distortion** is increased branching angles, excessive straightening or bowing of vessels. [figure 7 (A-D)].

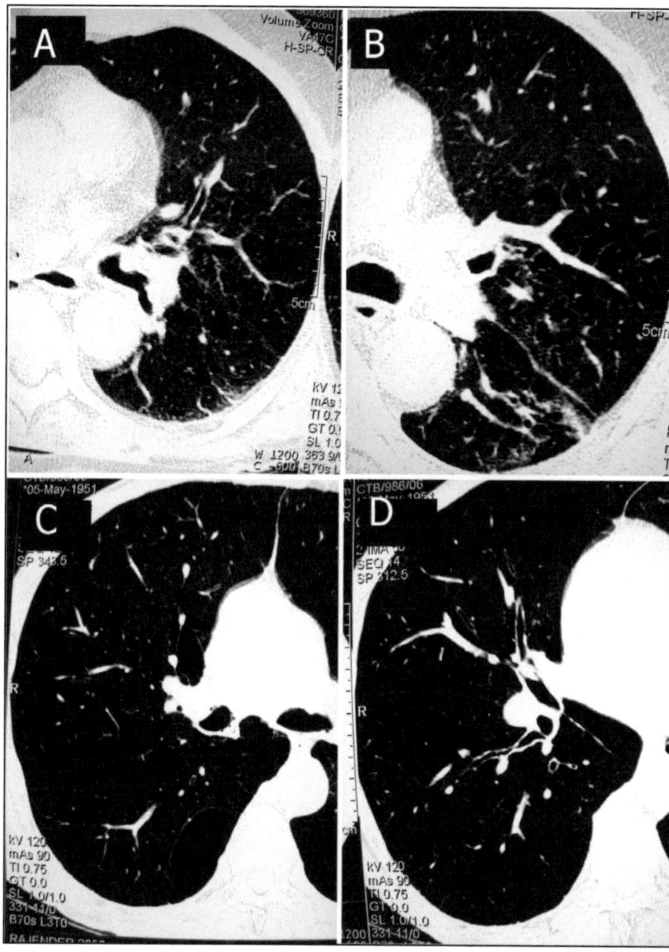

Fig. 7. (A-D): HRCT axial scans from COPD patients showing vascular distortion characterized by increased branching angles and excessive straightening of pulmonary vessels.

In a study, two radiologists and one chest physician assessed for destructive changes of emphysema manifested by low attenuation areas and disruption of vascular pattern (Kuwano et al 1990). Each slice was individually assessed using a modification of the **picture-grading system** of Thurlback (1994). CT scores correlated significantly with the pathological scores and it was concluded that HRCT can help to identify the presence and grading of mild emphysema. Other studies have found that vascular disruption in addition to areas of low attenuation is helpful in assessing and grading emphysema (Bergin et al 1986).

10. Saber-sheath trachea and tracheal index

In cross-section, the resting trachea is roughly horse-shoe shaped, with the open end of the cartilage rings closed by a compliant posterior sheath. In COPD patients, the coronal diameter is reduced and the saggital diameter correspondingly increased, a condition called **saber-sheath trachea** [Figure 8 (A-D)] . **Tracheal index** is a ratio of the coronal to the saggital length, measured 1 cm above the aortic arch.

In a study, it was found that patients with COPD had a reduced tracheal index. Saber-sheath trachea (tracheal index < 2/3) was observed to be a specific radiographic diagnostic parameter for the diagnosis of COPD (specificity, 92.9%), although sensitivity (39.1%) was low (Tsao et al 1994).

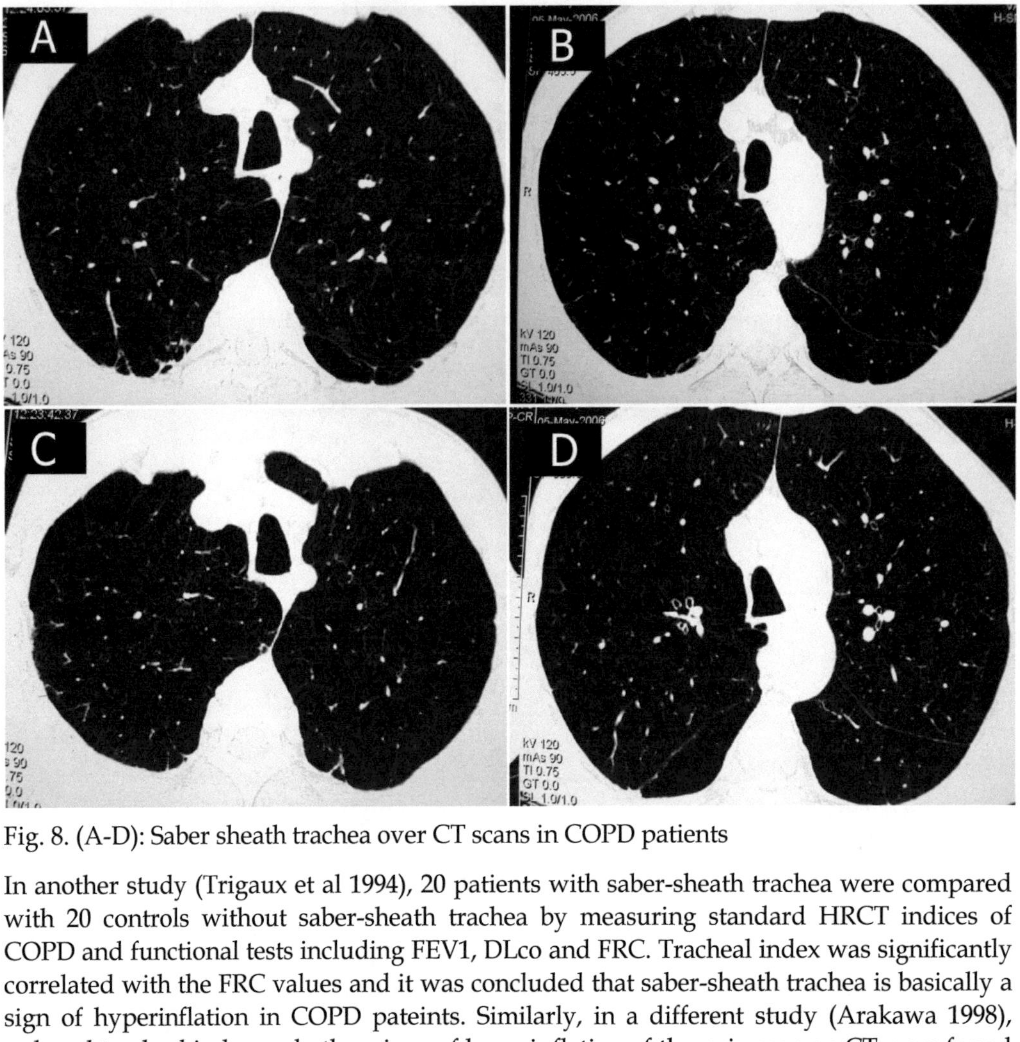

Fig. 8. (A-D): Saber sheath trachea over CT scans in COPD patients

In another study (Trigaux et al 1994), 20 patients with saber-sheath trachea were compared with 20 controls without saber-sheath trachea by measuring standard HRCT indices of COPD and functional tests including FEV1, DLco and FRC. Tracheal index was significantly correlated with the FRC values and it was concluded that saber-sheath trachea is basically a sign of hyperinflation in COPD pateints. Similarly, in a different study (Arakawa 1998), reduced tracheal index and other signs of hyperinflation of thoracic cage on CT were found to correlate significantly with pulmonary functions of chronic airway obstruction.

11. Sterno-aortic distance and mediastinal anterior junctional line

In retrosternal region, right and left lung with their corresponding pleural layers approach each other so closely that the area of contrast form a linear density. When present, the line is 1 to 2 mm wide and formed by two pleural layers on each side of a narrow zone of mediastinal connective tissue. This line is called **anterior junctional line** (AJL) [figure 9 (A-D)].

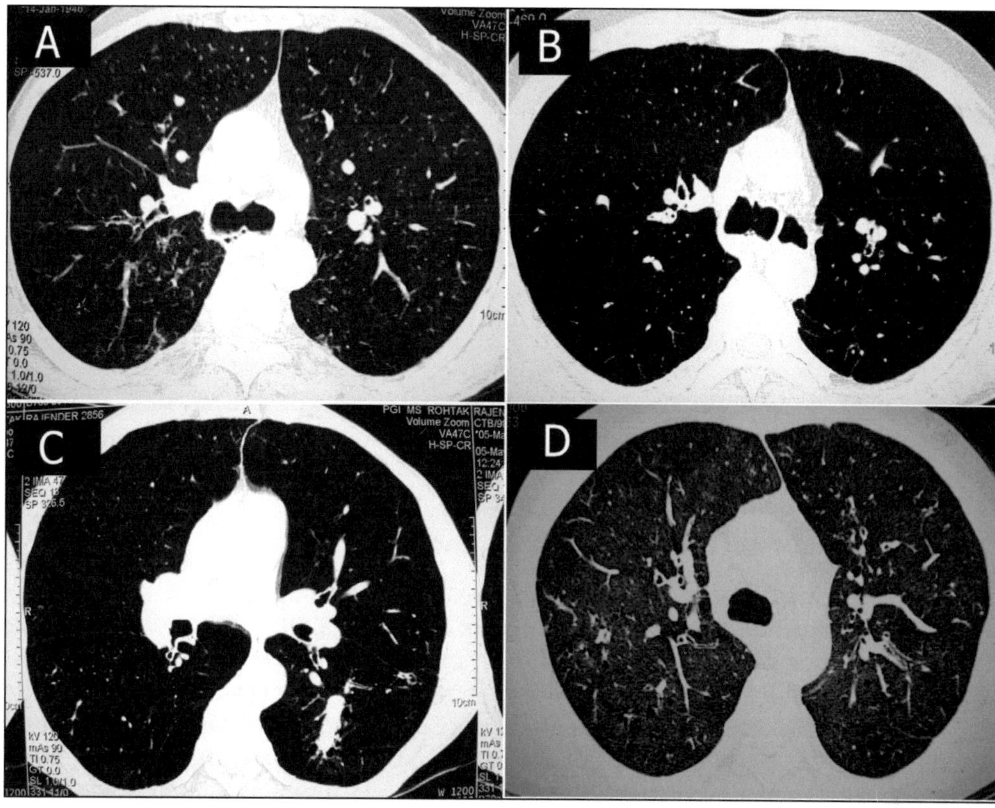

Fig. 9. (A-D): HRCT scans from COPD showing increased sterno-aortic distance and the anterior junctional line.

In a study, AJL and sterno-aortic distance (distance between sternum and ascending aorta) were measured in CT sections at carinal level in 22 patients with emphysema and 22 control subjects (Hagen & Kolebenstvedt 1993). The AJL could be measured in all emphysema patients. In the control group the line was non-existent in 11 of the 22 patients. The AJL was 3 cm or more in 10 of the emphysema patients, but in none of the controls. The sterno-aortic distance was 4 cm or more in 16 of the emphysema patients, but in none among control group. In another study, significant correlation was found between FEV1 / FVC and sterno-aortic distance (measured at tracheal carina on CT) in 74 patients who underwent thoracic surgery for lung cancer (Arakawa et al 1998).

12. Thoracic cage ratio and barrel chest

Arakawa et al (1998) measured thoracic cage ratios (anteroposterior/ transverse diameters) at carina and 5 cm below carina on CT in 74 patients. Other measurements of hyperinflation were also calculated and it was found that increased thoracic cage ratio correlated most significantly with a pulmonary functions of chronic airway obstruction.

In another study, normal thoracic cage ratio was 0.70 to 0.75 in adults. The thoracic cage ratio was found high in COPD patients and may reach upto > 0.9 which was called as **barrel chest** (Pierce et al 1958). Figure 10 (A-B) shows HRCT scans with barrel chest feature found in our studies (Gupta et al 2008, 2009).

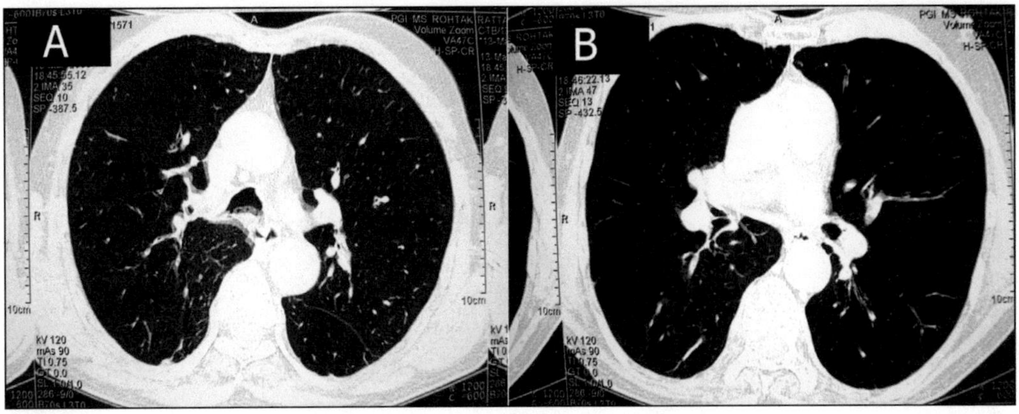

Fig. 10. (A-B): A marked increase in thoracic cage ratio above 0.9 described as barrel chest

13. Thoracic cross-sectional area (TCSA) index

The assessment of thoracic cross-sectional area (TCSA) is an important measure of thoracic cage hyperinflation commonly seen in advance COPD with air trapping and increased total lung capacity. TCSA is the area surrounded by the rib cage measured on CT scan made 1 cm below the top of the aortic arch. In a study (Kasai et al 2003) TCSA and pulmonary functions and dyspnea grade were measured in 24 COPD patients. In the group with grade IV dyspnea, the TCSA/ht^2 ratios were significantly greater than those in the groups with grade II and III dyspnea, combined. Analysis of data showed a good correlation between TCSA and total lung capacity, as well as functional residual capacity and residual volume.

14. HRCT characteristics observed in our studies

Our studies included 40 male patients with COPD. Their mean age was 58.55 years (range: 50-69 years). Total duration of illness due to COPD was in range from 2 to 25 years with a mean of 12.63 years. All subjects were significant smoker with mean smoking history of 33.25 pack years (range 20-74 pack years). They were evaluated for HRCT features including vascular attenuation and distortion, mosaic attenuation pattern, directly visible small airways, low attenuation areas of emphysema and measures of hyperinflation of lungs: tracheal index, sterno-aortic distance, thoracic cage ratio and thoracic cross-sectional area. Individual COPD patients having characteristics HRCT findings were as shown in table-1.

In our studies, tracheal index was observed to have significant inverse correlations with duration of illness, smoking pack years, and dyspnea scale; and had direct correlations with FEV1, PEFR, FEV1/FVC ratio, and FEV1/SVC ratio. Thoracic cage ratio at carina as well as thoracic cage ratio at 5 cm below carina had direct correlations with duration of illness, smoking pack years and dyspnea scale; and had inverse correlations with FEV1, FEV1/FVC ratio and FEV1/SVC ratio. Sterno-aortic distance and thoracic cross sectional area had correlations with duration of illness, smoking pack years and dyspnea scale; and they had inverse correlations with FEV1, FEV1/FVC ratio, and FEV1/SVC ratio.

HRCT features	Number of patients out of 40	Percentage of study subjects
Saber sheath trachea with tracheal index less than 0.67	14	35
Thoracic cage ratio over 0.75 at the level of carina	5	12.5
Thoracic cage ratio over 0.75 at the level 5 cm below carina	11	27.5
Sterno-aortic distance more than 4 cm	5	12.5
Thoracic cross-sectional area/ht^2 more than 80.00 cm^2/m^2	28	70
Vascular attenuation	25	62.5
Vascular distortion	8	20
Mosaic attenuation pattern	16	40
Directly visible small airways	36	90
Centriacinar emphysema	16	40
Panacinar emphysema	11	27.5
Paraseptal emphysema	13	32.5
Any type of emphysema	25	62.5

Table 1. HRCT features noted in individual COPD patients

Vascular attenuation had significant correlations with duration of illness, dyspnoea scale, smoking pack years, FEV1, FEV1/FVC ratio, and FEV1/SVC ratio. Vascular distortion had no significant correlation with any of the observed parameter. The mosaic attenuation pattern correlated significantly with duration of illness, dyspnea scale, smoking pack years, FEV1, FEV1/FVC ratio, and FEV1/SVC ratio. Correlation of presence of directly visible small airways was significant only with dyspnea scale. Centriacinar emphysema had significant correlations with PEFR, FEV1, FVC, FEV1/FVC ratio and FEV1/SVC ratio. Correlations of presence of any type of emphysema with age, duration, dyspnea scale, pack-years, PEFR, FEV1, FVC, FEV1/FVC ratio and FEV1/SVC ratio were statistically significant.

15. Recent advances

COPD is a heterogeneous group of disorders and needs to be evaluated by a combination of morphological and functional assessment. Recently, newer HRCT techniques as well as MRI have provided new insights to characterisation of various pulmonary components of COPD in term of morphology as well as functionality. Three-dimensional HRCT has been described as the technique of choice for morphological imaging. Inspiratory and expiratory 3D-HRCT with volumetric and texture analysis allows for deeper insights to regional hyperinflation and expiratory obstruction. Three-dimensional HRCT has also been described as the "gold standard" for non-invasive quantitative evaluation of airway dimensions. Newer generations of MRI allow for better visual assessment of the lung morphology as well as comprehensive functional imaging. The major advantage of MRI is the assessment of regional lung function including perfusion, respiratory dynamics and ventilation. The comprehensive diagnostic possibilities of CT complemented by MRI will allow for a more sensitive detection, phenotype-driven characterization and dedicated therapy monitoring of COPD.

16. Conclusion

While all this description appears voluminous, many things have not been discussed in detail due to want of space. The imaging techniques we are applying in day to day practice at present have opened new avenues for morphological and functional characterisation of various diseases incorporated under the heterogeneous group of COPD and helped in phenotyping as well as assessment of the progression of COPD. And, this is just beginning! In future we are definitely going to get more powerful equipments, supplemented with dedicated and advanced softwares that will provide deeper insight into the various diseases grouped under the umbrella of COPD.

17. Acknowledgments

The author wish to express his profound gratitude to Prof. Rohtas Yadav, Senior Professor, Radiodiagnosis; Dr Manish Verma, Ex-Resident, Respiratory Medicine; Prof. K B Gupta, Senior Professor, Respiratory Medicine; Dr Dipti Agarwal, Assistant Professor, Physiology; and Dr Manoj Kumar, Expert, Biostatistics - all from Postgraduate Institute of Medical Sciences, University of Health Sciences, Rohtak, India for their kind help, necessary inputs and critical review of the literature.

18. References

American Thoracic Society. (1995). Standards for the diagnosis and care of patients with chronic obstructive pulmonary disease. Am J Respir Crit Care Med 152 (5 pt 2): S77-121.

Arakawa H, Webb WR. (1998). Air trapping on expiratory high resolution CT scans in the absence of inspiratory scan abnormalities: correlation with pulmonary function tests and differential diagnosis. Am J Roentgenol 170: 1349-53.

Arakawa H, Kurihara Y, Nakajima Y, Niimi H, Ishikawa T, Tokuda M. (1998). Computed tomography measurements of overinflation in chronic obstructive pulmonary disease: evaluation of various radiographic signs. J Thorac Imaging 13 (3): 188-92.

Aziz ZA, Wells AU, Desai SR, et al. (2005). Functional impairment in emphysema: contribution of airway abnormalities and distribution of parenchymal disease. Am J Roentgenol 185: 1509–15

Bankier AA, De Maertelar V, Keyzer C, et al. (1999). Pulmonary emphysema: subjective visual grading versus objective quantification with macroscopic morphometry and thin-section CT densitometry. Radiology 211: 851–8.

Bergin C, Muller N, Nichols DM. (1986).The diagnosis of emphysema: a computed tomographic pathologic correlation. Am Rev Respir Dis 133: 541-6.

Blechschmidt RA, Werthschutzky R, Lorcher U. (2001). Automated CT image evaluation of the lung: a morphology-based concept. IEEE Trans Med Imaging 20: 434–42.

Boschetto P, Miniati M, Miotto D, et al. (2003). Predominant emphysema phenotype in chronic obstructive pulmonary. Eur Respir J 21: 450–4.

Boschetto P, Quintavalle S, Zeni E, et al. (2006). Association between markers of emphysema and more severe chronic obstructive pulmonary disease. Thorax 61: 1037–42.

Cooper JD, Trulock EP, Triantafillou AN, et al. (1995). Bilateral pneumectomy (volume reduction) for chronic obstructive pulmonary disease. J Thorac Cardiovasc Surg 109: 106-116. (discussion 116-109).

Copley SJ, Wells AU, Muller NL, et al. (2002). Thin-section CT in obstructive pulmonary disease: discriminatory value. Radiology 223: 812-19.

Dawkins PA, Dowson LJ, Guest PJ, et al. (2003). Predictors of mortality in alpha-1-antitrypsin deficiency. Thorax 58: 1020-6.

de Jong PA, Muller NL, et al. (2005). Computed tomographic imaging of the airways: relationship to structure and function. Eur Respir J 26: 140-52.

Desai SR, Hansell DM, Walker A, MacDonald SL, Chabat F, Wells AU. (2007). Quantification of emphysema: A composite physiologic index derived from CT estimation of disease extent. Eur Radiol 17: 911-8.

Deveci F, Murat A, Turgut T, Altuntas E, Muz MH. (2004). Airway wall thickness in patients with COPD and healthy current smokers and healthy non-smokers: assessment with high resolution computed tomographic scanning. Respiration 71: 602-10.

Fishman A, Martinez F, Naunheim K, et al. (2003). A randomized trial comparing lung-volume reduction surgery with medical therapy for severe emphysema. N Engl J Med 348: 2059-73.

Gevenois PA, De Vuyst P, de Maertelaer V, et al. (1996). Comparison of computed density and microscopic morphometry in pulmonary emphysema. Am J Respir Crit Care Med 154: 187-92.

Gevenois PA, Scillia P, De Maertelaer V, et al. (1996). The effects of age, sex, lung size, and hyperinflation on CT lung densitometry. Am J Roentgenol 167: 1169-73.

Gould GA, MacNee W, Mclean A. (1988). CT measurements of lung density in life can quantitate distal airspace enlargement: an essential defining feature of human emphysema. Am Rev Resp Dis 133: 380-92.

Grenier PA. (2005). Detection of altered lung physiology. Eur Radiol 15: 42-7.

Grenier PA, Beigelman-Aubry C, Fetita C, et al. (2004). Large airways at CT: Bronchiectasis, Asthma and COPD. In: Kauczor HU, editor. Functional imaging of the chest. Heidelberg: Springer; pp. 39-55.

Griffen CB, Primack SL. (2001). High resolution CT: Normal anatomy, techniques and pitfalls. Radiologic Clinic of North America 39 (6): 1073-90.

Group NETTR. (2001). Patients at high risk of death after lung-volume reduction surgery. N Engl J Med 345: 1075-83.

Gupta PP, Yadav R, Verma M, Gupta KB, Agarwal D. (2009). High resolution computed tomography features in patients with chronic obstructive pulmonary disease. Singapore Med J 50: 193-200.

Gupta PP, Yadav R, Verma M, Agarwal D, Kumar M. (2008). Correlation between high resolution computed tomography features and patients` characteristics in chronic obstructive pulmonary disease. Annals Thorac Med 3: 87-93.

Hagen G, Kolebenstvedt A. (1993). CT measurement of mediastinal anterior junction line in emphysema patients. Acta Radiologica 34: 194-5.

Hansell DM. (2001). Small airways diseases: detection and insights with computed tomography. Eur Respir J 17: 1294–1313.

Hoffman EA, Simon BA, McLennan G. (2006). State of the art. A structural and functional assessment of the lung via multidetector-row computed tomography: phenotyping chronic obstructive pulmonary disease. Proc Am Thorac Soc 3: 519–32.

Kasai T, Yamada M, Narushima M, Suzuki H. Relationship between thoracic cross-sectional area measured on CT and pulmonary function or dyspnea in patients with COPD. Nihon Kokyuki Gakkai Zasshi 2003; 41:526-30.

Klein JS, Gamsu G, Webb WR, Golden JA, Muller NL. (1992). High resolution CT diagnosis of emphysema in symptomatic patients with normal chest radiographs and isolated low diffusing capacity. Radiology 182: 817-21.

Kuhnigk JM, Dicken V, Zidowitz S, et al. (2005). Informatics in radiology (infoRAD): new tools for computer assistance in thoracic CT. Part 1. Functional analysis of lungs, lung lobes, and bronchopulmonary segments. Radiographics 25: 525–36.

Kurashima K, Takayanagi N, Sato N, et al. (2005). High resolution CT and bronchial reversibility test for diagnosing COPD. Respirology 2005; 10: 316–22.

Kuwano K, Matsuba K, Ikeda T, et al. (1990). The diagnosis of mild emphysema: correlation of computed tomography and pathology scores. Am Rev Respir Dis 141: 169-78.

Lamers RJ, Thelissen GR, Kessels AG, Wouters EF, van Engelshoven JM. (1994). Chronic obstructive pulmonary disease: evaluation with spirometrically controlled CT lung densitiometry. Radiology 193: 109-13.

MacNee W, Gould G, Lamb D. (1991). Quantifying emphysema by CT scanning: clinical-pathological correlates. Ann N Y Acad Sci 624: 179-194.

Martinez FJ, Foster G, Curtis JL, et al. (2006). Predictors of mortality in patients with emphysema and severe airflow obstruction. Am J Respir Crit Care Med 173: 1326–34.

Martinez FJ, Chang A. (2005). Surgical therapy for chronic obstructive pulmonary disease. Semin Respir Crit Care Med 26: 167–191.

Morgan MDL. (1992). Detection and quantification of pulmonary emphysema by computed tomography: a window of opportunity. Thorax 47: 1001-4.

Muller NL, Staples CA, Miller RR. (1998). "Density mask". An objective method to quantitate emphysema using computed tomography. Chest 94: 782-7.

Muller NL, Coxson H. (2002). Chronic obstructive pulmonary disease. 4: imaging the lungs in patients with chronic obstructive pulmonary disease. Thorax 57: 982–5.

Nakano Y, Sakai H, Muro S, et al. (1999). Comparison of low attenuation areas on computed tomographic scans between inner and outer segments of the lung in patients with chronic obstructive pulmonary disease: incidence and contribution to lung function. Thorax 54: 384–9.

Nakano Y, Muro S, Sakai H, et al. (2000). Computed tomographic measurements of airway dimensions and emphysema in smokers. Correlation with lung function. Am J Respir Crit Care Med 162: 1102–8.

Nakano Y, Wong JC, de Jong PA, et al. (2005). The prediction of small airway dimensions using computed tomography. Am J Respir Crit Care Med 171: 142–6.

Nowell Jr JD. CT of emphysema. (2002). Radiologic Clinics of North America 40 (1): 31-42.

O'Brien C, Guest PJ, Hill SL, et al. (2000). Physiological and radiological characterisation of patients diagnosed with chronic obstructive pulmonary disease in primary care. Thorax. 55: 635–42.

Orlandi I, Moroni C, Camiciottoli G, et al. (2005). Chronic obstructive pulmonary disease: thin section CT measurement of airway wall thickness and lung attenuation. Radiology 234: 604-10.

Patel IS, Vlahos I, Wilkinson TM, et al. (2004). Bronchiectasis, exacerbation indices, and inflammation in chronic obstructive pulmonary disease. Am J Respir Crit Care Med 170: 400–7.

Patel B, Make B, Coxson HO, et al. (2006). Airway and parenchymal disease in chronic obstructive pulmonary disease are distinct phenotypes. Proc Am Thorac Soc 3: 533.

Pauwels RA, Buist AS. (2001). Global strategy for the diagnosis, management, and prevention of chronic obstructive pulmonary disease. NHLBI/WHO Global Initiative for Chronic Obstructive Lung Disease (GOLD) Workshop summary. Am J Respir Crit Care Med 163: 1256–76.

Pierce JA, Ebert RV. (1958). The barrel deformity of the chest, the senile lung and obstructive pulmonary emphysema. Am J Med 25: 13-22.

Sanders C, Nath PH, Bailey WC. (1988). Detection of emphysema with computed tomography: correlation with pulmonary function tests and chest radiography. Invest Radio 23: 262-6.

Stern EJ, Frank MS. (1994). Small airway diseases of the lungs: Findings at expiratory CT. Am J Roentgenol 163: 37-41.

Sverzellati N, Molinari F, Pirronti T, Bonomo L, Spagnolo P, Zompatori M. (2007). New insights on COPD imaging via CT and MRI. Intern J COPD 2 (3): 301–12.

Teel GS, Engeler CE, Tashijian JH. (1996). Imaging of small airways disease. Radiographics 16: 27-41.

Thurlbeck WM. (1994). Emphysema then and now. Can Respir J 1: 21–39.

Trigaux JP, Hermes G, Dubois P, et al. (1994). CT of saber-sheath trachea. Correlation with clinical, chest radiographic and functional findings. Acta Radiol 35 (3): 247-50.

Tsao TC, Shieh WB. (1994). Intrathoracic tracheal dimensions and shape changes in chronic obstructive pulmonary disease. J Formos Med Assoc 93 (1): 30-4.

Uppaluri R, Mitsa T, Sonka M, et al. (1997). Quantification of pulmonary emphysema from lung computed tomography images. Am J Respir Crit Care Med 156: 248–54.

Uppaluri R, Hoffman EA, Sonka M, et al. (1999). Computer recognition of regional lung disease patterns. Am J Respir Crit Care Med 160: 648–54.

Zagiers H, Vrooman HA, Aarts NJM, et al. (1996). Assessment of the progression of emphysema by quantitative analysis of spirometrically gated computed tomography images. Invest Radiol 31: 761-7.

Zaporozhan J, Ley S, Eberhardt R, et al. (2005). Paired inspiratory/expiratory volumetric thin-slice CT scan for emphysema analysis: comparison of different quantitative evaluations and pulmonary function test. Chest 128: 3212–20.

Zompatori M, Sverzellati N, Gentile T, et al. (2006). Imaging of the patient with chronic bronchitis: an overview of old and new signs. Radiol Med 111: 634–9.

10

Bronchodilator Activity in Traditional Medicines: Gift of God Kingdom

Dinesh Kumar[1], Zulfiqar Ali Bhat[1], Ishtiaq Ahmad Chashoo[1], Ramesh S. Deoda[2], Satish C. Mudgade[3] and Vijender Kumar[1]
[1]*Department of Pharmaceutical sciences, University of Kashmir, Srinagar,*
[2]*Marathawada Mitra Mandal's, College of Pharmacy, Kalewadi, Pimpri, Pune,*
[3]*MBES college of Pharmacy, Barshi road Latur, Maharastra,*
India

1. Introduction

Since ancient times humanity has depended on the diversity of plant resources for food, clothing, shelter, and traditional medicine to cure myriads of ailments. Early humans recognized their dependence on nature in both health and illness. Physical evidence of the use of herbal remedies has been found some 60,000 years ago in a burial site of a Neanderthal man uncovered in 1960 in a cave in northern Iraq. Here, scientists found great quantities of plant pollen, some of which came from medicinal plants still used today. The first written records detailing the use of herbs in the treatment of illness are in the form of Mesopotamian clay tablet writings and Egyptian papyrus. Led by instinct, taste and experience, primitive men and women treated illness by using plants, animal parts, and minerals that were not part of their usual diet. Primitive people learned by trial and error to distinguish useful plants with beneficial effects from those that were toxic or non-active, and also which combinations or processing methods had to be used to gain consistent and optimal results. Even in ancient cultures, tribal people methodically collected information on herbs and developed well-defined herbal pharmacopeias. Traditional medicine evolved over centuries, depending on local flora, culture, and religion.

Nature has been a source of medicinal agents for thousands of years, and an impressive number of modern drugs have been isolated from natural sources, particularly plants and with many based on their use in traditional medicine. By using medicinal chemistry and combinatorial chemical and biosynthetic technology, novel natural product leads will be optimized on the basis of their biological activities to yield effective chemotherapeutic and other bioactive agents (Cragg et. al. 2005).

During the past decades, public interest in natural therapies, namely herbal medicine, has increased dramatically not only in developing countries but mainly in industrialized countries (Calixto, 2000). The market for ayurvedic medicines is estimated to be expanding at 20% annually. Sales of medicinal plants have grown by nearly 25% in India during 1987-96, the highest rate of growth in the world. The global trade in medicinal plants is of the order of US$ 800 million per year. Export statistics available between 1992 and 1995 indicate that India exported about 32,600 tonnes of crude drugs valued at $US 46 million. China with exports of over 120,000 tons per annum (US$ 264.5 million) and India with over 32,000 tons per annum dominate the international market. The annual export of medicinal plants from India is valued at Rs. 1200 million. Two of the largest users of medicinal plants are China and India. Traditional Chinese Medicine (TCM) uses over 5000 plant species, India uses about 7000. According to Export Import Bank, the international market for medicinal plant related trade is to the tune of US$ 60 billion having a growth rate of 7% per annum. China's share in world herbal market is US$ 6 billion while India's share is only US$1 billion. The World Bank estimated global trade in medicinal and aromatic plants and their products at US $ 5 trillion by 2050 AD. Global herbal market is around $ 70.5 billion with an average annual growth of 10-12% per annum. In European union, it contributes to around 45%($ 32 billion), rest of the Europe 4% (2.8 billion), North America 10% (7.8 billion), Asia 19% (12.2 billion) and others 7% (4.6 billion) (Handa, 2007).

Complimentary alternative medicine therapies continue to gain popularity as modalities for the treatment of atopic disorders, such as asthma, allergic rhinitis, and atopic dermatitis. In Chinese, Japanese, Korean, Indian, and Western cultures, herbal therapies are commonly used for allergies. Although well controlled scientific studies have been performed for many of the Asian herbal therapies, and some basic studies have been performed for various herbal components (active ingredients), more needs to be done to assess the composite effects of many of these remedies (Zuckerman et al., 2002) Complementary and alternative medicines (CAMs) are used in more than 80% of the world's population and are becoming an increasing component of the US health care system, with more than 70% of the population using CAM at least once and annual spending reaching as much as $34 billion.

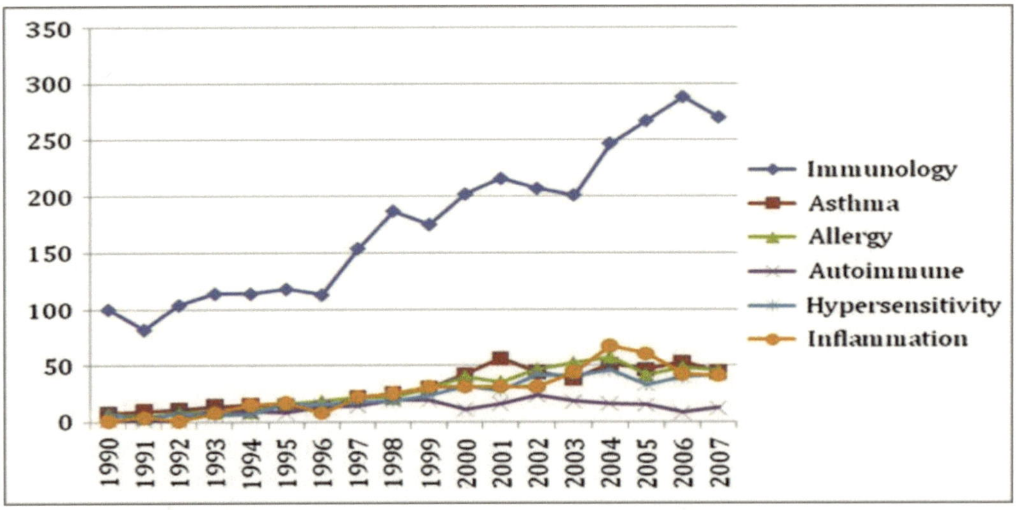

Fig. 1. Annual CAM publications related to allergy and immunology. The numbers of articles published and available for search through PubMed using the search terms complementary medicine and immunology, asthma, allergy, autoimmune, hypersensitivity, or inflammation are shown.

Since the inception of the National Centre for Complementary and Alternative Medicine, there has been an enormous increase in the number of basic science and therapy-based clinical trials exploring CAM. The subspecialty of allergy and immunology represents a particularly fertile area with a large number of CAM therapies that have been shown to affect the immune system. Research has shown that phytoconstituents such as resveratrol, quercetin, and magnolol may affect transcription factors such as nuclear factor-kB and the signal transducer and activator of transcription/Janus kinase pathways with resultant changes in cytokines and inflammatory mediators. Clinically, there have been hundreds of trials looking at the effect of CAM on asthma, allergic rhinitis, and atopic dermatitis.

2. Bronchitis and related diseases

Bronchitis is described as the inflammation of the bronchial tubes (inflammation = itis). The inflammation causes swelling of the lining of these breathing tubes, narrowing the tubes and promoting secretion of inflammatory fluid.

Bronchiolitis is a term that describes inflammation of the smaller bronchi referred to as bronchioles. In infants, this is usually caused by respiratory syncytial viruses (RSV) and affects the small bronchi and bronchioles more than the large. In adults, other viruses as well as some bacteria can cause bronchiolitis and often manifest as persistent cough and at times production of small plugs of mucus.

Acute bronchitis describes the inflammation of the bronchi usually caused by a viral infection, although bacteria and chemicals may also cause acute bronchitis. Acute bronchitis is a cough that begins suddenly, usually due to a viral infection involving the larger airways. Colds (also known as viral upper airway infections) often involve the throat (pharyngitis) and nasal passages, and at times the larynx (resulting in a diminished hoarse voice, also known as laryngitis). Symptoms can include a runny nose, nasal stuffiness, and sore throat. Croup usually occurs in infants and young children and involves the voice box and upper large airways (the trachea and large bronchi).

Chronic bronchitis for research purposes is defined as a daily cough with sputum production for at least three months, two years in a row. Chronic bronchitis is a diagnosis usually made on the basis of clinical findings of a long term persistent cough usually associated with tobacco abuse. From a pathologic standpoint, characteristic microscopic findings involving inflammatory cells seen in airway tissue samples make the diagnosis. When referring to pulmonary function testing, a decrease in the ratio of the volume of airflow at 1 second when compared to total airflow is less than 70%. This confirms the presence of obstructive airways disease of which chronic bronchitis is one type. Certain findings can be seen on imaging studies (chest X-ray, and CT or MRI of the lungs) to suggest the presence of chronic bronchitis; usually this involves an appearance of thickened tubes.

Asthma: Asthma is a chronic inflammatory disease that affects about 300 million people worldwide, a total that is expected to rise to about 400 million over the next 15–20 years. Most asthmatic individuals respond well to the currently available treatments of inhaled corticosteroids and β-adrenergic agonists; however, 5–10% has severe disease that responds poorly. Asthma is a life threatening respiratory condition that causes:

1. The lining of the airways to become swollen
2. The body produces thick mucous

3. Tightness of the muscle around the airways.

This combination of problems interferes with the exchange of oxygen and carbon dioxide in the lungs **Figure 2**.

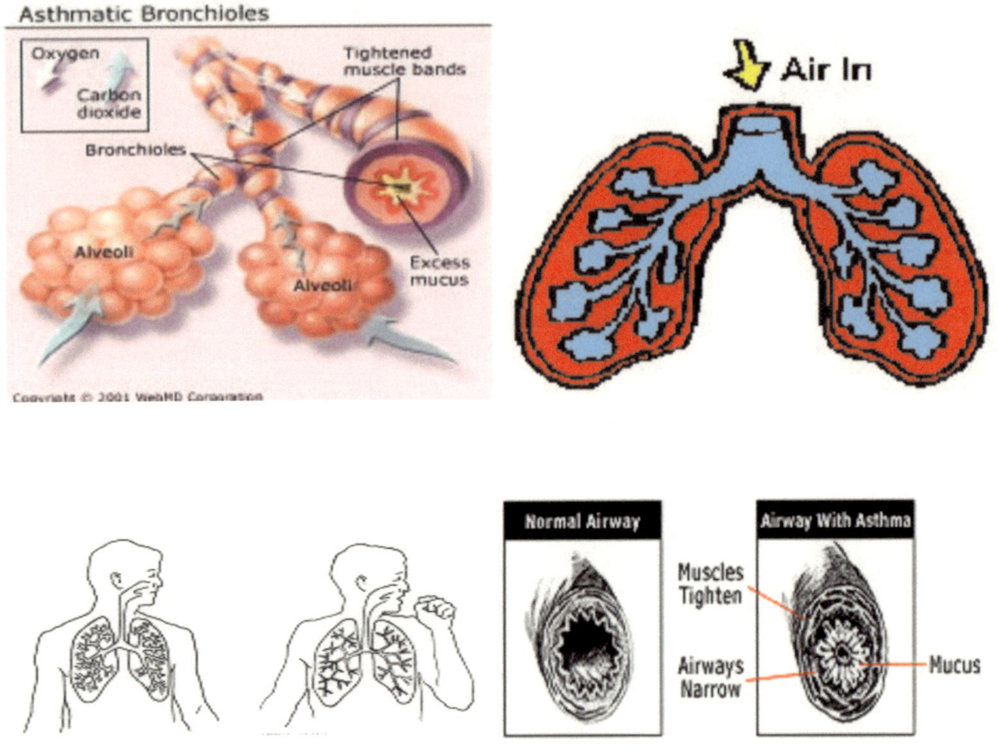

Fig. 2. Bronchitis and related diseases

3. Symptoms

- Breathlessness
- Wheezing
- Sputum Production
- Difficulty in talking
- Dyspnoea
- Tightness of Neck Muscle
- Coughing after physical activity
- Whistling Sound while breathing
- Frequent coughing
- Feeling Frightened, exhaustion
- Chest Tightness
- Greyish or bluish colouring of lips

4. Trigors or mediators responsible for bronchitis and related diseases

List of agents	Events triggering asthma
Respiratory infection	Respiratory syncytial virus (RSV), Rhinovirus, Influenza and Para-influenza virus, Mycoplasma pneumonia bacteria
Allergens	Airborne pollens (grass, trees, weeds), house-dust, mites, animal dander, cockroaches, fungal spores
Environment	Cold air, fog, ozone, sulfur dioxide, nitrogen, tobacco smoke, wood smoke
Emotions	Anxiety, stress, laughter
Exercise	particularly in cold, dry climate
Drugs/preservatives	Aspirin, NSAIDs, Sulfites, Benzalkonium chloride, β blockers,
Occupational stimuli	Bakers (flour dust), farmers (hay mold), spice and enzyme workers, printers (Arabic gum), chemical workers (azodyes, anthraquinone, ethylenediamine, toluene, diisocyanates, PVC), plastics, rubber and wood workers (formaldehyde, western cedar, dimethylethanolamine, anhydrides)

Table 1. List of agents responsible as triggers in **bronchitis and related diseases**

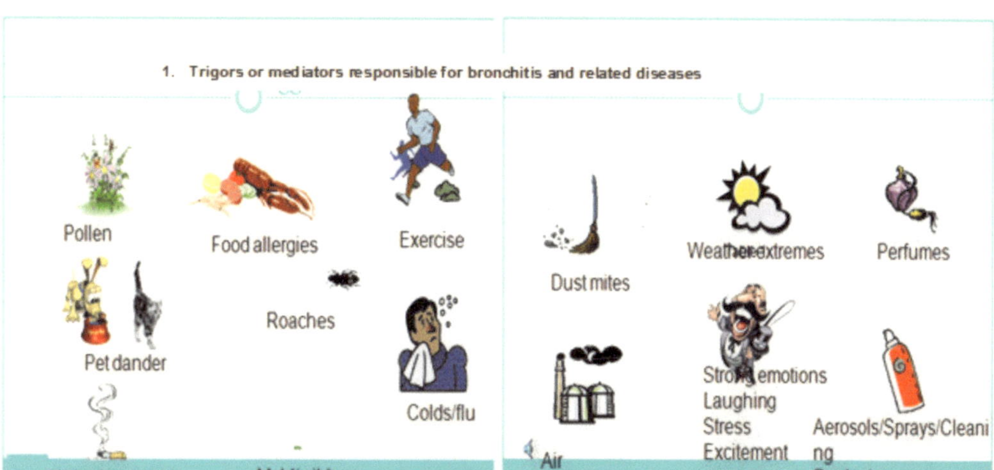

Fig. 3. Agents responsible as triggers in bronchitis and related diseases

5. Tradtional medicines as bronchodilator and used in related diseases

Plants	Vernacular name	Traditional Uses
Adhatoda zeylanica Medic. F: Acanthaceae	Addasaramu	2-3 spoonfuls of leaf extract given for about a month.
Ailanthus excelsa Roxb. F: Simaroubaceae	Peddamanu	Bark decoction administered orally in 2 spoonfuls thrice a day for about one month
Azima tetracantha Lamk. F:Salvadoraceae	Uppi Teega	Leaf juice administered orally,2 spoonfuls, twice a day for about 20 days.
Bambusa arundinacea (Retz.) Willd. F: Gramineae	Veduru	Leaf decoction administered orally, 3 spoonfuls, twice a day for about one month.
Barleria cuspidata Heyne.ex Nees F: Acanthaceae	Nelambram	Root decoction administered orally, 2 spoonfuls 3-4 times a day for 7days.
Barleria prionitis L. F: Acanthaceae	Mulla Gorinta	Stem ground with honey and ginger ,made into dry pillets and administered , 2 pillets, twice a day for amonth.
Blumea mollis (D.Don.) Merr. F: Compositae	Kukka Pogaku	Dried leaves smoked with wrapping leaves of *Diospyros mealanoxylon*
Boerhavia diffusa L. F: Nyctaginaceae	Atika Mamidi	Root extract is administered orally, one spoonful a day for 15days.
Calotropis procera (Ait.) R.Br. F: Asclepiadaceae	Jilledu	Flower powder mixed with honey and administered, 2 spoonfuls, twice a day for a month
Cassia fistula L. F: Leguminosae, Sf; Caesalpinoideae	Rela	Fruits ground with roots of ***Hemidesmus*** and the paste administered in 10g twice a day about 20 d.
Curculigo orchioides Gaertn. F: Hypoxidaceae	Nela Tadi	Rhizome extract administered, 2 spoonfuls, twice a day for about 2 months or till cure.
Datura metal L. F: Solanaceae	Erri Ummetta	Fruits ground and made into small pills with honey and 2 pills taken twice a day for about 3 months
Desmodium triflorum (L.) DC. F:Leguminosae, Sf; Papilionatae	Munta Manda	Root decoction given in 2 spoonfuls twice a day for about 10d.
Lepidagathis cristata Willd. F: Acanthaceae	Suryakanta	Powder of shade dried whole plant mixed with honey in 2 spoonfuls is administered twice a day for a bout 20d.

Plants	Vernacular name	Traditional Uses
Nerium oleander (L.) F: Apocynaceae	Ganneru.	Flowers ground with jaggery and the extract administered in 2 spoonfuls twice a day for about 2 months.
Opuntia stricta (Haw.) Haw. F: Cactaceae	Naga Phanni	Fruits are warmed and the juice given in 2 spoonfuls thrice a day for about 2 weeks.
Passiflora foetida L. F: Passifloraceae	Tella Jumiki	Leaf decoction administered in 2 spoonfuls with fruit juice of ***Terminalia chebula*** thrice a day for about one month.
Pergularia daemia (Forssk.) Chiov. F: Asclepiadaceae	Dustapa teega	Leaf decoction taken in 2 spoonfuls 2-3 times a day for about 15d.
Phyllanthus emblica L. F: Euphorbiaceae	Pedda Usiri	Fruits ground with tubers of *Cyperus rotundus* and leaves of *Tinospora cordifolia* and the paste administered with honey in 2 spoonfuls twice a day for about one month.
Phyllanthus reticulatus Poir. F: Euphorbiaceae,	Puli Chettu	Root decoction with honey administered in 2 spoonfuls twice a day for one month.
Piper longum L. F: Piperaceae	Pippallu	Whole plant ground with leaves of *Adhatoda zeylanica* and made into powder. A spoonful of powder is taken once in day for 20d.
Portulaca quadrifida L. F: Portulacaceae	Sanna pappu koora	Whole plant extract mixed with honey and administered in 2 spoonfuls thrice a day for about 20d.
Solanum surattense Burm.f. F: Solanaceae	Mulla	Root decoction administered in 2-3 times a day for about one month.
Tragia involucrata L. F: Euphorbiaceae	Durada gondi	Root powder cigared with leaves if ***Diospyros melanoxylon*** and smoked to reduce suffering
Tylophora fasciculata Ham. F:ASclepiadaceae	Veripala teega	Tender leaf juice administered in 2 spoonfuls twice a day for 20 – 30d.
Vicoa indica (L.) DC. F: Compositae	Adavi poddu tirugudu	Leaf juice administered in 2 spoonfuls twice a day for 15d
Vitex negundo L. F: Verbenaceae	Vavili	Leaf juice with dried powder of *Zingiber officinale* given in 2 spoonfuls twice a day for about 20d.
Zaleya decandra (L.) Burm.f.F: Aizoaceae	Tella garijelu	Root juice administered in 2 spoonfuls twice a day for about 20d.

Table 2. List of traditional medicinal plant drugs for the treatment of bronchial diseases (Madhu et al., 2010).

6. Reported bronchodilators from medicinal plant drugs

Plant	Part used	Extract/Active principle	Probable action in asthma
Achyranthus aspera	Roots	Oily preparation	Decreased ESR, Decreased total Eosinophil count. (Sharadini,1985)
Adhathoda vasica	Leaves Roots	Alkaloids	Bronchodilator, Anti- anaphylactic (Sharadini,1985)
Albizzia lebbeck	Flower, Bark	Decoction	Anaphylaxis, Histamine Induced Bronchospsm (Tripathi & Das,1977)
Belamcand chinensis	Leaves, Rhizome	50% Ethanolic Extract	Histamine Induced Bronchospasm (Singh & Agrawal, 1990)
Bupleurum falcatum	Roots	saikosaponin-A (SSA), triterpenoid glycoside.	Inhibited the passive cutaneous anaphylaxis reaction in rats & antagonism of the histamine action and inhibition of allergic mediators (Park et al., 2002).
Benincasa hispida	Fruit Pulp	Metanolic Extract	Histamine & Ach Induced Bronchospasm(Anilkumar D., Ramu,2002)
Boswellia serrata	Root	Boswellin, boswellic acids	Inhibit LT biosynthesis and block synthesis of 5-HETE & LTB4 (Gupta,1998)
Curcuma longa	Rhizome	Tumerones, curcuminoids	Inhibits histamine release from rat peritoneal mast cells (Ammon & Wahl,1991)
Eugenia caryophylis	Flower buds, leaves	Eugenol	Antianaphylaxis, inhibits C 48/80 induced anaphylaxis(Sharadini,1985)
Picrorhiza kurroa	Roots	Picrorrhizin	Inhibits release of histamine and SRS-A (Doshi & Shetge, 1983)
Solanum xanthocarpum	Herb	Salasodin	Bronchodilator (Govindan & Viswanathan, 1999)
Tenospora. cardoifofia	Stem	Aqueous extract	Mast cell stabilizing activity (Nayampalli & Desai,1986)
Tamarandus indica	Whole plant	Indolizidine alkaloid.	Bronchodilatory, membrane stabilizing (Sharadini,1985)
Vitex. negundo	Leaves	Alcoholic extract	Bronchodilatory, membrane stabilizing (Saraf & Nair,1995)
Calotropis gigantea	Flower	α&β calotropeol, β-amyrin, ,giganteol	Bronchodilator anti-inflammatory (Sangraula and Kumar 1999)
Calotropis procera	Flower	α&β calotropeol, β-amyrin, giganteol	Bronchodilator anti-inflammatory (Sangraula and Kumar 1999)

Plant	Part used	Extract/Active principle	Probable action in asthma
Cedrus deodara	Wood	Himacholol	Mast cell stabilizing activity (Shinde *et al.*, 1999)
Centipeda minima	Whole plant	Pseudoguainolid,sesquiterpen,lactones, flavonoids	Inhibits passive cutaneous anaphylaxis in rats (Wu *et al.*, 1985)
Clerodendrum serratum	Leaves	Aqueous extract.	Bronchodilator (Gupta, S.S., 1994)
Inula. racemosa	Roots	Aqueous, alcoholic	Anti-histaminic, Anti-serotonergic (Srivastava *et al.*, 1999)
Sarcostemm brevistigma	Twigs	Alkaloid fraction	Inhibits passive cutaneous anaphylaxis in rates (Saraf and Patwardhan,1998)
Tephrosia purpurea	Whole plant	Ethanolic extract	Bronchodilatory, antianaphylactic (Gokhale and Saraf,2000)

Table 3.

7. Bronchodilator activity of two combined component of alkaloidal fraction of Ailanthus excelsa Roxb

Asthma is a chronic inflammatory disease that affects about 300 million people worldwide, a total that is expected to rise to about 400 million over the next 15-20 years (Kumar et al., 2010_a) *Ailanthus* is a deciduous tree belonging to the family Simarubaceae, and widely distributed in Asia and North Australia. Commonly it is known as a Plant of Heaven. The bark of this plant is used as an anthelminthic, expectorant, antiasthmic, antispasmodic and antipyretic (Kumar et al., 2010_b). *Ailanthus excelsa* is reported to be useful in a many ailments like asthma, allergy, bronchoconstriction etc. In the present study two combined Component of alkaloidal fraction of stem bark of *Ailanthus excelsa* Roxb.(AFAE) was for the first time evaluated for its bronchodilator activity.

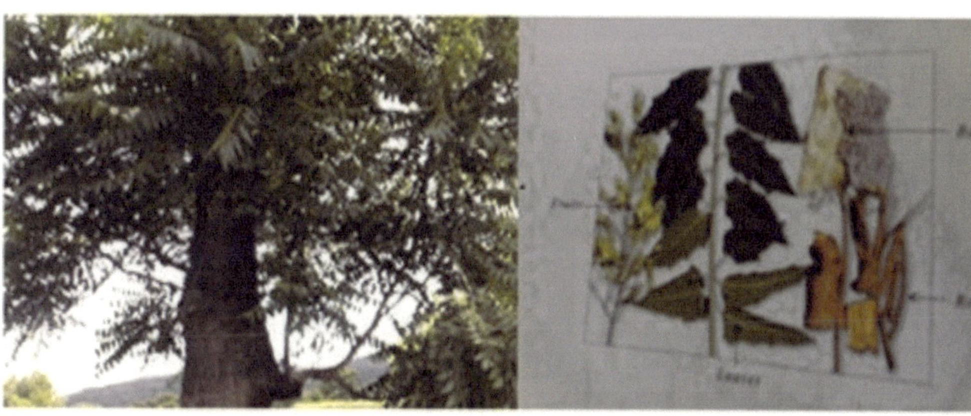

Plant *A. excelsa* Roxb. Flowers, Leaves and Barks of *A. excelsa* Roxb.

Fig. 4.

7.1 Materials and methods

Plant material: Stem barks of *Ailanthus excelsa* Roxb were collected in Aug. 2008 from local area of Pimpri, pune-18 (INDIA) and identified by the RRI of Ayurveda Kothrude, Pune (INDIA). A voucher specimen - 899 was authenticated. Stem barks were dried, powdered, passed through 40 mesh sieve. The powdered material was extracted with methanol (95%) using soxhlet apparatus (10%). The brown extract (2gm) of stem bark of *Ailanthus excelsa* roxb. was used to prepare an alkaloidal rich fraction. The alkaloidal fraction was 500 mg and this Alkaloidal fraction was subjected to column chromatography for isolation of pure constituents using different polarity solvent and silica (60-120) as adsorbent. The component was isolated in chloroform: methanol (4:1) proportion (50 mg) and the same was checked for its purity by performing TLC in Beznene: methanol (4:1) solvent system. A single spot with Rf value of 0.56 was recorded. The isolated sample was then subjected to GC-MS which however showed the same to be a mixure of two components having close resemblance to each other and the fragmentation pattern was almost same and the retention time gap was very small. The molecular weights were 413 and 429. Alkaoidal tests were positive for the constituents.

Animal: Albino rats (Wistar strain) and mice (musmusculus strain) of either sex weighing 150-200gm rats and 20-25gm mice respectively were used. They were housed in microlon boxes with standard laboratory diet and water *ad libitum*. The study was conducted after obtaining Institutional Animal Ethical Committee clearance (198/99/CPCSEA).

Acute toxicity studies: AFAE was safe upto 1000mg/kg and based on the results of preliminary toxicity testing the doses of 10, 20 and 40mg/kg p.o were chosen for further experiments.

7.2 Bronchodilator activity

Effect of test drug on isolated goat trachea chain preparation: Isolated adult Goat tracheal tissue was obtained immediately after slaughter of the animals. Trachea was cut into individual rings and tied together in series to form a chain. Trachea was suspended in bath of Kreb's solution which was continuously aerated and maintained at 37 ± 0.5 °C. Tissue was allowed to equilibrate for 45 min. under a load of 400 mg. A dose response curve for histamine was taken in variant molar concentrations, by maintaining 15 min time cycle. After obtaining a dose response curve of histamine on trachea, the AFAE was added to the respective reservoir and same doses of histamine were repeated. Graph of percentage of maximum contractile response on ordinate and negative logarithm of molar concentration of histamine on abscissa were plotted to record dose response curve of histamine, in absence and in presence AFAE (Bhujbal et al., 2009).

Milk induced leukocytosis and eosinophilia: Mice were divided into five groups, six animals in each group. Animals belonging to group-I received distilled water (DW) 10 ml/kg, (p.o.). Animals belonging to group II, III, IV, V received boiled and cooled milk injection in dose of 4 ml/kg, (s.c.). Animals belonging to groups III, IV and V received AFAE in dose 10, 20 and 400 mg/kg, p. o. respectively, 1 hr before milk injection. Blood samples were collected from each mouse from the retro orbital plexus, under light ether anaesthesia. Total leukocyte count and total eosinophilia count was done in each group before drug administration and 24 hr after milk injection. Difference in Total leukocyte count and total eosinophilia count before and 24hr after drug administration was calculated.

Clonidine-induced Mast Cell Degranulation: Rats were divided into five groups, six animals in each group. Animals belonging to group-I received vehicles 5 ml/kg, (p.o.) Animals belonging to group-II received Sodium cromoglycate 50 mg/kg, (i.p.). Animals belonging to group-III, IV and V received AFAE in dose (10, 20 and 40mg/kg, p.o.) respectively. The treatment was continued for 7 days. On day 7 th, 2 hour after the assigned treatment mast cells were collected from the peritoneal cavity. 10 ml of normal saline solution was injected into peritoneal cavity and abdomen was gently massaged for 90 second. The peritoneal cavity was carefully opened and the fluid containing mast cells was aspirated and collected in siliconised test tube containing 7 to 10 ml of RPMI-1640 Medium (pH 7.2- 7.4). The mast cells were then washed thrice by centrifugation at low speed (400-500 rpm) and the pallet of mast cells were taken in the medium. The mast cells suspension approximately (1×10^6 cells/ml) was challenged with 0.5 μg/ml of clonidine solution and stained with 1 % toluidine blue and observed under high power microscope field (400 X). Total 100 cells were counted from different visual areas and the number of intact and degranulated cells was counted. The percent protection was calculated (Kumar et al., 2009).

Bronchoalveolar lavage and lung histology in rats: Animals were divided into five groups each group containing six animals. All the animals were sensitized by an intraperitoneal injection of 1ml alum precipitate antigen containing 20μg of ovaalbumin and 8mg of alum suspended in 0.9% sodium chloride solution. A booster injection of this alum-ovalbumin mixture was given 7 days later. Non sensitized animals were injected with alum only. Seven days after (15th day) second injection animals were exposed to aerosolized ovaalbumin(1%) for 30 min. Standard & test group was received Dexamethasone (1mg/kg, i.p.) as standard and AFAE 10, 20, 40mg/kg as test drug, 5 hr before antigen challenge. The rats were sacrificed at the end of study (24 hr after sensitization) and tracheal catheter was inserted in trachea. Bronchoalveolar lavage fluid was collected by lavaging the lung with 2 aquilots of 5 ml of 0.9% sodium chloride solution total recovery volume per rat was approximately 8ml. Total leukocytes and eosinophiles, neutrophiles were counted under microscope and Histopathological evaluation of lung tissue was carried out (Kumar et al, 2010_c).

7.3 Statistical analysis

All values were expressed as mean± S.E.M. and data were analysed by ANOVAs followed by dennest.

8. Results

Fraction quantity	Solvent proportion	Yield (mg)	colour	Identification test	TLC benzene: methanol (4:1)
500mg	Chloroform: methanol (80:20)	50 mg	brown	UV- 365 flurosent, positive for alkaloids	Single spot with Rf value - 0.56.

Table 4. Isolation and Characterization of AFAE

a. **Alkaloidal fraction:** U.V spectroscopy: UV λ max. –282, 242, 220, IR range:

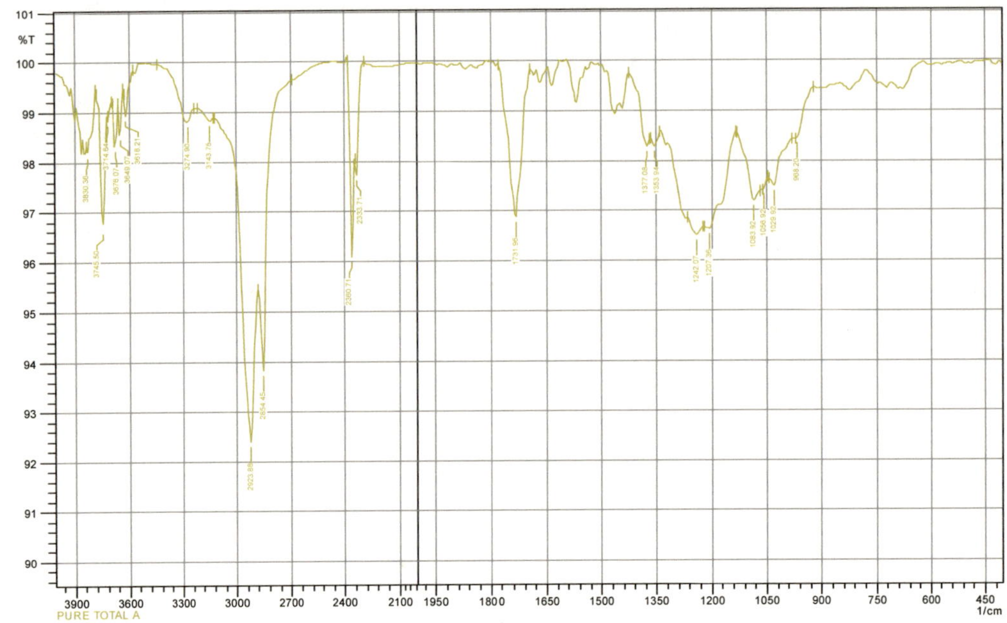

968.20 1029.92 1056.92 1083.92 1207.36 1242.07 1353.94 1377.08 1731.96 2333.71 2360.71 2854.45 2923.88 3143.75 3274.90 3618.21 3649.07 3676.07 3714.64 3745.50 3830.36.

Fig. 5.

b. **AFAE:** U.V spectroscopy: UV λ max. – 209, 220, IR range:

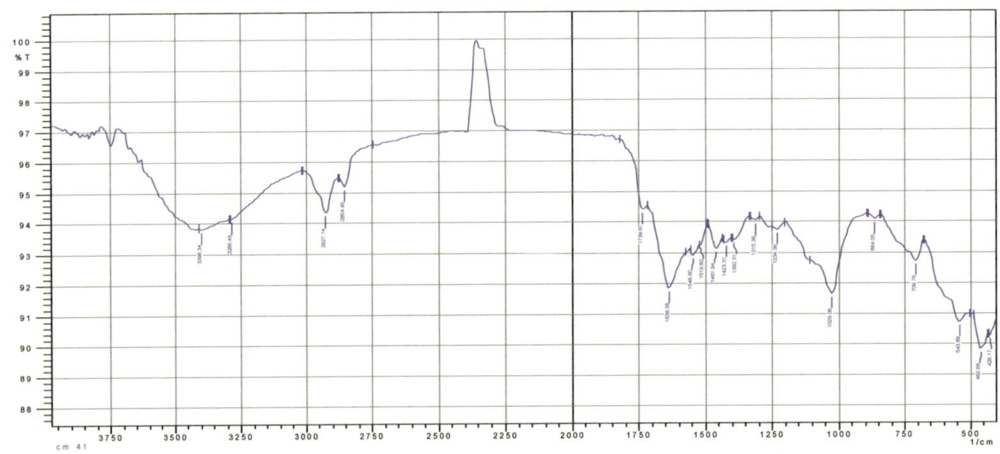

428.17 462.88 543.89 709.76 864.05 1026.06 1234.36 1315.36 1392.51 1423.37 1461.94 1519.80 1546.80 1639.38 1739.67 2854.45 2927.74 3286.48 3398.34.

Fig. 6.

SATC
Department of Chemistry
University of Pune
Pune 411007

Chromatogram HC13 C:\GCMSsolution\Data\GCMS2009\Other Dept\HC13.QGD

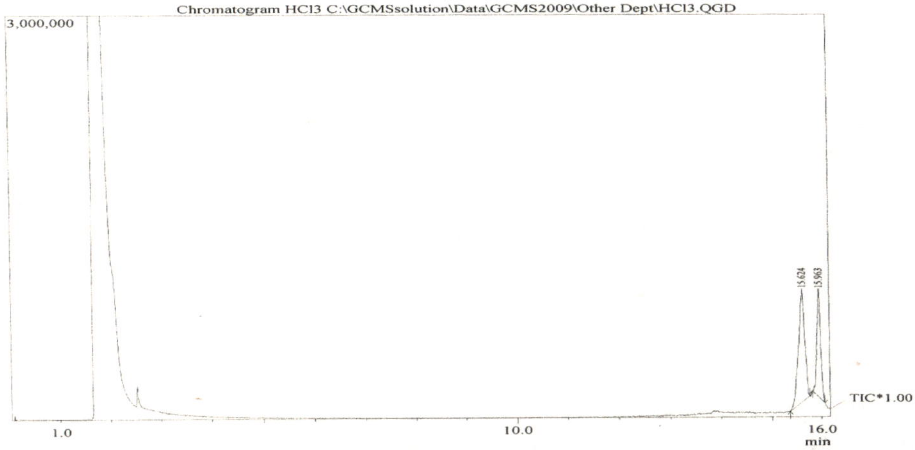

Peak Report TIC

Peak#	R.Time	Area	Area%	Height	Height%
1	15.624	7582106	63.98	842811	50.77
2	15.963	4268686	36.02	817323	49.23
		11850792	100.00	1660134	100.00

Chromatogram (Zoom)

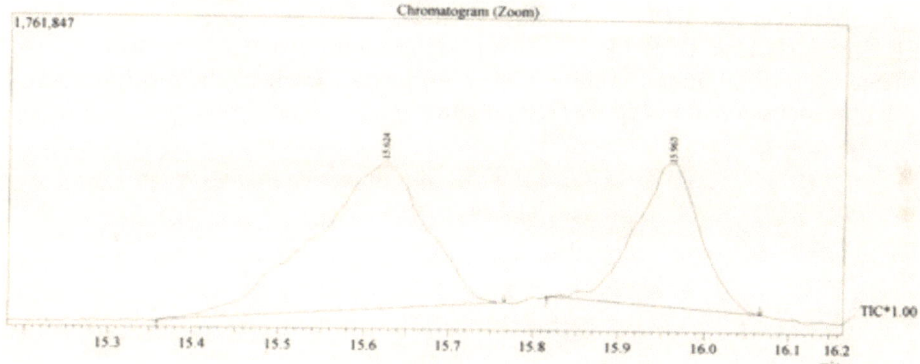

Spectrum

Line#:1 R.Time:15.617(Scan#:1874)
MassPeaks:120
RawMode:Single 15.617(1874) BasePeak:57.15(107212)
BG Mode:None

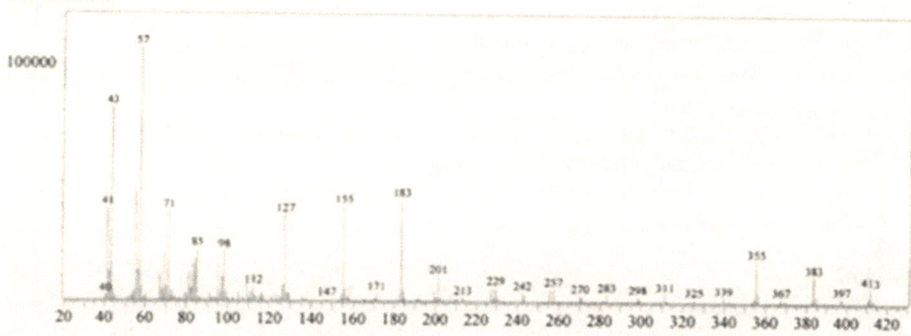

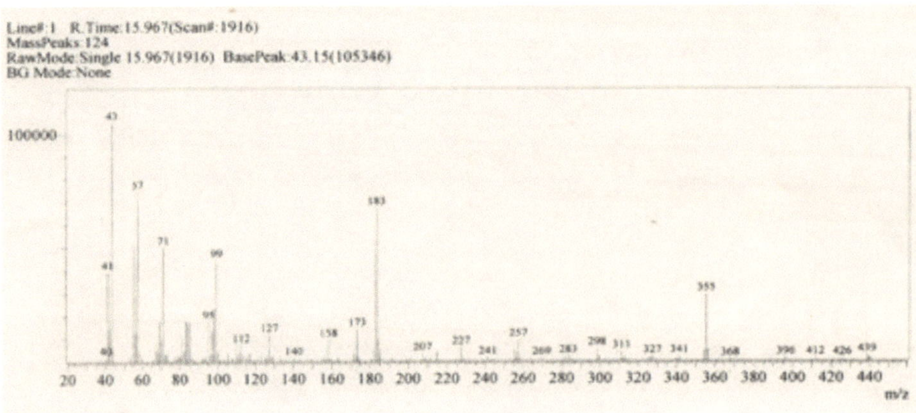

GC-MS

Fig. 7. The above compounds having very less retention time and they have similar ion peaks so in their structure there may be the possibilities of similarity.

8.1 Bronchodilator activity: In vitro

Effect of AFEA (30µg/ml) on Histamine induced contraction of isolated goat tracheal chain preparation: In the present study, it was observed that AFAE inhibits the contraction produced by histamine in these tissue preparations. Histamine (10µg/ml) was taken in different dose level and DRC was plotted in absence and in presence of *Ailanthus excelsa* extract. Study showed that AFAE inhibits significantly (*p<0.05, **p<0.01, ***p<0.001) percentage contraction at concentration 30µg/ml in goat tracheal chain preparation. Dose dependent response relationship was seen (Figure 8).

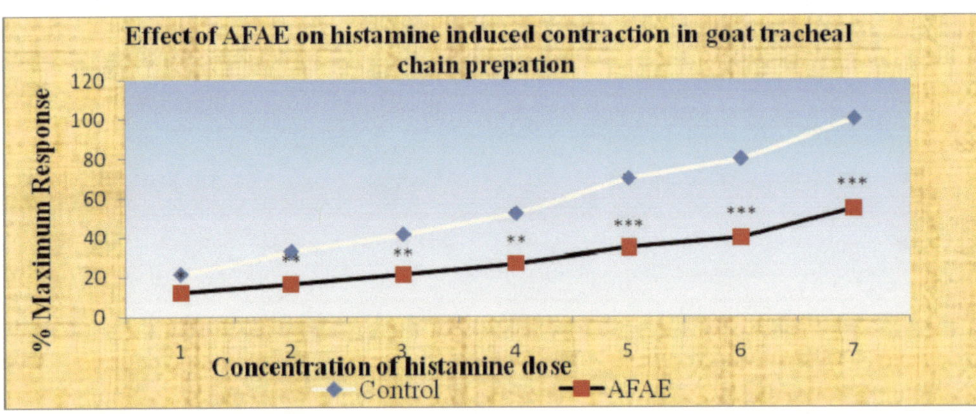

n = 6, Values are in Mean ± SEM. Control = D.R.C. of Histamine in absence of AFAE. AFAE = D.R.C. of Histamine in presence of AFAE (30µg/ml). Statistical analysis done by using Student's't'-test. (*p<0.05, **p<0.01, ***p<0.001), significantly different from control.

Fig. 8.

8.2 In - vivo

Milk induced leukocytosis and eosinophilia: Subcutaneous injection of milk at dose of 4 ml/kg produced a significant (***p< 0.001) increase in the leucocytes and eosinophiles count after 24 hr of its administration. In the groups of mice pretreated with AFAE at dose (10 mg/kg, 20 mg/kg and 40 mg/kg, p.o.), there was significant (*p<0.05, **p<0.01) inhibition of milk-induced Leucocytosis and eosinophilia (Figure 9 & 10).

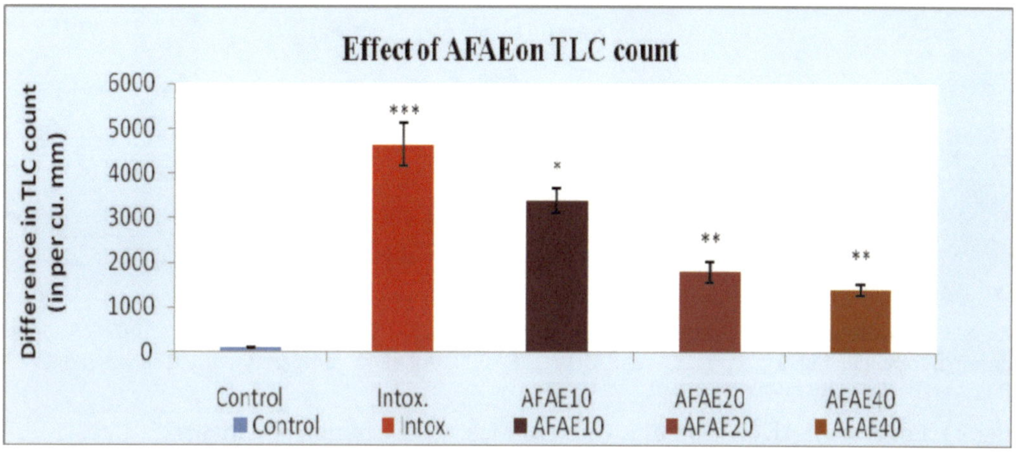

n= 6, values are expressed in mean±SEM. Control = Vehicle (10 ml/kg, p.o.). Intox. = milk 4 ml/kg, ***p<0.001, Intox. group compared with control group using student't, test and *p< 0.05, **p<0.01, AFAE compared to intox. Group using Statistical analysis done by ANOVA followed by Dunnet's test.

Fig. 9. Effect of AFAE on TLC count

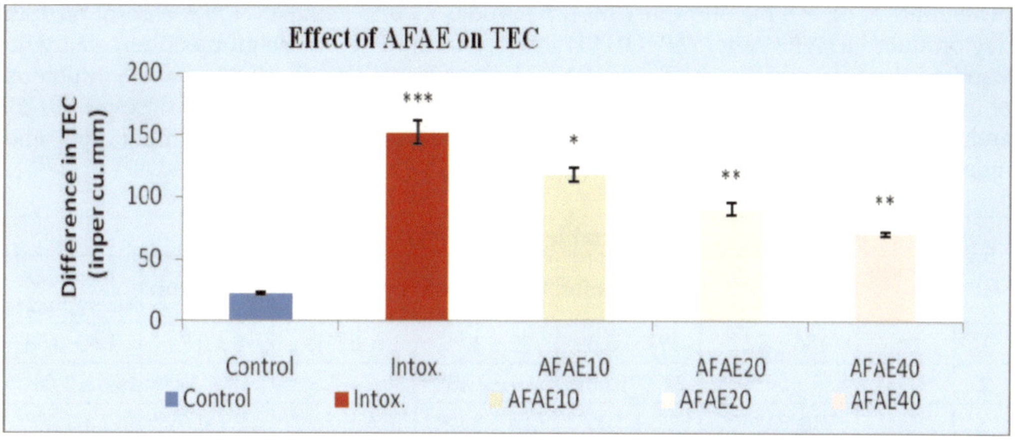

n= 6, values are expressed in mean±SEM. Control = Vehicle (10 ml/kg, p.o.). Intox. = milk 4 ml/kg, ***p<0.001, Intox. group compared with control group using student't, test and *p< 0.05, **p<0.01, AFAE compared to intox. Group using Statistical analysis done by ANOVA followed by Dunnet's test.

Fig. 10. Effect of AFAE on TEC

Effect of AFAE on clonidine-induced mast cell degranulation in rats: Clonidine induced mast cell degranulation was significantly (**p<0.01) inhibited by sodium cromoglycate (50 mg/kg, i.p.) and percent protection was found to be 68.42%. In the groups pre-treated AFAE (10, 20, 40 mg/kg, p.o) there was significant protection (**p< 0.01) of mast cells and the percent protection was 37.89, 54.21, and 61.42 % respectively (Figure 11).

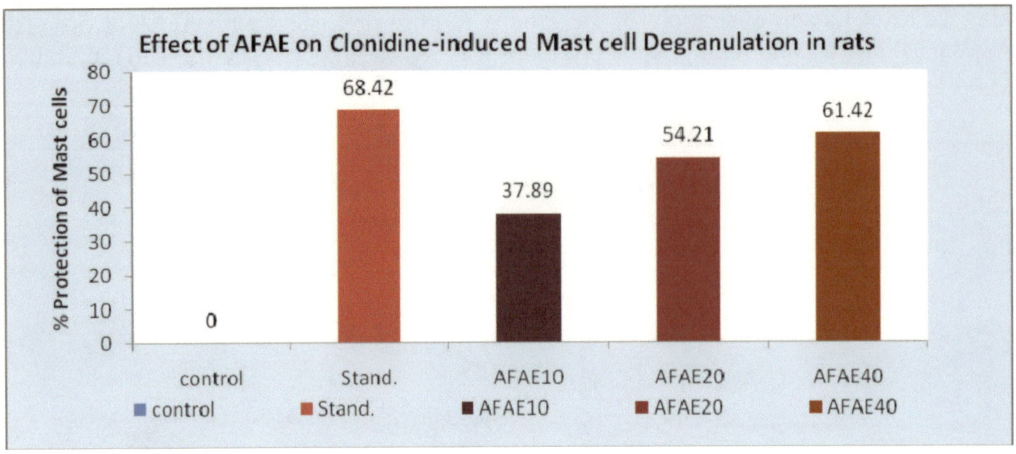

n= 6, values are expressed in mean±SEM. Control = Distilled water (5 ml/kg, p.o.). Std. = Sodium cromoglycate (50 mg/kg, i.p.), Std., AFAE10, AFAE20, AFAE40 compared with Control (ANOVA followed by Dunnett's test), **p < 0.01.

Fig. 11. Effect of AFAE on Clonidine-induced Mast cell Degranulation in rats

Effect of AFAE on Bronchoalveolar lavage in rats: Persistent mucosal airway inflammation, associated with an increase in T helper type 2 (Th2) cytokine levels, eosinophil infiltration into the airways, and mucus and immunoglobulin (IgE) production, are the main features of allergic asthma. The infiltration of cells like eosinophils, neutrophils, monocytes, macrophages, lymphocytes, etc., increases the allergic asthmatic effect. Injection of ovalbumin 20 μg + 8 mg alum in 1 ml (i.p.) on days 1 and 7 and 1% OVA aerosol on 15th day produced a significant (***$P < 0.001$) increase in the TLC. In the groups pretreated with standard drug dexamethasone (1 mg/kg i.p.), there was a significant (**$P < 0.01$) inhibition of ovalbumin-induced TLC and differential leukocyte count. The AFAE at doses of 10, 20, and 40mg/kg showed significant decrease in TLC and neutrophils, lymphocytes and monocytes, macrophages and eosinophils (*$P < 0.05$, **$P < 0.01$ [Table 5]. **AFAE40**

Sr. No.	Groups	Recoverable BAL Cells (×10³/μl)(Mean ± SEM)					
		Total Cells	Neutrophile	Eosinophils	Lymphoctes	Monocytes	Alveolar Macrophages
1.	NS	186 ± 8.12	19.6 ± 3.69	13 ± 1.55	6 ± 1.34	4 ± 0.71	4.8 ± 0.58
2.	S	820 ± 57.09***	122 ± 10.08***	79.8 ± 4.13***	39.2 ± 3.8***	19.8 ± .74***	16.6 ± 1.08***
3.	Std	218 ±7.84**	52.6 ± 1.17**	32.4 ± 3.98**	10.6 ± 0.66**	6.8 ± 0.66**	6.2 ± 1.36**
4.	AFAE10	384 ± 24.97**	98.4 ± 7.17*	66 ± 4.44	18.4 ± 2.06**	13 ± 1.05**	12 ± 0.71
5.	AFAE20	322 ± 26.91**	76.8 ± 3.61**	56.2 ± 2.71**	18.6 ± 1.03**	12 ± 0.95**	13.2 ± 0.97**
6.	AFAE40	246 ± 12.39**	66.2 ± 3.64**	45.2 ± 4.83**	13.3 ± 1.50**	9.4 ± 0.86**	9.6 ± 0.81**

n= 6, values are expressed in mean±SEM. NS = Non Sensitized group, Distilled water + 8mg alum in 1 ml (i.p.). S = Sensitized group, Ovaalbumin20μg+8mg alum in 1ml (i.p.) 1,7 day and 1% OVA aerosol on 15 day. Std. = Dexamethasone (1mg/kg, i.p.). NS compared with S by using student't, test***p < 0.001 and Std., AFAE10, AFAE20, AFAE40 compared with S (ANOVA followed by Dunnett's test), *p < 0.05, **p < 0.01.

Table 5. Effect of AFAE on Bronchoalveolar lavage in rats

Effect of AFAE on Histopathological evaluation of Lung Tissue: The histopathological evaluation of lung tissue showed the reduction of inflateration and mediators of brnchoconstruction. The AFAE showed significant bronchodilator activity. Light micrograph of rat lungs collected from different treatment groups and the lungs were fixed in formalin and embedded in paraffin wax. Section of lung tissue were cut at 5µm thickness, mounted on glass slides, stained with hematoxylin and eosin (H × E) and cells were identified as either eosinophils, neutrophils or mononuclear cells by standard morphology and 200 cells counted under 400X magnification (Figure 12).

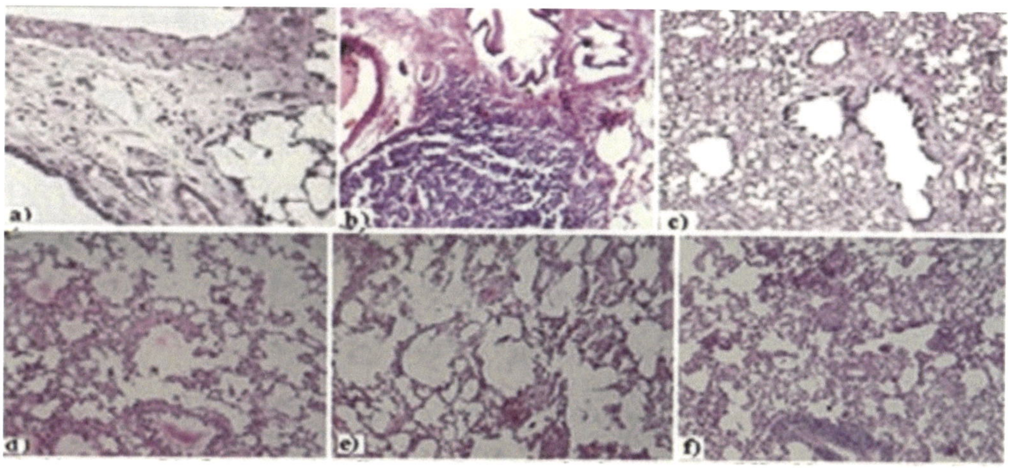

Fig. 12. Effect of AFAE on histopathological evaluation of lung tissue.
Where a) = Abscence of imfalmmatory cells, no edema in the lung tissue (NS- Non sensitized). b) = Abscess formation, fluid accumulation along with inflammatory cells, blood cells, edema (S- Sensitized). c) = a low magnification lung section from an antigen-challenged animals received (standard) dexamethasone (1mg/kg i.p.) showing abscence of fluid accumulaton around the blood vessel. d) = AFAE10 showing haemorrhages, emphysema, MNC and edema. e) = AFAE20 showing emphysema, MNC and haemorrhages. f) = AFAE40 showing emphysema.

9. Discussion

The role of plants serving as purifiers of air has been known to us, since times immemorial. To cope with the gradually increasing levels of toxic pollutants, tree plantation programs have been undertaken in different countries of the world to help in environmental cleanup. Ailanthus excelsa Roxb. (Simaroubaceae) is one such exotic avenue tree, the plantation of which has been encouraged under social forestry programs for large-scale tree plantation in different densely populated cities and towns of India [Mondal et al., 2007]. Histamine contracts the tracheobronchial muscle of guinea pig, goat, horse, dog and man. Goat tracheal chain is easier to handle and to prepare; it is also much more sensitive than guinea pig tracheal chain. Therefore, the dose relative contractile responses of different agonists like ACh, histamine, 5hydroxytryptamine and bradykinin can be observed in isolated goat trachea. In the present study the isolated goat tracheal chain preparation; there is right side shift of Dose Response Curve (DRC) of histamine in the presence of AFAE indicating Bronchodilation [Bhujbal et al., 2009]. In the rat mast cell granules, the histamine concentration has been calculated to be around 0.3 M. Both clonidine and compound 48/80 act through the dynamic expulsion of granules without causing any damage to the cell wall. Clonidine releases histamine from mast cells in a similar manner to a selective liberator like compound 48/80 [Lakdawala et al., 1980]. It is known that sodium cromoglycate; a standard mast cell stabilizer prevents degranulation of mast cells by raising the cyclic adenosine monophosphate. It has been known that all pharmacological agents that increase intracellular levels of cAMP relax airway smooth muscle and inhibit the release of autocoids from the tissue and basophils. The groups of animals pre-treated with AFAE resulted in a significant reduction in degranulation of mast cells and offered significant protection when challenged with clonidine indicating mast cell stabilizing activity which ultimately produces bronchodilation. The inflammatory response is characterized by an increase in the numbers of eosinophils and mast cells, mucus hypersecretion, and activation of T cells. Several studies have shown that T-helper type (Th2) cells play a major role in the initiation and maintenance of allergic airway inflammation and asthma through their increased production of Th2-type cytokines (IL-4, IL-5, and IL- 13). These inflammatory cytokines also produced in the bronchial tissue by mast cells, alveolar macrophages, and epithelial cells, play a significant role in the pathogenesis of airway inflammation. The inflammatory mediators produce bronchoconstriction and the PAE helps to reduce the mediator which leads to bronchodilation. Ovalbumin increases the neutrophils, eosinophils, macrophages, monocytes, leukocytes, lymphocytes, epithelial cells, mucus etc., in BALF and AFAE helps to reduce all the allergic factors [Kumar ett al., 2010_c].

Thus, it can be concluded from the results obtained in the present investigation that AFAE possesses significant bronchodilating activity. Hence, further detailed study needs to be conducted to separate the constituents and individually evaluate these phytoconstituent responsible to produce the above result and their clinical efficacy in the treatment of asthmatic patients.

10. Acknowledgement

I would like to thank Dr. R. K. Nanda, Santosh S. Bhujbal and other staff members of Dr. D. Y. Patil IPSR Pune for guiding me to conduct this valuable work.

I would like to thank NCL- Pune scientists and library staff members for their sport and help for literature review.

I would like to thank NTC- Pune for providing animals and Dr. Surayawanshi for provinding histopathological evaluation (Omega labs. Pvt. Ltd.).

I would like to thank Dr. Rajesh Dabur for authentication of Plant in RRI-Pune, India.

would like to attribute special thank to Late Popinder singh, Department of Pharmaceutical Sciences University of Kashmir-190006 for his content support and enouragement.

11. References

Ammon HP, Wahl MA. (1991). Pharmacology of *Curcuma longa*. Planta Medica, 57, pp. 11-7.

Anilkumar D, Ramu P. (2002). Effect of Methanolic extract of *Benincasa hispida* against histamine & acetycholine induced bronchoplasm in Guinea pigs. Indian J. Pharmacology, 34, pp. 365-366.

Bhujbal SS, Kumar D, Deoda RS, Deore TK, Patil MJ. (2009). Antiasthmatic activity of roots of *Hemidesmus indicus* R. Br. Pharmacologyonline, 1, pp. 209-216.